Diet and Nutrition

SOURCEBOOK

Fifth Edition

Health Reference Series

Fifth Edition

Diet and Nutrition

SOURCEBOOK

Basic Consumer Health Information about Dietary Guidelines, Servings and Portions, Recommended Daily Nutrient Intakes and Meal Plans, Vitamins and Supplements, Weight Loss and Maintenance, Nutrition for Different Life Stages and Medical Conditions, and Healthy Food Choices

Along with Details about Government Nutrition Support Programs, a Glossary of Nutrition and Dietary Terms, and a Directory of Resources for More Information

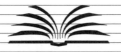

OMNIGRAPHICS

615 Griswold, Ste. 901, Detroit, MI 48226

Bibliographic Note
Because this page cannot legibly accommodate all the copyright notices, the Bibliographic
Note portion of the Preface constitutes an extension of the copyright notice.

* * *

Health Reference Series
Keith Jones, *Managing Editor*
***
OMNIGRAPHICS
A PART OF RELEVANT INFORMATION
***

Copyright © 2016 Omnigraphics
ISBN 978-0-7808-1383-0
E-ISBN 978-0-7808-1412-7

Library of Congress Cataloging-in-Publication Data
Names: Omnigraphics, Inc., issuing body.

Title: Diet and nutrition sourcebook : basic consumer health information about dietary
guidelines, servings and portions, recommended daily nutrient intakes and meal
plans, vitamins and supplements, weight loss and maintenance, nutrition for different life stages and medical conditions, and healthy food choices; along with details
about government nutrition support programs, a glossary of nutrition and dietary
terms, and a directory of resources for more information.

Description: Fifth edition. | Detroit, MI : Omnigraphics, [2016] | Series: Health
reference series | Includes bibliographical references and index.

Identifiers: LCCN 2016024893 (print) | LCCN 2016026051 (ebook) | ISBN
9780780813830 (hardcover : alk. paper) | ISBN 9780780814127 (ebook) | ISBN
9780780814127 (eBook)

Subjects: LCSH: Nutrition--Popular works. | Diet--Popular works. | Health--Popular
works. | Consumer education.

Classification: LCC RA784 .D534 2016 (print) | LCC RA784 (ebook) | DDC 613.2-
-dc23

LC record available at https://lccn.loc.gov/2016024893

Table of Contents

Part II: The Elements of Good Nutrition

Part III: Nutrition through the Life Span

Part IV: Lifestyle and Nutrition

Part V: Nutrition-Related Health Concerns

Part VII: Nutrition for People with Other Medical Concerns

Part VIII: Additional Help and Information

Preface

About This Book

Nutrition affects health, well-being, quality of life, and longevity, yet according to the *2015-2020 Dietary Guidelines* (health.gov), about half of all American adults—117 million individuals—have one or more preventable diet-related chronic diseases many of which are related to poor quality eating patterns and physical inactivity. This, along with increasingly sedentary lifestyles and busy schedules, can lead to obesity, heart disease, certain cancers, and diabetes. The direct medical costs associated with these diet-related health problems are significant. The continued high rates of overweight and obesity and low levels of progress toward meeting *Dietary Guideline* recommendations highlight the need to improve dietary and physical activity education and behaviors across the U.S. population.

Diet and Nutrition Sourcebook, Fifth Edition, provides up-to-date data on nutrition and health, including information from the recently updated *Dietary Guidelines for Americans* and facts about the new MyPlate food guidance system. It details how children, seniors, vegetarians, athletes, and others can benefit from good nutrition. It offers tips for smart grocery shopping, healthy food preparation, and the consumption of a varied, balanced, and nutritious diet. It also discusses strategies for maintaining healthy eating patterns in restaurants, fast food establishments, and other places where meals are consumed away from home. People with certain medical concerns will learn how dietary choices play a role in disease management practices, and a special section discusses the link between nutrition and weight loss and weight maintenance. The book concludes with a glossary, information about government nutrition programs, and a directory of related organizations.

How to Use This Book

This book is divided into parts and chapters. Parts focus on broad areas of interest. Chapters are devoted to single topics within a part.

Part I: Guidelines for Healthy Food Consumption introduces basic concepts from the recently updated Dietary Guidelines for Americans and the new MyPlate food guidance system. It also discusses the key elements of healthy eating patterns, portions and serving sizes, and food labeling information.

Part II: The Elements of Good Nutrition presents details about basic food groups, fluids, vitamins, minerals, and functional foods. Individual chapters describe the importance of protein, carbohydrates, fats, fruits and vegetables, dairy products, and grains. Other chapters explain why vitamins, minerals, phytonutrients, and antioxidants are important dietary components.

Part III: Nutrition through the Life Span provides dietary information for people in different age groups. These include infants and toddlers, children and tweens, teens and college students, pregnant and menopausal women, and older persons.

Part IV: Lifestyle and Nutrition presents nutrition statistics and explores ways for Americans to make healthy food choices when shopping for food, when cooking at home, or when eating out. It also discusses vegetarian eating patterns, organic food choices, sports nutrition, and alcohol use.

Part V: Nutrition-Related Health Concerns describes the most common dietary issues facing Americans, such as metabolic syndrome and other concerns about added sugars, food additives, excess sodium, and high-calorie beverage consumption. Food safety and the health consequences of nutrition misinformation are also discussed.

Part VI: Nutrition and Weight Control focuses on the health risks faced by those who are overweight, and a special chapter addresses weight concerns in children. Other chapters provide tips for healthy weight loss and evaluate popular diet plans, diet medications and supplements, and low-fat foods.

Part VII: Nutrition for People with Other Medical Concerns discusses healthy eating patterns for people with diabetes, heart disease, lactose intolerance, food allergies, celiac disease, eating disorders, and cancer. It also describes the role nutrition plays in oral health.

Part VIII: Additional Help and Information includes a glossary of nutrition terms and details about government-sponsored nutrition programs for people who lack access to affordable food, including programs for women and infants, school-aged children, and seniors. It concludes with a directory of sources for more information.

Bibliographic Note

This volume contains documents and excerpts from publications issued by the following U.S. government agencies:

Agricultural Marketing Service (AMS); Agricultural Research Service (ARS); Centers for Disease Control and Prevention (CDC); ChooseMyPlate.gov; Early Childhood Learning and Knowledge Center (ECLKC); Economic Research Service (ERS); Food and Nutrition Service (FNS); FoodSafety.gov; Kids.gov; National Agricultural Library (NAL); National Cancer Institute (NCI); National Center for Complementary and Integrative Health (NCCIH); National Heart, Lung, and Blood Institute (NHLBI); National Institute of Arthritis and Musculoskeletal and Skin Diseases (NIAMS); National Institute of Dental and Craniofacial Research (NIDCR); National Institute of Diabetes and Digestive and Kidney Diseases (NIDDK); National Institute of Mental Health (NIMH); National Institute on Aging (NIA); National Institutes of Health (NIH); NIH Director's Blog; *NIH News in Health*; NIHSeniorHealth; Office of Disease Prevention and Health Promotion (ODPHP); Office of Research Services (ORS); Office on Dietary Supplements (ODS); Office on Women's Health (OWH); Social Security Administration (SSA); U.S. Department of Agriculture (USDA); U.S. Department of Health and Human Services (HHS); U.S. Department of Veterans Affairs (VA); and U.S. Food and Drug Administration (FDA).

In addition, this volume contains copyrighted documents from the following organization: The Nemours Foundation

It may also contain original material produced by Omnigraphics and reviewed by medical consultants.

About the Health Reference Series

The *Health Reference Series* is designed to provide basic medical information for patients, families, caregivers, and the general public. Each volume takes a particular topic and provides comprehensive coverage. This is especially important for people who may be dealing with a newly diagnosed disease or a chronic disorder in themselves or in a family member. People looking for preventive guidance, information about disease warning signs, medical statistics, and risk factors for health problems will also find answers to their questions in the *Health Reference Series*. The *Series*, however, is not intended to serve as a tool for diagnosing illness, in prescribing treatments, or as a substitute for the physician/patient relationship. All people concerned about medical symptoms or the possibility of disease are encouraged to seek professional care from an appropriate health care provider.

A Note about Spelling and Style

Health Reference Series editors use *Stedman's Medical Dictionary* as an authority for questions related to the spelling of medical terms and the *Chicago Manual of Style* for questions related to grammatical structures, punctuation, and other editorial concerns. Consistent adherence is not always possible, however, because the individual volumes within the *Series* include many documents from a wide variety of different producers, and the editor's primary goal is to present material from each source as accurately as is possible. This sometimes means that information in different chapters or sections may follow other guidelines and alternate spelling authorities.

Medical Review

Omnigraphics contracts with a team of qualified, senior medical professionals who serve as medical consultants for the *Health Reference Series*. As necessary, medical consultants review reprinted and originally written material for currency and accuracy. Citations including the phrase, "Reviewed (month, year)" indicate material reviewed by this team. Medical consultation services are provided to the *Health Reference Series* editors by:

Dr. Vijayalakshmi, MBBS, DGO, MD
Dr. Senthil Selvan, MBBS, DCH, MD
Dr. K. Sivanandham, MBBS, DCH, MS (Research), PhD

Our Advisory Board

We would like to thank the following board members for providing initial guidance on the development of this series:

- Dr. Lynda Baker, Associate Professor of Library and Information Science, Wayne State University, Detroit, MI

- Nancy Bulgarelli, William Beaumont Hospital Library, Royal Oak, MI

- Karen Imarisio, Bloomfield Township Public Library, Bloomfield Township, MI

- Karen Morgan, Mardigian Library, University of Michigan-Dearborn, Dearborn, MI

- Rosemary Orlando, St. Clair Shores Public Library, St. Clair Shores, MI

Health Reference Series *Update Policy*

The inaugural book in the *Health Reference Series* was the first edition of *Cancer Sourcebook* published in 1989. Since then, the *Series* has been enthusiastically received by librarians and in the medical community. In order to maintain the standard of providing high-quality health information for the layperson the editorial staff at Omnigraphics felt it was necessary to implement a policy of updating volumes when warranted.

Medical researchers have been making tremendous strides, and it is the purpose of the *Health Reference Series* to stay current with the most recent advances. Each decision to update a volume is made on an individual basis. Some of the considerations include how much new information is available and the feedback we receive from people who use the books. If there is a topic you would like to see added to the update list, or an area of medical concern you feel has not been adequately addressed, please write to:

Managing Editor
Health Reference Series
Omnigraphics
615 Griswold, Ste. 901
Detroit, MI 48226

Part One

Guidelines for Healthy Food Consumption

Chapter 1

Federal Dietary Guidelines and Food Guidance System

Chapter Contents

Section 1.1

Dietary Guidelines and Key Recommendations 2015–2020

This section includes text excerpted from "Dietary Guidelines for
Americans 2015–2020 Eighth Edition—Executive Summary,"
Office of Disease Prevention and Health Promotion (ODPHP), U.S.
Department of Health and Human Services (HHS), December 2015.

Dietary Guidelines for Americans at a Glance

Over the past century, deficiencies of essential nutrients have dramatically decreased, many infectious diseases have been conquered, and the majority of the U.S. population can now anticipate a long and productive life. At the same time, rates of chronic diseases—many of which are related to poor quality diet and physical inactivity—have increased. About half of all American adults have one or more preventable, diet-related chronic diseases, including cardiovascular disease, type 2 diabetes, and overweight and obesity.

However, a large body of evidence now shows that healthy eating patterns and regular physical activity can help people achieve and maintain good health and reduce the risk of chronic disease throughout all stages of the lifespan. *The 2015–2020 Dietary Guidelines for Americans* reflects this evidence through its recommendations.

The *Dietary Guidelines* is designed for professionals to help all individuals ages two years and older and their families consume a healthy, nutritionally adequate diet. The information in the *Dietary Guidelines* is used in developing Federal food, nutrition, and health policies and programs. It also is the basis for Federal nutrition education materials designed for the public and for the nutrition education components of U.S. Department of Health and Human Services (HHS) and U.S. Department of Agriculture (USDA) food programs. It is developed for use by policymakers and nutrition and health professionals. Additional audiences who may use *Dietary Guidelines* information to develop programs, policies, and communication for the general public include businesses, schools, community groups, media, the food industry, and State and local governments.

Previous editions of the *Dietary Guidelines* focused primarily on individual dietary components such as food groups and nutrients. However, people do not eat food groups and nutrients in isolation but rather in combination, and the totality of the diet forms an overall eating pattern. The components of the eating pattern can have interactive and potentially cumulative effects on health. These patterns can be tailored to an individual's personal preferences, enabling Americans to choose the diet that is right for them. A growing body of research has examined the relationship between overall eating patterns, health, and risk of chronic disease, and findings on these relationships are sufficiently well established to support dietary guidance. As a result, eating patterns and their food and nutrient characteristics are a focus of the recommendations in the *2015–2020 Dietary Guidelines*.

The *2015–2020 Dietary Guidelines* provides five overarching Guidelines that encourage healthy eating patterns, recognize that individuals will need to make shifts in their food and beverage choices to achieve a healthy pattern, and acknowledge that all segments of our society have a role to play in supporting healthy choices. These Guidelines also embody the idea that a healthy eating pattern is not a rigid prescription, but rather, an adaptable framework in which individuals can enjoy foods that meet their personal, cultural, and traditional preferences and fit within their budget. Several examples of healthy eating patterns that translate and integrate the recommendations in overall healthy ways to eat are provided.

The Guidelines

1. **Follow a healthy eating pattern across the lifespan**. All food and beverage choices matter. Choose a healthy eating pattern at an appropriate calorie level to help achieve and maintain a healthy body weight, support nutrient adequacy, and reduce the risk of chronic disease.

2. **Focus on variety, nutrient density, and amount.** To meet nutrient needs within calorie limits, choose a variety of nutrient-dense foods across and within all food groups in recommended amounts.

3. **Limit calories from added sugars and saturated fats and reduce sodium intake**. Consume an eating pattern low in added sugars, saturated fats, and sodium. Cut back on foods and beverages higher in these components to amounts that fit within healthy eating patterns

4. **Shift to healthier food and beverage choices**. Choose nutrient-dense foods and beverages across and within all food groups in place of less healthy choices. Consider cultural and personal preferences to make these shifts easier to accomplish and maintain.

5. **Support healthy eating patterns for all**. Everyone has a role in helping to create and support healthy eating patterns in multiple settings nationwide, from home to school to work to communities.

Key recommendations provide further guidance on how individuals can follow the five Guidelines:

Key Recommendations

- The *Dietary Guidelines* key recommendations for healthy eating patterns should be applied in their entirety, given the interconnected relationship that each dietary component can have with others.

- **Consume a healthy eating pattern that accounts for all foods and beverages within an appropriate calorie level.**

- **A healthy eating pattern includes:**

- A variety of vegetables from all of the subgroups—dark green, red and orange, legumes (beans and peas), starchy, and other

- Fruits, especially whole fruits

- Grains, at least half of which are whole grains

- Fat-free or low-fat dairy, including milk, yogurt, cheese, and/or fortified soy beverages

- A variety of protein foods, including seafood, lean meats and poultry, eggs, legumes (beans and peas), and nuts, seeds, and soy products

- Oils

A Healthy Eating Pattern Limits:

- Saturated fats and *trans* fats, added sugars, and sodium

Key recommendations that are quantitative are provided for several components of the diet that should be limited. These components are of particular public health concern in the United States, and the specified limits can help individuals achieve healthy eating patterns within calorie limits:

- Consume less than 10 percent of calories per day from added sugars

- Consume less than 10 percent of calories per day from saturated fats

- Consume less than 2,300 milligrams (mg) per day of sodium

- If alcohol is consumed, it should be consumed in moderation—up to one drink per day for women and up to two drinks per day for men—and only by adults of legal drinking age.

In tandem with the recommendations above, Americans of all ages—children, adolescents, adults, and older adults—should meet the *Physical Activity Guidelines for Americans* to help promote health and reduce the risk of chronic disease. Americans should aim to achieve and maintain a healthy body weight. The relationship between diet and physical activity contributes to calorie balance and managing body weight. As such, the *Dietary Guidelines* includes a Key Recommendation to

- Meet the *Physical Activity Guidelines for Americans*

Section 1.2

Key Elements of Healthy Eating Patterns

This section includes text excerpted from "Dietary Guidelines for Americans 2015–2020 Eighth Edition—Key Elements of Healthy Eating Patterns," Office of Disease Prevention and Health Promotion (ODPHP), U.S. Department of Health and Human Services (HHS), December 2015.

Over the course of any given day, week or year, individuals consume foods and beverages in combination—an eating pattern. An eating pattern is more than the sum of its parts; it represents the totality of what individuals habitually eat and drink, and these dietary components act synergistically in relation to health. As a result, the eating pattern may be more predictive of overall health status and disease risk than individual foods or nutrients. Thus, eating patterns, and their food and nutrient components, are at the core of the *2015–2020 Dietary Guidelines for Americans.* The goal of the *Dietary Guidelines* is for individuals throughout all stages of the lifespan to have eating patterns that promote overall health and help prevent chronic disease.

Healthy Eating Patterns: Dietary Principles

Healthy eating patterns support a healthy body weight and can help prevent and reduce the risk of chronic disease throughout periods of growth, development, and aging as well as during pregnancy. The following principles apply to meeting the key recommendations:

An eating pattern represents the totality of all foods and beverages consumed. All foods consumed as part of a healthy eating pattern fit together like a puzzle to meet nutritional needs without exceeding limits, such as those for saturated fats, added sugars, sodium, and total calories. All forms of foods, including fresh, canned, dried, and frozen, can be included in healthy eating patterns.

Nutritional needs should be met primarily from foods. Individuals should aim to meet their nutrient needs through healthy eating patterns that include nutrient-dense foods. Foods in nutrient-dense forms contain essential vitamins and minerals and also dietary fiber and other naturally occurring substances that may have positive health effects. In some cases, fortified foods and dietary supplements may be useful in providing one or more nutrients that otherwise may be consumed in less than recommended amounts.

Healthy eating patterns are adaptable. Individuals have more than one way to achieve a healthy eating pattern. Any eating pattern can be tailored to the individual's socio-cultural and personal preferences.

The Science Behind Healthy Eating Patterns

The components of healthy eating patterns recommended in this edition of the *Dietary Guidelines* were developed by integrating findings from systematic reviews of scientific research, food pattern modeling, and analyses of current intake of the U.S. population:

- Systematic reviews of scientific research examine relationships between the overall diet, including its constituent foods, beverages, and nutrients, and health outcomes.

- Food pattern modeling assesses how well various combinations and amounts of foods from all food groups would result in healthy eating patterns that meet nutrient needs and accommodate limits, such as those for saturated fats, added sugars, and sodium.

- Analyses of current intakes identify areas of potential public health concern.

Together, these complementary approaches provide a robust evidence base for healthy eating patterns that both reduce risk of diet-related chronic disease and ensure nutrient adequacy.

Scientific evidence supporting dietary guidance has grown and evolved over the decades. Previous editions of the *Dietary Guidelines* relied on the evidence of relationships between individual nutrients, foods, and food groups and health outcomes. Although this evidence base continues to be substantial, foods are not consumed in isolation, but rather in various combinations over time—an "eating pattern." As previously noted, dietary components of an eating pattern can have interactive, synergistic, and potentially cumulative relationships, such that the eating pattern may be more predictive of overall health status and disease risk than individual foods or nutrients. However, each identified component of an eating pattern does not necessarily have the same independent relationship to health outcomes as the total eating pattern, and each identified component may not equally contribute (or may be a marker for other factors) to the associated health outcome. An evidence base is now available that evaluates overall eating patterns and various health outcomes.

Associations Between Eating Patterns and Health

Evidence shows that healthy eating patterns, as outlined in the guidelines and key recommendations, are associated with positive health outcomes. The evidence base for associations between eating patterns and specific health outcomes continues to grow. Strong evidence shows that healthy eating patterns are associated with a reduced risk of cardiovascular disease (CVD). Moderate evidence indicates that healthy eating patterns also are associated with a reduced risk of type 2 diabetes, certain types of cancers (such as colorectal and postmenopausal breast cancers), overweight, and obesity. Emerging evidence also suggests that relationships may exist between eating patterns and some neurocognitive disorders and congenital anomalies.

Within this body of evidence, higher intakes of vegetables and fruits consistently have been identified as characteristics of healthy eating patterns; whole grains have been identified as well, although with slightly less consistency. Other characteristics of healthy eating patterns have been identified with less consistency and include fat-free or low-fat dairy, seafood, legumes, and nuts. Lower intakes of meats, including processed meats; processed poultry; sugar-sweetened foods, particularly beverages; and refined grains have often been identified as characteristics of healthy eating patterns.

Associations Between Dietary Components and Health

The evidence on food groups and various health outcomes that is reflected in this 2015–2020 edition of the *Dietary Guidelines* complements and builds on the evidence of the previous 2010 edition. For example, research has shown that vegetables and fruits are associated with a reduced risk of many chronic diseases, including CVD, and may be protective against certain types of cancers. Additionally, some evidence indicates that whole grain intake may reduce risk for CVD and is associated with lower body weight. Research also has linked dairy intake to improved bone health, especially in children and adolescents.

Section 1.3

Introduction to the MyPlate Food Guidance System

This section includes text excerpted from "Build a Healthy Eating Style," Office of Disease Prevention and Health Promotion (ODPHP), U.S. Department of Health and Human Services (HHS), January 7, 2016.

MyPlate is a reminder to find your healthy eating style and build it throughout your lifetime. Everything you eat and drink matters. The right mix can help you be healthier now and in the future. This means:

- Focus on variety, amount, and nutrition.

- Choose foods and beverages with less saturated fat, sodium, and added sugars.

- Start with small changes to build healthier eating styles.

- Support healthy eating for everyone.

Eating healthy is a journey shaped by many factors, including our stage of life, situations, preferences, access to food, culture, traditions, and the personal decisions we make over time. All your food and beverage choices count. MyPlate offers ideas and tips to help you create a healthier eating style that meets your individual needs and improves your health.

All Food and Beverage Choices Matter–Focus on Variety, Amount, and Nutrition

- Focus on making healthy food and beverage choices from all five food groups including fruits, vegetables, grains, protein foods, and dairy to get the nutrients you need.

- Eat the right amount of calories for you based on your age, sex, height, weight, and physical activity level.

- Building a healthier eating style can help you avoid overweight and obesity and reduce your risk of diseases such as heart disease, diabetes, and cancer.

11

Choose an Eating Style Low in Saturated Fat, Sodium, and Added Sugars

- Use Nutrition Facts labels and ingredient lists to find amounts of saturated fat, sodium, and added sugars in the foods and beverages you choose.

- Look for food and drink choices that are lower in saturated fat, sodium, and added sugar.

  - Eating fewer calories from foods high in saturated fat and added sugars can help you manage your calories and prevent overweight and obesity. Most of us eat too many foods that are high in saturated fat and added sugar.

  - Eating foods with less sodium can reduce your risk of high blood pressure.

Make Small Changes to Create a Healthier Eating Style

- Think of each change as a personal "win" on your path to living healthier. Each MyWin is a change you make to build your healthy eating style. Find little victories that fit into your lifestyle and celebrate as a MyWin!

- Start with a few of these small changes.

  - Make half your plate fruits and vegetables.

  - Focus on whole fruits.

  - Vary your veggies.

  - Make half your grains whole grains.

  - Move to low-fat and fat-free dairy.

  - Vary your protein routine.

  - Eat and drink the right amount for you.

Support Healthy Eating for Everyone

- Create settings where healthy choices are available and affordable to you and others in your community.

- Professionals, policymakers, partners, industry, families, and individuals can help others in their journey to make healthy eating a part of their lives.

Chapter 2

Portion Sizes and Servings

Chapter Contents

Section 2.1

Food Servings and Food Exchange Lists

This section contains text excerpted from the following sources: Text in this section begins with excerpts from "Does Portion Size Matter?" Office of Research Services (ORS), National Institutes of Health (NIH), January 2014; Text under the heading "Serving Sizes and Portions" is excerpted from "Serving Sizes and Portions," National Heart, Lung, and Blood Institute (NHLBI), September 30, 2013.

Does Portion Size Matter?

Portion size is almost always part of conversations about eating well, but why is portion size so important? If eating well were as simple as just eating the right amount, we would all be very healthy. Right?

What Is Portion Size?

When we say portion size we are usually talking about the amount of a food that we eat at a given time. This is often different from serving size, which refers to the "recommended" or "usual" amount of a food that is included on the nutrition label or in messages about eating better. For example, a serving of cooked pasta is 1/2 cup, but the portion we eat at dinner may be 1 1/2 cups of spaghetti.

How Does Portion Size Impact How We Eat?

Most of us are not very good at estimating how much food we are eating unless we are measuring in some way. Influences such as the color of a plate, the size of a plate and even whether a plate has a rim can alter how much food we perceive is on the plate. We also tend to eat more when we start with a larger portion on our plates, leading us to eat more than we thought or wanted.

Better Portioning

To familiarize yourself with standard serving sizes and what they look like on a plate, practice with measuring cups at home. Start

14

meals by serving yourself a measured amount that you think will be enough and only go back for more if you are not satisfied. This practice can help you get better at estimating portion size and can also help you understand how much food you actually need. When eating out, you can practice your portioning too. Many of our cafes have signs and marked serving utensils that can help you better estimate your portion sizes.

Serving Sizes and Portions

A **portion** is the amount of food that you choose to eat for a meal or snack. It can be big or small, you decide.

A **serving** is a measured amount of food or drink, such as one slice of bread or one cup (eight ounces) of milk.

Many foods that come as a **single portion** actually contain **multiple** *servings*. The Nutrition Facts label on packaged foods, on the backs of cans, sides of boxes, etc. tells you the number of servings in the container.

For example, look at the label of a 20-ounce soda (usually consumed as one portion). It has 2.5 servings in it. A 3-ounce bag of chips, which some would consider a single portion, contains 3 servings.

Portion Distortion

Average portion sizes have grown so much over the past 20 years that sometimes the plate arrives and there's enough food for two or even three people on it. Growing portion sizes are changing what Americans think of as a "normal" portion at home too. We call it **portion distortion**.

Check out these examples of how **larger portions** lead to **increased calories**:

Table 2.1. Comparison of Portions and Calories 20 Years Ago to Present Day

20 Years Ago			Today	
	Portion	Calories	Portion	Calories
Bagel	3" diameter	140	6" diameter	350
Cheeseburger	1	333	1	590

Table 2.1. Continued

20 Years Ago			Today	
Spaghetti w/ meatballs	1 cup sauce 3 small meatballs	500	2 cups sauce 3 large meatballs	1020
Soda	6.5 ounces	82	20 ounces	250
Blueberry muffin	1.5 ounces	210	5 ounces	500

Section 2.2

Food Exchange Lists

This section includes text excerpted from "Food Exchange Lists," National Heart, Lung, and Blood Institute (NHLBI), July 26, 2014.

You can use the American Dietetic Association food exchange lists to check out serving sizes for each group of foods and to see what other food choices are available for each group of foods.

- Vegetables
- Fat-Free and Very Low-Fat Milk
- Very Lean Protein
- Fruits
- Lean Protein
- Medium-Fat Proteins
- Starches
- Fats

Vegetables contain 25 calories and 5 grams of carbohydrate. One serving equals:

Table 2.2. Serving Sizes and Food Choices for Vegetables

½ C	Cooked vegetables (carrots, broccoli, zucchini, cabbage, etc.)
1 C	Raw vegetables or salad greens
½ C	Vegetable juice

If you're hungry, eat more fresh or steamed vegetables.

Fat-Free and Very Low-Fat Milk contain 90 calories per serving. One serving equals:

Table 2.3. Serving Sizes and Food Choices for Fat-Free and Very Low-Fat Milk

1 C	Milk, fat-free or 1% fat
¾ C	Yogurt, plain nonfat or low-fat
1 C	Yogurt, artificially sweetened

Very Lean Protein choices have 35 calories and 1 gram of fat per serving. One serving equals:

Table 2.4. Serving Sizes and Food Choices for Very Lean Protein

1 oz	Turkey breast or chicken breast, skin removed
1 oz	Fish fillet (flounder, sole, scrod, cod, etc.)
1 oz	Canned tuna in water
1 oz	Shellfish (clams, lobster, scallop, shrimp)
¾ C	Cottage cheese, nonfat or low-fat
2	Egg whites
¼ C	Egg substitute
1 oz	Fat-free cheese
½ C	Beans, cooked (black beans, kidney, chickpeas or lentils): count as 1 starch/bread and 1 very lean protein

Fruits contain 15 grams of carbohydrate and 60 calories. One serving equals:

Table 2.5. Serving Sizes and Food Choices for Fruits

1 small	Apple, banana orange, nectarine
1 med.	Fresh peach
1	Kiwi
½	Grapefruit
½	Mango
1 C	Fresh berries (strawberries, raspberries or blueberries)
1 C	Fresh melon cubes
1/8th	Honeydew melon
4 oz	Unsweetened juice
4 tsp	Jelly or jam

 Lean Protein choices have 55 calories and 2–3 grams of fat per serving. One serving equals:

Table 2.6. Serving Sizes and Food Choices for Lean Protein

1 oz	Chicken—dark meat, skin removed
1 oz	Turkey—dark meat, skin removed
1 oz	Salmon, swordfish, herring
1 oz	Lean beef (flank steak, London broil, tenderloin, roast beef)*
1 oz	Veal, roast or lean chop*
1 oz	Lamb, roast or lean chop*
1 oz	Pork, tenderloin or fresh ham*
1 oz	Low-fat cheese (with 3 g or less of fat per ounce)
1 oz	Low-fat luncheon meats (with 3 g or less of fat per ounce)
¼ C	4.5% cottage cheese
2 med.	Sardines

* Limit to 1–2 times per week

 Medium-Fat Proteins have 75 calories and 5 grams of fat per serving. One serving equals:

Table 2.7. Serving Sizes and Food Choices for Medium-Fat Proteins

1 oz	Beef (any prime cut), corned beef, ground beef**
1 oz	Pork chop
1	Whole egg (medium)**
1 oz	Mozzarella cheese
¼ C	Ricotta cheese
4 oz	Tofu (note this is a heart healthy choice)

 **Starches contain 15 grams of carbohydrate and 80 calories per serving. One serving equals:

Table 2.8. Serving Sizes and Food Choices for Starches

1 slice	Bread (white, pumpernickel, whole wheat, rye)
2 slices	Reduced-calorie or "lite" bread
¼ (1 oz)	Bagel (varies)
½	English muffin

Table 2.8. Continued

½	Hamburger bun
¾ C	Cold cereal
1⁄3 C	Rice, brown or white, cooked
1⁄3 C	Barley or couscous, cooked
1⁄3 C	Legumes (dried beans, peas or lentils), cooked
½ C	Pasta, cooked
½ C	Bulgar, cooked
½ C	Corn, sweet potato or green peas
3 oz	Baked sweet or white potato
¾ oz	Pretzels
3 C	Popcorn, hot air popped or microwave (80% light)

Fats contain 45 calories and 5 grams of fat per serving. One serving equals:

Table 2.9. Serving Sizes and Food Choices for Fats

1 tsp	Oil (vegetable, corn, canola, olive, etc.)
1 tsp	Butter
1 tsp	Stick margarine
1 tsp	Mayonnaise
1 Tbsp	Reduced-fat margarine or mayonnaise
1 Tbsp	Salad dressing
1 Tbsp	Cream cheese
2 Tbsp	Lite cream cheese
1/8th	Avocado
8 large	Black olives
10 large	Stuffed green olives
1 slice	Bacon

Section 2.3

Estimated Calorie Requirements and Energy Balance

This section contains text excerpted from the following sources: Text beginning with the heading "What Is Energy Balance?" is excerpted from "Balance Food and Activity," National Heart, Lung, and Blood Institute (NHLBI), February 13, 2013; Text under the heading "Estimated Calorie Needs per Day, by Age, Sex, and Physical Activity Level" is excerpted from *"Dietary Guidelines for Americans 2015– 2020 Eighth Edition*—Estimated Calorie Needs per Day, by Age, Sex, and Physical Activity Level," Office of Disease Prevention and Health Promotion (ODPHP), U.S. Department of Health and Human Services (HHS), December 2015.

What Is Energy Balance?

Energy is another word for "calories." Your energy balance is the balance of calories consumed through eating and drinking compared to calories burned through physical activity. What you eat and drink is ENERGY IN. What you burn through physical activity is ENERGY OUT.

You burn a certain number of calories just by breathing air and digesting food. You also burn a certain number of calories (ENERGY OUT) through your daily routine. For example, children burn calories just being students—walking to their lockers, carrying books, etc.— and adults burn calories walking to the bus stop, going shopping, etc. A chart of estimated calorie requirements for children and adults is available at the link below; this chart can help you maintain a healthy calorie balance.

An important part of maintaining energy balance is the amount of ENERGY OUT (physical activity) that you do. People who are more **physically active** burn **more** calories than those who are not as physically active.

The same amount of ENERGY IN (calories consumed) and ENERGY OUT
(calories burned) over time = weight stays the same

More IN than OUT over time = weight gain
More OUT than IN over time = weight loss

Your ENERGY IN and OUT don't have to balance every day. It's having a balance **over time** that will help you stay at a healthy weight for the long term. Children need to balance their energy, too, but they're also growing and that should be considered as well. Energy balance in children happens when the amount of ENERGY IN and ENERGY OUT supports natural growth without promoting excess weight gain.

That's why you should take a look at the Estimated Calorie Requirement chart, to get a sense of how many calories (ENERGY IN) you and your family need on a daily basis.

Estimated Calorie Needs per Day, by Age, Sex, and Physical Activity Level

The total number of calories a person needs each day varies depending on a number of factors, including the person's age, sex, height, weight, and level of physical activity. In addition, a need to lose, maintain or gain weight and other factors affect how many calories should be consumed. Estimated amounts of calories needed to maintain calorie balance for various age and sex groups at three different levels of physical activity are provided in Table 2.10. These estimates are based on the Estimated Energy Requirements (EER) equations, using reference heights (average) and reference weights (healthy) for each age-sex group. For children and adolescents, reference height and weight vary. For adults, the reference man is 5 feet 10 inches tall and weighs 154 pounds. The reference woman is 5 feet 4 inches tall and weighs 126 pounds.

Estimates range from 1,600 to 2,400 calories per day for adult women and 2,000 to 3,000 calories per day for adult men. Within each age and sex category, the low end of the range is for sedentary individuals; the high end of the range is for active individuals. Due to reductions in basal metabolic rate that occur with aging, calorie needs generally decrease for adults as they age. Estimated needs for young children range from 1,000 to 2,000 calories per day, and the range for older children and adolescents varies substantially from 1,400 to 3,200 calories per day, with boys generally having higher calorie needs than girls. These are only estimates, and approximations of individual calorie needs can be aided with online tools such as those available at www.supertracker.usda.gov.

Table 2.10. Estimated Calorie Needs per Day, by Age, Sex, and Physical Activity Level

MALES				FEMALES			
AGE	Sedentary	Moderately Active	Active	AGE	Sedentary	Moderately Active	Active
2	1000	1000	1000	2	1000	1000	1000
3	1000	1400	1400	3	1000	1200	1400
4	1200	1400	1600	4	1200	1400	1400
5	1200	1400	1600	5	1200	1400	1600
6	1400	1600	1800	6	1200	1400	1600
7	1400	1600	1800	7	1200	1600	1800
8	1400	1600	2000	8	1400	1600	1800
9	1600	1800	2000	9	1400	1600	1800
10	1600	1800	2200	10	1400	1800	2000
11	1800	2000	2200	11	1600	1800	2000
12	1800	2200	2400	12	1600	2000	2200
13	2000	2200	2600	13	1600	2000	2200
14	2000	2400	2800	14	1800	2000	2400
15	2200	2600	3000	15	1800	2000	2400
16	2400	2800	3200	16	1800	2000	2400
17	2400	2800	3200	17	1800	2000	2400
18	2400	2800	3200	18	1800	2000	2400
19–20	2600	2800	3000	19–20	2000	2200	2400
21–25	2400	2800	3000	21–25	2000	2200	2400
26–30	2400	2600	3000	26–30	1800	2000	2400
31–35	2400	2600	3000	31–35	1800	2000	2200
36–40	2400	2600	2800	36–40	1800	2000	2200
41–45	2200	2600	2800	41–45	1800	2000	2200
46–50	2200	2400	2800	46–50	1800	2000	2200
51–55	2200	2400	2800	51–55	1600	1800	2200
56–60	2200	2400	2600	56–60	1600	1800	2200
61–65	2000	2400	2600	61–65	1600	1800	2000
66–70	2000	2200	2600	66–70	1600	1800	2000
71–75	2000	2200	2600	71–75	1600	1800	2000
76 and up	2000	2200	2400	76 and up	1600	1800	2000

Energy Balance in Real Life

Think of it as balancing your "lifestyle budget." For example, if you know you and your family will be going to a party and may eat more high-calorie foods than normal, then you may wish to eat fewer calories for a few days before so that it balances out. Or, you can increase your physical activity level for the few days before or after the party, so that you can burn off the extra energy.

The same applies to your kids. If they'll be going to a birthday party and eating cake and ice cream—or other foods high in fat and added sugar—help them balance their calories the day before and/or after by providing ways for them to be more physically active.

Here's another way of looking at energy balance in real life.

Eating just **150 calories more a day** than you burn can lead to an **extra 5 pounds** over **6 months**. That's a **gain of 10 pounds a year**. If you don't want this weight gain to happen or you want to lose the extra weight, you can either reduce your ENERGY IN or increase your ENERGY OUT. Doing both is the best way to achieve and maintain a healthy body weight.

- Here are some ways to **cut** 150 calories (ENERGY IN):

- Drink water instead of a 12-ounce regular soda

- Order a small serving of French fries instead of a medium or order a salad with dressing on the side instead

- Eat an egg-white omelet (with three eggs), instead of whole eggs

- Use tuna canned in water (6-ounce can), instead of oil

- Here are some ways to **burn** 150 calories (ENERGY OUT), **in just 30 minutes** (for a 150 pound person):
  - Shoot hoops
  - Walk two miles
  - Do yard work (gardening, raking leaves, etc.)
  - Go for a bike ride
  - Dance with your family or friends

Chapter 3

Food Labels

Chapter Contents

Section 3.1

How to Use Nutrition Labels?

This section contains text excerpted from the following sources: Text
in this section begins with excerpts from "How to Understand and
Use the Nutrition Facts Label?" U.S. Food and Drug Administration
(FDA), May 25, 2016; Text beginning with the heading "FDA
Modernizes Nutrition Facts Label for Packaged Food" is excerpted
from "Changes to the Nutrition Facts Label," U.S. Food and
Drug Administration (FDA), June 17, 2016.

People look at food labels for different reasons. But whatever the
reason, many consumers would like to know how to use this information more effectively and easily. The following label-building skills
are intended to make it easier for you to use nutrition labels –to make
quick, informed food choices that contribute to a healthy diet.

Nutrition Facts Panel: An Overview

The information in this section, can vary with each food product;
it contains product-specific information (serving size, calories, and
nutrient information). The bottom part contains a footnote with Daily
Values (DVs) for 2,000 and 2,500 calorie diets. This footnote provides
recommended dietary information for important nutrients, including
fats, sodium and fiber. The footnote is found only on larger packages
and does not change from product to product.

The Serving Size

The first place to start when you look at the Nutrition Facts label
is the serving size and the number of servings in the package. Serving
sizes are standardized to make it easier to compare similar foods; they
are provided in familiar units, such as cups or pieces, followed by the
metric amount, e.g., the number of grams.

The size of the serving on the food package influences the number
of calories and all the nutrient amounts listed on the top part of the
label. **Pay attention to the serving size, especially how many
servings there are in the food package. Then ask yourself, "How**

26

many servings am I consuming"? (e.g., 1/2 serving, 1 serving or more). In the sample label, one serving of macaroni and cheese equals one cup. If you ate the whole package, you would eat **two** cups. That doubles the calories and other nutrient numbers, including the % Daily Values as shown in the sample label.

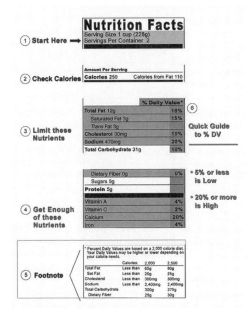

Figure 3.1. *Sample Label for Macaroni and Cheese*

Figure 3.2. *Serving Size*

Table 3.1. The Serving Size

Example				
	Single Serving	**%DV**	**Double Serving**	**%DV**
Serving Size	1 cup (228g)		2 cups (456g)	
Calories	250		500	
Calories from Fat	110		220	

Table 3.1. Continued

Example				
	Single Serving	**%DV**	**Double Serving**	**%DV**
Total Fat	12g	18.00%	24g	36.00%
Trans Fat	1.5g		3g	
Saturated Fat	3g	15.00%	6g	30.00%
Cholesterol	30mg	10.00%	60mg	20.00%
Sodium	470mg	20.00%	940mg	40.00%
Total Carbohydrate	31g	10.00%	62g	20.00%
Dietary Fiber	0g	0.00%	0g	0.00%
Sugars	5g		10g	
Protein	5g		10g	
Vitamin A		4.00%		8.00%
Vitamin C		2.00%		4.00%
Calcium		20.00%		40.00%
Iron		4.00%		8.00%

Calories (and Calories from Fat)

Calories provide a measure of how much energy you get from a serving of this food. Many Americans consume more calories than they need without meeting recommended intakes for a number of nutrients. The calorie section of the label can help you manage your weight (i.e., gain, lose or maintain.)

Remember: the number of servings you consume determines the number of calories you actually eat (your portion amount).

In the example, there are 250 calories in one serving of this macaroni and cheese. How many calories from fat are there in ONE serving? Answer: 110 calories, which means almost half the calories in a single serving come from fat. What if you ate the whole package content? Then, you would consume two servings or 500 calories, and 220 would come from fat.

Amount Per Serving

Calories 250   Calories from Fat 110

Figure 3.3. *Amount per Serving*

General Guide to Calories

- 40 Calories is low

- 100 Calories is moderate

- 400 Calories or more is high

The General Guide to Calories provides a general reference for calories when you look at a Nutrition Facts label. This guide is based on a 2,000 calorie diet.

Eating too many calories per day is linked to overweight and obesity.

The Nutrients: How Much?

Limit These Nutrients

The nutrients listed first are the ones Americans generally eat in adequate amounts or even too much. They are identified as **Limit these Nutrients.** Eating too much fat, saturated fat, trans fat, cholesterol or sodium may increase your risk of certain chronic diseases, like heart disease, some cancers or high blood pressure.

Total Fat 12g	**18%**
Saturated Fat 3g	**15%**
Trans Fat 3g	
Cholesterol 30mg	**10%**
Sodium 470mg	**20%**

Figure 3.4. *Limit These Nutrients*

Important: Health experts recommend that you keep your intake of saturated fat, trans fat and cholesterol as low as possible as part of a nutritionally balanced diet.

Get Enough of These

Most Americans don't get enough dietary fiber, vitamin A, vitamin C, calcium, and iron in their diets. They are identified as **Get Enough of these Nutrients**. Eating enough of these nutrients can improve your health and help reduce the risk of some diseases and conditions. For example, getting enough calcium may reduce the risk of osteoporosis, a condition that results in brittle bones as one ages. Eating a diet high in dietary fiber promotes healthy bowel function. Additionally, a diet rich in fruits, vegetables, and grain products that contain dietary fiber, particularly soluble fiber, and low in saturated fat and cholesterol may reduce the risk of heart disease.

Dietary Fiber 0g	0%
Vitamin A	4%
Vitamin C	2%
Calcium	20%
Iron	4%

Figure 3.5. *Get Enough of These*

Understanding the Footnote on the Bottom of the Nutrition Facts Label

Note the * used after the heading "%Daily Value" on the Nutrition Facts label. It refers to the Footnote in the lower part of the nutrition label, which tells you "**%DVs are based on a 2,000 calorie diet**". This statement must be on all food labels. But the remaining information in the full footnote may not be on the package if the size of the label is too small. When the full footnote does appear, it will always be the same. It doesn't change from product to product, because it shows recommended dietary advice for all Americans—it is not about a specific food product.

*Percent Daily Values are based on a 2,000 calorie diet. Your Daily Values may be higher or lower depending on your calorie needs.

	Calories:	2,000	2,500
Total Fat	Less than	65g	80g
Sat Fat	Less than	20g	25g
Cholesterol	Less than	300mg	300mg
Sodium	Less than	2,400mg	2,400mg
Total Carbohydrate		300g	375g
Dietary Fiber		25g	30g

Figure 3.6. *Get Enough of These*

Look at the amounts circled in red in the footnote—these are the Daily Values (DV) for each nutrient listed and are based on public health experts' advice. DVs are recommended levels of intakes. DVs in the footnote are based on a 2,000 or 2,500 calorie diet. Note how the DVs for some nutrients change, while others (for cholesterol and sodium) remain the same for both calorie amounts.

How the Daily Values Relate to the %DVs

Look at the example below for another way to see how the Daily Values (DVs) relate to the %DVs and dietary guidance. For each nutrient listed there is a DV, a %DV, and dietary advice or a goal. If you follow this dietary advice, you will stay within public health experts' recommended upper or lower limits for the nutrients listed, based on a 2,000 calorie daily diet.

Examples of DVs versus %DVs

Table 3.2. Based on a 2,000 Calorie Diet

Nutrient	DV	%DV	Goal
Total Fat	65g	#N/A	Less than
Sat Fat	20g	#N/A	Less than
Cholesterol	300mg	#N/A	Less than
Sodium	2400mg	#N/A	Less than
Total Carbohydrate	300g	#N/A	At least
Dietary Fiber	25g	#N/A	At least

Upper Limit-Eat "Less Than"

The nutrients that have "upper daily limits" are listed first on the footnote of larger labels and on the example above. Upper limits means it is recommended that you stay below-eat "less than"-the Daily Value nutrient amounts listed per day. For example, the DV for Saturated fat is 20g. This amount is 100%DV for this nutrient. What is the goal or dietary advice? To eat "less than" 20 g or 100%DV for the day.

Lower Limit-Eat "At Least"

Now look at the section where dietary fiber is listed. The DV for dietary fiber is 25g, which is 100%DV. This means it is recommended that you eat "at least" this amount of dietary fiber per day.

The DV for Total Carbohydrate (section in white) is 300g or 100%DV. This amount is recommended for a balanced daily diet that is based on 2,000 calories, but can vary, depending on your daily intake of fat and protein.

The Percent Daily Value (%DV)

The % Daily Values (%DVs) are based on the Daily Value recommendations for key nutrients but only for a 2,000 calorie daily diet—not 2,500 calories. You, like most people, may not know how many calories you consume in a day. But you can still use the %DV as a frame of reference whether or not you consume more or less than 2,000 calories.

The %DV helps you determine if a serving of food is high or low in a nutrient.

Do you need to know how to calculate percentages to use the %DV? No, the label (the %DV) does the math for you. It helps you interpret the numbers (grams and milligrams) by putting them all on the same scale for the day (0–100%DV). The %DV column doesn't add up vertically to 100%. Instead each nutrient is based on 100% of the daily requirements for that nutrient (for a 2,000 calorie diet). This way you can tell high from low and know which nutrients contribute a lot or a little, to your **daily** recommended allowance (upper or lower).

Quick Guide to %DV

5%DV or less is low and 20%DV or more is high

This guide tells you that **5%DV or less is low** for all nutrients, those you want to limit (e.g., fat, saturated fat, cholesterol, and sodium) or for those that you want to consume in greater amounts (fiber, calcium, etc). As the **Quick Guide** shows, **20%DV or more is high** for all nutrients.

Example: Look at the amount of Total Fat in one serving listed on the sample nutrition label. Is 18%DV contributing a lot or a little to your fat limit of 100%DV? **Check the Quick Guide to %DV.** 18%DV, which is below 20%DV, is not yet high, but what if you ate the whole package (two servings)? You would double that amount, eating 36% of your daily allowance for Total Fat. Coming from just one food, that amount leaves you with 64% of your fat allowance (100%-36%=64%) for all of the other foods you eat that day, snacks and drinks included.

	% Daily Value*
Total Fat 12g	18%
Saturated Fat 3g	15%
Trans Fat 3g	
Cholesterol 30mg	10%
Sodium 470mg	20%
Total Carbohydrate 31g	10%
Dietary Fiber 0g	0%
Sugars 5g	
Protein 5g	
Vitamin A	4%
Vitamin C	2%
Calcium	20%
Iron	4%

Figure 3.7. *Quick Guide to %DV*

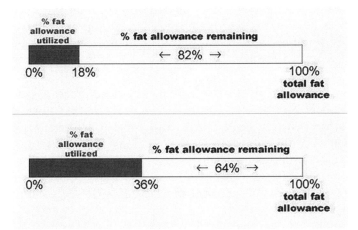

Figure 3.8. *Serving list*

Using the %DV

Comparisons: The %DV also makes it easy for you to make comparisons. You can compare one product or brand to a similar product.

Just make sure the serving sizes are similar, especially the weight (e.g. gram, milligram, ounces) of each product. It's easy to see which foods are higher or lower in nutrients because the serving sizes are generally consistent for similar types of foods, except in a few cases like cereals.

Nutrient Content Claims: Use the %DV to help you quickly distinguish one claim from another, such as "reduced fat" vs. "light" or "nonfat." Just compare the %DVs for Total Fat in each food product to see which one is higher or lower in that nutrient—there is no need to memorize definitions. This works when comparing all nutrient content claims, e.g., less, light, low, free, more, high, etc.

Dietary Trade-Offs: You can use the %DV to help you make dietary trade-offs with other foods throughout the day. You don't have to give up a favorite food to eat a healthy diet. When a food you like is high in fat, balance it with foods that are low in fat at other times of the day. Also, pay attention to how much you eat so that the total amount of fat for the day stays below 100%DV.

Nutrients with a %DV but No Weight Listed-Spotlight on Calcium

Calcium: Look at the %DV for calcium on food packages so you know how much one serving contributes to the *total amount you need* per day. Remember, a food with 20%DV or more contributes a lot of calcium to your daily total, while one with 5%DV or less contributes a little.

Experts advise adult consumers to consume adequate amounts of calcium, that is, 1,000mg or 100%DV in a daily 2,000 calorie diet. This advice is often given in milligrams (mg), but the Nutrition Facts label only lists a %DV for calcium.

For certain populations, they advise that adolescents, especially girls, consume 1,300mg (130%DV) and postmenopausal women consume 1,200mg (120%DV) of calcium daily. The DV for calcium on food labels is 1,000mg.

Don't be fooled—always check the label for calcium because you can't make assumptions about the amount of calcium in specific food categories. Example: the amount of calcium in milk, whether skim or whole, is generally the same per serving, whereas the amount of calcium in the same size yogurt container (8oz) can vary from 20–45 %DV.

Nutrition Facts

Serving Size 1 cup (236ml)
Servings Per Container 1

Amount Per Serving

Calories 80	Calories from Fat 0

	% Daily Value*
Total Fat 0g	0%
Saturated Fat 0g	0%
Trans Fat 0g	
Cholesterol Less than 5mg	0%
Sodium 120mg	5%
Total Carbohydrate 11g	4%
Dietary Fiber 0g	0%
Sugars 11g	
Protein 9g	17%

Vitamin A 10%	•	Vitamin C 4%
Calcium 30%	• Iron 0%	•Vitamin D 25%

*Percent Daily Values are based on a 2,000 calorie diet. Your daily values may be higher or lower depending on your calorie needs.

Figure 3.9. *Nutrition Facts*

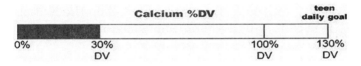

Figure 3.10. *Calcium %DV*

Table 3.3. Equivalencies

Equivalencies
30%DV = 300mg calcium = one cup of milk
100%DV = 1,000mg calcium
130%DV = 1,300mg calcium

Nutrients without a %DV: Trans Fats, Protein, and Sugars:

Note that Trans-fat, Sugars and, Protein do not list a %DV on the Nutrition Facts label.

Trans Fat: Experts could not provide a reference value for trans-fat nor any other information that FDA believes is sufficient to establish a Daily Value or %DV. Scientific reports link trans-fat (and saturated fat) with raising blood LDL ("bad") cholesterol levels, both of which increase your risk of coronary heart disease, a leading cause of death in the United States.

Protein: A %DV is required to be listed if a claim is made for protein, such as "high in protein". Otherwise, unless the food is meant for use by infants and children under 4 years old, none is needed. Current scientific evidence indicates that protein intake is not a public health concern for adults and children over 4 years of age.

Sugars: No daily reference value has been established for sugars because no recommendations have been made for the total amount to eat in a day. Keep in mind, the sugars listed on the Nutrition Facts label include naturally occurring sugars (like those in fruit and milk) as well as those added to a food or drink. Check the ingredient list for specifics on added sugars.

Take a look at the Nutrition Facts label for the two yogurt examples. The plain yogurt on the left has 10g of sugars, while the fruit yogurt on the right has 44g of sugars in one serving.

Now look below at the ingredient lists for the two yogurts. Ingredients are listed in descending order of weight (from most to least). Note that no added sugars or sweeteners are in the list of ingredients for the plain yogurt, yet 10g of sugars were listed on the Nutrition Facts label. This is because there are no added sugars in plain yogurt, only naturally occurring sugars (lactose in the milk).

Nutrition Facts		
Serving Size 1 container (226g)		
Amount Per Serving		
Calories 110 Calories from Fat 0		
		% Daily Value*
Total Fat 0g		0 %
Saturated Fat 0g		0 %
Trans Fat 0g		
Cholesterol Less than 5mg		1 %
Sodium 160mg		7 %
Total Carbohydrate 15g		5 %
Dietary Fiber 0g		0 %
Sugars 10g		
Protein 13g		
Vitamin A 0 % • Vitamin C		4 %
Calcium 45 % • Iron		0 %
*Percent Daily Values are based on a 2,000 calorie diet. Your Daily Values may be higher or lower depending on your calorie needs.		

Figure 3.11. *Plain Yogurt*

Nutrition Facts		
Serving Size 1 container (227g)		
Amount Per Serving		
Calories 240 Calories from Fat 25		
		% Daily Value*
Total Fat 3g		4 %
Saturated Fat 1.5g		9 %
Trans Fat 0g		
Cholesterol 15mg		5 %
Sodium 140mg		6 %
Total Carbohydrate 46g		15 %
Dietary Fiber Less than 1g		3 %
Sugars 44g		
Protein 9g		
Vitamin A 2 % • Vitamin C		4 %
Calcium 35 % • Iron		0 %
*Percent Daily Values are based on a 2,000 calorie diet. Your Daily Values may be higher or lower depending on your calorie needs.		

Figure 3.12. *Fruit Yogurt*

Plain Yogurt—contains no added sugars

INGREDIENTS: CULTURED PASTEURIZED GRADE A NONFAT MILK, WHEY PROTEIN CONCENTRATE, PECTIN, CARRAGEENAN.

Figure 3.13. *Ingredients for Plain Yogurt*

Fruit Yogurt—contains added sugars

INGREDIENTS: CULTURED GRADE A REDUCED FAT MILK, APPLES, HIGH FRUCTOSE CORN SYRUP, CINNAMON, NUTMEG, NATURAL FLAVORS, AND PECTIN. CONTAINS ACTIVE YOGURT AND L. ACIDOPHILUS CULTURES.

Figure 3.14. *Ingredients for Fruit Yogurt*

If you are concerned about your intake of sugars, make sure that added sugars are not listed as one of the first few ingredients. Other names for added sugars include: corn syrup, high-fructose corn syrup, fruit juice concentrate, maltose, dextrose, sucrose, honey, and maple syrup.

To limit nutrients that have no %DV, like trans-fat and sugars, compare the labels of similar products and choose the food with the lowest amount.

Nutrition Facts

Serving Size 1 cup (236ml)
Servings Per Container 1

Amount Per Serving

Calories 120	Calories from Fat 45

	% Daily Value*
Total Fat 5g	8%
Saturated Fat 3g	15%
Trans Fat 0g	
Cholesterol 20mg	7%
Sodium 120mg	5%
Total Carbohydrate 11g	4%
Dietary Fiber 0g	0%
Sugars 11g	
Protein 9g	17%

Vitamin A 10%	•	Vitamin C 4%
Calcium 30% • Iron 0% • Vitamin D 25%		

*Percent Daily Values are based on a 2,000 calorie diet. Your daily values may be higher or lower depending on your calorie needs.

Figure 3.15. *Reduced Fat Milk— 2% Milk fat*

Nutrition Facts

Serving Size 1 cup (236ml)
Servings Per Container 1

Amount Per Serving

Calories 80	Calories from Fat 0

	% Daily Value*
Total Fat 0g	0%
Saturated Fat 0g	0%
Trans Fat 0g	
Cholesterol Less than 5mg	0%
Sodium 120mg	5%
Total Carbohydrate 11g	4%
Dietary Fiber 0g	0%
Sugars 11g	
Protein 9g	17%

Vitamin A 10%	•	Vitamin C 4%
Calcium 30% • Iron 0% • Vitamin D 25%		

*Percent Daily Values are based on a 2,000 calorie diet. Your daily values may be higher or lower depending on your calorie needs.

Figure 3.16. *Non-fat Milk*

Comparison Example

Below are two kinds of milk-one is "Reduced Fat," the other is "Non-fat" milk. Each serving size is one cup. Which has more calories and more saturated fat? Which one has more calcium?

FDA Modernizes Nutrition Facts Label for Packaged Food

Features a Refreshed Design

- The "iconic" look of the label remains, but we are making important updates to ensure consumers have access to the information they need to make informed decisions about the foods they eat. These changes include increasing the type size for "Calories," "servings per container," and the "Serving size" declaration, and bolding the number of calories and the "Serving size" declaration to highlight this information.

- Manufacturers must declare the actual amount, in addition to percent Daily Value of vitamin D, calcium, iron, and potassium. They can voluntarily declare the gram amount for other vitamins and minerals.

- The footnote is changing to better explain what percent Daily Value means. It will read: "*The % Daily Value tells you how much a nutrient in a serving of food contributes to a daily diet. 2,000 calories a day is used for general nutrition advice."

Reflects Updated Information about Nutrition Science

- "Added sugars," in grams and as percent Daily Value, will be included on the label. Scientific data shows that it is difficult to meet nutrient needs while staying within calorie limits if you consume more than 10 percent of your total daily calories from added sugar, and this is consistent with the 2015–2020 *Dietary Guidelines* for Americans.

- The list of nutrients that are required or permitted to be declared is being updated. Vitamin D and potassium will be required on the label. Calcium and iron will continue to be required. Vitamins A and C will no longer be required but can be included on a voluntary basis.

- While continuing to require "Total Fat," "Saturated Fat," and "Trans Fat" on the label, "Calories from Fat" is being removed because research shows the type of fat is more important than the amount.

- Daily values for nutrients like sodium, dietary fiber and vitamin D are being updated based on newer scientific evidence from the Institute of Medicine and other reports such as the 2015 *Dietary Guidelines* Advisory Committee Report, which was used in developing the 2015–2020 *Dietary Guidelines* for Americans. Daily values are reference amounts of nutrients to consume or not to exceed and are used to calculate the percent Daily Value (%DV) that manufacturers include on the label. The %DV helps consumers understand the nutrition information in the context of a total daily diet.

Updates Serving Sizes and Labeling Requirements for Certain Package Sizes

- By law, serving sizes must be based on amounts of foods and beverages that people are actually eating, not what they should be eating. How much people eat and drink has changed since the previous serving size requirements were published in 1993. For example, the reference amount used to set a serving of ice cream was previously ½ cup but is changing to ⅔ cup. The reference amount used to set a serving of soda is changing from 8 ounces to 12 ounces.

- Package size affects what people eat. So for packages that are between one and two servings, such as a 20 ounce soda or a 15-ounce can of soup, the calories and other nutrients will be required to be labeled as one serving because people typically consume it in one sitting.

- For certain products that are larger than a single serving but that could be consumed in one sitting or multiple sittings, manufacturers will have to provide "dual column" labels to indicate the amount of calories and nutrients on both a "per serving" and "per package" / "per unit" basis. Examples would be a 24-ounce bottle of soda or a pint of ice cream. With dual-column labels available, people will be able to easily understand how many calories and nutrients they are getting if they eat or drink the entire package/unit at one time.

Section 3.2

Understanding Claims on Food Labels

This section includes text excerpted from "Understanding Food Labels," Office on Women's Health (OWH), U.S. Department of Health and Human Services (HHS), November 5, 2013.

The Nutrition Facts Label

The U.S. government has rules for the information that is in the Nutrition Facts box on food packages. All packages have to include the same facts, so you can compare the packages to see which choice is best for you. For example, let's say you want to try to eat more fiber. You can look at two boxes of cereal to see which offers the most. You also can use the label to keep track of nutrients you should eat, like calcium. And you can see how much you're eating of nutrients you should limit, like sodium.

Ingredients Lists

The ingredients list on a food package tells you what items are used to make the product. The ingredients are listed in order from most to least, so the product has the largest amount of those items at the start of the list. You can use the ingredients list to look for items you want to limit, such as added sugars or items that you need to avoid because of food allergies.

Other Food Label Terms

In addition to the Nutrition Facts label, you may see lots of other words describing packaged foods. The government has rules for certain claims that food companies make. These include things like "fat-free," "reduced calorie," or "light." Here is what some of those terms mean:

Calorie Claims

- **Low-calorie** means 40 calories or less per serving.

- **Reduced-calorie** means at least 25% fewer calories per serving compared with the full calorie food.

- **Light or lite** means the food has half as much fat (or even less) than a similar food. If the food gets less than half its calories from fat, "light" or "lite" means it has half as much fat as a similar food or 30% fewer calories.

Sugary Words

- **Sugar-free** means less than 1/2 gram of sugar per serving.

- **Reduced sugar** means a product has at least 25 percent less sugar per serving compared with the regular-sugar food. So, the product still could have a lot of sugar even though it has less than a similar one.

Fat Facts

- **Fat-free or 100% fat-free** means less than 1/2 gram of fat per serving.

- **Low-fat** means 3 grams of fat or less per serving.

- **Reduced-fat** means at least 25% less fat when compared with the regular-fat food. So, the product still could have a lot of fat in it.

What's "Organic"?

- **The USDA organic seal means that the U.S. Department of Agriculture certifies that a food is organic**, which means that it is made without using things like pesticides, fertilizers made from sewerage, and antibiotics. You can learn more about the USDA organic program.

- **100% organic** means that all the ingredients in the food are organic.

- **Organic** means that if a food has more than one ingredient in it, at least 95% of the ingredients are organic.

- **Made with organic ingredients** means that 70% of the item is organic.

Sodium and Salt Sayings

- **Low-sodium** means the food has 140 milligrams (mg) or less of sodium per serving.

- **Very low-sodium** means a food has 35 mg or less of sodium per serving.

- **Reduced or less salt or sodium** means that a product has 25% less than a similar food.

- **Light in sodium or lightly salted** means the product has less than 50% salt or sodium than a similar product.

Part Two

The Elements of Good Nutrition

Chapter 4

Carbohydrates

What Are Carbohydrates?

Carbohydrates are the body's main source of energy. They are some-times called "carbs" for short. If you have heard of low-carb diets, you may think carbs are bad for you. Well, eating some carbohydrates is important. They help your body store energy for later use. Keep read-ing to learn more about:

- Types of carbohydrates
- Choosing carbohydrates

What Are the Types of Carbohydrates?

The carbohydrate group includes simple carbohydrates, complex carbohydrates, and fiber.

Simple carbohydrates are "simple" because they are in the most basic form. They are also sometimes called simple sugars. They include the sugar in sugar bowls and in candy. They also include the kinds of sugar that are naturally in fruits, vegetables, and milk. So, if fruit and candy both have sugar, why should you pick the fruit? Fruit has

This chapter includes text excerpted from "Carbohydrates," Office on Wom-en's Health (OWH), U.S. Department of Health and Human Services (HHS), November 5, 2013.

lots of other nutrients that are great for your health. An orange, for example, has vitamin C that is good for your skin.

Complex carbohydrates are "complex" because they are made of lots of simple sugars strung together. They are also called starches. They include bread, cereal, and pasta. They also include certain vegetables, like potatoes, peas, and corn. Your body needs to break starches down into sugars to use them for energy.

Fiber comes in many forms, like the outer parts of rice and other grains. Fiber offers a lot of health benefits, including helping with digestion. Also, because your body can't break it down, fiber helps you feel full. That means you may be less likely to overeat.

Choosing Carbohydrates

Sure, you may want to have some sweet treats from time to time. Try to choose carbohydrates that offer the best boost for your health. Here's some useful info to help you choose:

When Eating Grains, Choose Mostly Whole Grains

Grains are foods like wheat, rice, oats, and cornmeal. There are two main types of grains: whole grains and refined grains.

- **Whole grains** are foods like whole wheat bread, brown rice, whole cornmeal, and oatmeal. They offer lots of nutrients that your body needs, like vitamins, minerals, and fiber.

- At least half the grains you eat should be whole grains.

- It's not hard to figure out whether a product has a lot of whole grain. Just check the ingredients list on the package and see if a whole grain is one of the first few items listed.

- Keep in mind that "multi grain," "100% wheat," and brown-looking bread are not necessarily whole grain breads.

- **Refined grains** mean that the food company has removed some of the grain—and, along with it, some of the great nutrients. That's why your best bet is whole grain.

- **Enriched products** means some of the nutrients have been added back in. If you eat products with refined grains, try to eat ones that are enriched.

Try to Eat Foods with Dietary Fiber

Foods that contain good amounts of fiber include fruits, veggies, beans, nuts, seeds, and whole grains.

- The Nutrition Facts label on the back of food packages tells you how much fiber a product has. Aim to eat a total of around 25 grams of fiber per day.

Try to Avoid Foods with a Lot of Added Sugar

- Foods with a lot of sugar can have many calories but not much nutrition.

- Eating a lot of calories can lead to being an unhealthy weight, which can cause health problems such as diabetes and heart disease.

- Aim to keep added sugars to less than 10% of your calories. If you eat around 2,000 calories a day, that means you want no more than 200 calories to come from added sugar. A can of regular soda might have around 150 calories from added sugar.

- Things that have a lot of added sugars include fruit drinks, energy or sports drinks, cakes, cookies, donuts, and ice cream.

- You can tell if a food or drink has added sugars by looking at the list of ingredients. The ingredients are listed from the greatest amount to the least amount. If a type of sugar comes early in the list, it means the product has a lot of sugar. Types of added sugars include:

- Corn sweetener and corn syrup

- Fructose and high-fructose corn syrup

- Dextrose

- Glucose

- Maltose

- Sucrose

- Honey

- Sugar and brown sugar

- Molasses

- Syrup and malt syrup

- If you are thinking about using a sugar substitute, you may wonder if they are safe. The U.S. Food and Drug Administration (FDA) approves their safety before they can be sold in foods and drinks like diet sodas. They can be used "in moderation," so try not to eat and drink them all day long, and focus instead on foods that are packed with nutrients, such as fruits and vegetables. Some sugar substitutes you can buy include:

- Aspartame, in products such as Equal

- Sucralose, in products such as Splenda

- Saccharin, in products such as Sweet'N Low

- Acesulfame potassium, in products such as Sweet One

- Stevia, in products such as Truvia

Chapter 5

Protein

Learning about Proteins

You probably know you need to eat protein, but what is it? Many foods contain protein, but the best sources are beef, poultry, fish, eggs, dairy products, nuts, seeds, and legumes like black beans and lentils.

Protein builds, maintains, and replaces the tissues in your body. Your muscles, your organs, and your immune system are made up mostly of protein.

Your body uses the protein you eat to make lots of specialized protein molecules that have specific jobs. For instance, your body uses protein to make **hemoglobin**, the part of red blood cells that carries oxygen to every part of your body.

Other proteins are used to build cardiac muscle. What's that? Your heart! In fact, whether you're running or just hanging out, protein is doing important work like moving your legs, carrying oxygen to your body, and protecting you from disease.

All about Amino Acids

When you eat foods that contain protein, the digestive juices in your stomach and intestine go to work. They break down the protein in food into basic units, called amino acids. The amino acids then can be reused to make the proteins your body needs to maintain muscles, bones, blood, and body organs.

This chapter includes excerpts from "Learning about Proteins," © 1995–2016. The Nemours Foundation/KidsHealth®. Reprinted with permission.

Proteins are sometimes described as long necklaces with differently shaped beads. Each bead is a small amino acid. These amino acids can join together to make thousands of different proteins. Scientists have found many different amino acids in protein, but 22 of them are very important to human health.

Of those 22 amino acids, your body can make 13 of them without you ever thinking about it. Your body can't make the other nine amino acids, but you can get them by eating protein-rich foods. They are called essential amino acids because it's **essential** that you get them from the foods you eat.

Different Kinds of Protein

Protein from animal sources, such as meat and milk, is called complete, because it contains all nine of the essential amino acids. Most vegetable protein is considered incomplete because it lacks one or more of the essential amino acids. This can be a concern for someone who doesn't eat meat or milk products. But people who eat a vegetarian diet can still get all their essential amino acids by eating a wide variety of protein-rich vegetable foods.

For instance, you can't get all the amino acids you need from peanuts alone, but if you have peanut butter on whole-grain bread, you're set. Likewise, red beans won't give you everything you need, but red beans and rice will do the trick.

The good news is that you don't have to eat all the essential amino acids in every meal. As long as you have a variety of protein sources throughout the day, your body will grab what it needs from each meal.

How Much Is Enough?

You can figure out how much protein you need if you know how much you weigh. Each day, kids need to eat about 0.5 grams of protein for every pound (0.5 kilograms) they weigh. That's a gram for every 2 pounds (1 kilogram) you weigh. Your protein needs will grow as you get bigger, but then they will level off when you reach adult size. Adults, for instance, need about 60 grams per day.

To figure out your protein needs, multiply your weight in pounds times 0.5 or you can just take your weight and divide by 2. For instance, a 70-pound (or 32-kilogram) kid should have about 35 grams of protein every day. If you only know your weight in kilograms, you need about 1 gram of protein each day for every kilogram you weigh.

You can look at a food label to find out how many protein grams are in a serving. But if you're eating a balanced diet, you don't need to keep track of it. It's pretty easy to get enough protein. Here's an example of how a kid might get about 35 grams of protein in a day:

- 2 tablespoons (15 milliliters) peanut butter (7 grams protein)
- 1 cup (240 milliliters) low-fat milk (8 grams protein)
- 1 ounce (30 grams) or two domino-size pieces of cheddar cheese (7 grams protein)
- 1.5 ounces (90 grams) chicken breast (10.5 grams protein)
- ½ cup (80 grams) broccoli (2 grams protein)

Of course, you can choose your own favorite combination of protein-rich foods—now that you're a pro at protein!

Chapter 6

Fats

Chapter Contents

Section 6.1

Dietary Fats: An Overview

This section contains text excerpted from documents published
by two public domain sources. Text under headings marked 1
are excerpted from "All about Oils," ChooseMyPlate.gov, U.S.
Department of Agriculture (USDA), February 3, 2016; Text under
headings marked 2 are excerpted from "What Are Solid Fats?,"
ChooseMyPlate.gov, U.S. Department of Agriculture
(USDA), September 30, 2015.

What Are "Oils"?[1]

Oils are fats that are liquid at room temperature, like the vegetable
oils used in cooking. Oils come from many different plants and from
fish. Oils are NOT a food group, but they provide essential nutrients.
Therefore, oils are included in U.S. Department of Agriculture (USDA)
food patterns.

Some **commonly eaten oils** include: canola oil, corn oil, cottonseed
oil, olive oil, safflower oil, soybean oil, and sunflower oil. Some oils
are used mainly as **flavorings**, such as walnut oil and sesame oil. A
number of foods are naturally high in oils, like nuts, olives, some fish,
and avocados.

Foods that are mainly oil include: mayonnaise, certain salad
dressings, and soft (tub or squeeze) margarine with no trans fats.
Check the Nutrition Facts label to find margarines with 0 grams of
trans fat. Amounts of trans fat are required to be listed on labels.

Most oils are high in monounsaturated or polyunsaturated fats,
and low in saturated fats. Oils from plant sources (vegetable and nut
oils) do not contain any cholesterol. In fact, no plant foods contain
cholesterol. A few plant oils, however, including coconut oil, palm oil,
and palm kernel oil, are high in saturated fats and for nutritional
purposes should be considered to be solid fats.

Solid fats are fats that are solid at room temperature, like butter
and shortening. Solid fats come from many animal foods and can be
made from vegetable oils through a process called hydrogenation. Some

common fats are: butter, milk fat, beef fat (tallow, suet), chicken fat, pork fat (lard), stick margarine, shortening, and partially hydrogenated oil.

How Much Is My Allowance for Oils?[1]

Some Americans consume enough oil in the foods they eat, such as:

- nuts
- fish
- cooking oil
- salad dressing

Others could easily consume the recommended allowance by substituting oils for some solid fats they eat. A person's allowance for oils depends on age, sex, and level of physical activity. Daily allowances for oils are shown in the table below.

Table 6.1. Daily Allowance

Daily Allowance		
Children	2–3 years old 4–8 years old	3 teaspoons 4 teaspoons
Girls	9–13 years old 14–18 years old	5 teaspoons 5 teaspoons
Boys	9–13 years old 14–18 years old	5 teaspoons 6 teaspoons
Women	19–30 years old 31–50 years old 51+ years old	6 teaspoons 5 teaspoons 5 teaspoons
Men	19–30 years old 31–50 years old 51+ years old	7 teaspoons 6 teaspoons 6 teaspoons

How Do I Count the Oils I Eat?[1]

The table below gives a quick guide to the amount of oils in some common foods.

Table 6.2. Oil Table

Oil table				
	Amount of food	Amount of oil	Calories from oil	Total calories
		Teaspoons/grams	Approximate calories	Approximate calories

Table 6.2. Continued

Oil table				
	Amount of food	**Amount of oil**	**Calories from oil**	**Total calories**
Oils:				
Vegetable oils (such as canola, corn, cottonseed, olive, peanut, safflower, soybean, and sunflower)	1 Tbsp	3 tsp/14 g	120	120
Foods rich in oils:				
Margarine, soft (trans fat free)	1 Tbsp	2 ½ tsp/11 g	100	100
Mayonnaise	1 Tbsp	2 ½ tsp/11 g	100	100
Mayonnaise-type salad dressing	1 Tbsp	1 tsp/5 g	45	55
Italian dressing	2 Tbsp	2 tsp/8 g	75	85
Thousand Island dressing	2 Tbsp	2 ½ tsp/11 g	100	120
Olives*, ripe, canned	4 large	½ tsp/ 2 g	15	20
Avocado*	½ med	3 tsp/15 g	130	160
Peanut butter*	2 T	4 tsp/16 g	140	190
Peanuts, dry roasted*	1 oz	3 tsp/14 g	120	165
Mixed nuts, dry roasted*	1 oz	3 tsp/14 g	130	170
Cashews, dry roasted*	1 oz	3 tsp/14 g	115	165
Almonds, dry roasted*	1 oz	3 tsp/14 g	130	170
Hazelnuts*	1 oz	4 tsp/ 18 g	160	185
Sunflower seeds*	1 oz	3 tsp/14 g	120	165

Avocados and olives are part of the Vegetable Group; nuts and seeds are part of the Protein Foods Group. These foods are also high in oils. Soft margarine, mayonnaise, and salad dressings are mainly oil and are not considered to be part of any food group.

What Are Solid Fats?[2]

Solid fats are fats that are solid at room temperature, like beef fat, butter, and shortening. Solid fats mainly come from animal foods and can also be made from vegetable oils through a process called hydrogenation. Some common solid fats are:

- butter
- milk fat
- beef fat (tallow, suet)
- chicken fat
- cream
- pork fat (lard)
- stick margarine
- shortening
- hydrogenated and partially hydrogenated oils*
- coconut oil*
- palm and palm kernel oils*

* The starred items are called "oils" because they come from plant sources. Even though they are called "oils," they are considered to be solid fats because they are high in saturated or trans fatty acids.

Most solid fats are high in saturated fats and/or trans fats and have less monounsaturated or polyunsaturated fats. Animal products containing solid fats also contain cholesterol. Saturated fats and trans fats tend to raise "bad" Low-density lipoprotein (LDL) cholesterol levels in the blood. This, in turn increases the risk for heart disease. To lower risk for heart disease, cut back on foods containing saturated fats and trans fats. Some foods that contain solid fats include:

- many desserts and baked goods, such as cakes, cookies, donuts, pastries, and croissants
- many cheeses and foods containing cheese, such as pizza
- sausages, hot dogs, bacon, and ribs
- ice cream and other dairy desserts
- fried potatoes (French fries)-if fried in a solid fat or hydrogenated oil

- regular ground beef and cuts of meat with marbling or visible fat

- fried chicken and other chicken dishes with the skin

In some cases, the fat in foods is not visible. For example, the fat in fluid milk is a solid fat. Milk fat (butter) is solid at room temperature but it is suspended in the fluid milk by the process of homogenization.

In contrast to solid fats, oils are fats that are liquid at room temperature, like the vegetable oils used in cooking. Oils come from many different plants-such as corn and peanuts-and from fish. A few plant oils, including coconut oil and palm oil, are high in saturated fats and for nutritional purposes are considered solid fats.

Solid fats and oils provide the same number of calories per gram. However, oils are generally better for your health than solid fats because they contain less saturated fats and/or trans fats. Foods containing partially hydrogenated vegetable oils usually contain trans fats. Trans fats can be found in many cakes, cookies, crackers, icings, margarines, and microwave popcorns.

How Are Oils Different from Solid Fats?[1]

All fats and oils are a mixture of saturated fatty acids and unsaturated fatty acids. Unsaturated fatty acids include monounsaturated and polyunsaturated fats.

Oils are fats that are liquid at room temperature, like the vegetable oils used in cooking. Oils come from many different plants and from fish. Oils contain more monounsaturated and polyunsaturated fats.

Solid fats are fats that are solid at room temperature, like beef fat, butter, and shortening. Solid fats mainly come from animal foods and can also be made from vegetable oils through a process called hydrogenation. Solid fats contain more saturated fats and/or trans fats than oils. Saturated fats and trans fats tend to raise "bad" (LDL) cholesterol levels in the blood, which in turn increases the risk for heart disease. To lower risk for heart disease, cut back on foods containing saturated fats and trans fats.

Why Is It Important to Consume Oils?[1]

Oils are not a food group, but they do provide essential nutrients and are therefore included in USDA recommendations for what to eat. Note that only small amounts of oils are recommended.

Most of the fats you eat should be polyunsaturated (PUFA) or monounsaturated (MUFA) fats. Oils are the major source of MUFAs and

PUFAs in the diet. PUFAs contain some fatty acids that are necessary for health–called "essential fatty acids." Because oils contain these essential fatty acids, there is an allowance for oils in the food guide.

The MUFAs and PUFAs found in fish, nuts, and vegetable oils do not raise LDL ("bad") cholesterol levels in the blood. In addition to the essential fatty acids they contain, oils are the major source of vitamin E in typical American diets.

While consuming some oil is needed for health, oils still contain calories. In fact, oils and solid fats both contain about 120 calories per tablespoon. Therefore, the amount of oil consumed needs to be limited to balance total calorie intake. The Nutrition Facts label provides information to help you make smart choices.

Section 6.2

Types of Fats

This section includes text excerpted from "What Are the Types of Fat?" U.S. Department of Veterns Affairs (VA), March 22, 2014.

Most foods contain several different kinds of fat. Some are better for your health than others. It is wise to choose healthier types of fat, and enjoy them in moderation. Keep in mind that even healthier fats contain calories and should be **used sparingly** for weight management. Here is some information about healthy and harmful dietary fats.

The four major types of fats are:

1. Monounsaturated fats

2. Polyunsaturated fats

3. Saturated fats

4. Trans fats

Monounsaturated and polyunsaturated fats are known as "healthy fats" because they are good for your heart, cholesterol levels, and overall health. These fats tend to be "liquid" at room temperature. Consider beneficial polyunsaturated fats containing Omega-3 fatty acids found in fatty fish, flaxseed, and walnuts.

Harmful Dietary Fats

Table 6.3. Harmful Dietary Fats

Saturated Fat	Trans Fat
High-fat cuts of meat (beef, lamb, pork)	Commercially baked pastries, cookies, doughnuts, muffins, cakes, pizza dough, pie crusts
Chicken with the skin	Packaged snack foods (crackers, microwave popcorn, chips)
Whole-fat dairy products (cream/milk)	Stick margarine
Butter	Vegetable shortening
Palm and coconut oil (snack foods, nondairy creamers, whipped toppings)	Fried foods (French fries, fried chicken, chicken nuggets, breaded fish)
Ice cream	Candy bars
Cheese	Pre-mixed products (cake mix, pancake mix, chocolate drink mix)

Healthy Dietary Fats

Table 6.4. Healthy Dietary Fats

Monounsaturated Fat	Polyunsaturated Fat
Olive oil	Soybean oil
Canola oil	Corn oil
Sunflower oil	Safflower oil
Peanut oil	Walnuts
Olives	Sunflower, sesame, and pumpkin seeds; flaxseed
Nuts (almonds, peanuts, hazelnuts, macadamia nuts, pecans, cashews)	Fatty fish (salmon, tuna, mackerel, herring, trout, anchovies, sardines, and eel)
Avocados	Soymilk
Peanut butter	Tofu

Tips for Increasing Healthy Fats in Your Diet:

- Cook with olive oil.

- Plan snacks of nuts or olives.

- Eat more avocados.

- Dress your own salads instead of using commercial dressings.

Saturated fats and trans fats are known as the "harmful fats." They increase your risk of disease and elevate cholesterol. Saturated fats tend to be solid at room temperature, but they are also found in liquid tropical oils (palm and coconut). Trans fats (partially hydrogenated or hydrogenated fats) are oils that have been modified for longer shelf life. Trans fats are very bad for you. No amount of trans fats is healthy.

Tips for Decreasing Harmful Fats in Your Diet:

- Read food labels and avoid trans fats and hydrogenated/partially hydrogenated oils.

- Avoid fried products.

- Avoid fast food.

- When eating out, ask that foods be prepared with olive oil.

Section 6.3

Omega-3 Supplements

This section includes text excerpted from "Omega-3 Supplements: In Depth," National Center for Complementary and Integrative Health (NCCIH), August 2015.

Omega-3 fatty acids (omega-3s) are a group of polyunsaturated fatty acids that are important for a number of functions in the body. Some types of omega-3s are found in foods such as fatty fish and shellfish. Another type is found in some vegetable oils. Omega-3s are also available as dietary supplements. This section provides basic information about omega-3s—with a focus on dietary supplements, summarizes scientific research on effectiveness and safety, and suggests sources for additional information.

Key Facts

- There has been a substantial amount of research on supplements of omega-3s, particularly those found in seafood and fish oil, and heart disease. The findings of individual studies have been inconsistent. In 2012, two combined analyses of the results of these studies did not find convincing evidence these omega-3s protect against heart disease.

- There is some evidence that omega-3s found in seafood and fish oil may be modestly helpful in relieving symptoms in rheumatoid arthritis. For most other conditions for which omega-3s have been studied, definitive conclusions cannot yet be reached or studies have not shown omega-3s to be beneficial.

- Omega-3 supplements may interact with drugs that affect blood clotting.

- It is uncertain whether people with fish or shellfish allergies can safely consume fish oil supplements.

- Fish liver oils (which are not the same as fish oils) contain vitamins A and D as well as omega-3 fatty acids; these vitamins can be toxic in high doses.

- Tell all your healthcare providers about any complementary health approaches you use. Give them a full picture of what you do to manage your health. This will help ensure coordinated and safe care.

About Omega-3 Fatty Acids

The three principal omega-3 fatty acids are alpha-linolenic acid (ALA), eicosapentaenoic acid (EPA), and docosahexaenoic acid (DHA). The main sources of ALA in the U.S. diet are vegetable oils, particularly canola and soybean oils; flaxseed oil is richer in ALA than soybean and canola oils but is not commonly consumed. ALA can be converted, usually in small amounts, into EPA and DHA in the body. EPA and DHA are found in seafood, including fatty fish (e.g., salmon, tuna, and trout) and shellfish (e.g., crab, mussels, and oysters).

Commonly used dietary supplements that contain omega-3s include fish oil (which provides EPA and DHA) and flaxseed oil (which provides ALA). Algae oils are a vegetarian source of DHA.

Omega-3 fatty acids are important for a number of bodily functions, including muscle activity, blood clotting, digestion, fertility, and cell division and growth. DHA is important for brain development and function. ALA is an "essential" fatty acid, meaning that people must obtain it from food or supplements because the human body cannot manufacture it.

Safety

- Omega-3 fatty acid supplements usually do not have negative side effects. When side effects do occur, they typically consist of minor gastrointestinal symptoms, such as belching, indigestion or diarrhea.

- It is uncertain whether people with fish or shellfish allergies can safely consume fish oil supplements.

- Omega-3 supplements may extend bleeding time (the time it takes for a cut to stop bleeding). People who take drugs that affect bleeding time, such as anticoagulants ("blood thinners") or non-steroidal anti-inflammatory drugs (NSAIDs), should discuss the use of omega-3 fatty acid supplements with a healthcare provider.

- Fish liver oils, such as cod liver oil, are not the same as fish oil. Fish liver oils contain vitamins A and D as well as omega-3 fatty acids. Both of these vitamins can be toxic in large doses. The amounts of vitamins in fish liver oil supplements vary from one product to another.

- There is conflicting evidence about whether omega-3 fatty acids found in seafood and fish oil might increase the risk of prostate cancer. Additional research on the association of omega-3 consumption and prostate cancer risk is under way.

If You Are Considering Omega-3 Supplements

- Do not use omega-3 supplements to replace conventional care or to postpone seeing a healthcare provider about a health problem.

- Consult your healthcare provider before using omega-3 supplements. If you are pregnant, trying to become pregnant or breastfeeding; if you take medicine that affects blood clotting; if you are allergic to fish or shellfish; or if you are considering giving a child an omega-3 supplement, it is especially important to consult your (or your child's) healthcare provider.

- Look for published research studies on omega-3 supplements for the health condition that interests you. Information on evidence-based studies is available from NCCIH.

- Tell all your healthcare providers about any complementary health approaches you use. Give them a full picture of what you do to manage your health. This will help ensure coordinated and safe care.

Chapter 7

Dietary Fiber

Fit More Fiber into Your Day

Fiber—you know it's good for you. But if you're like many Americans, you don't get enough. In fact, most of us get less than half the recommended amount of fiber each day.

Dietary fiber is found in the plants you eat, including fruits, vegetables and whole grains. It's sometimes called bulk or roughage. You've probably heard that it can help with digestion. So it may seem odd that fiber is a substance that your body can't digest. It passes through your digestive system practically unchanged.

"You might think that if it's not digestible then it's of no value. But there's no question that higher intake of fiber from all food sources is beneficial," says Dr. Joanne Slavin, a nutrition scientist at the University of Minnesota.

Fiber can relieve constipation and normalize your bowel movements. Some studies suggest that high-fiber diets might also help with weight loss and reduce the risk for cardiovascular disease, diabetes, and cancer.

The strongest evidence of fiber's benefits is related to cardiovascular health. Several large studies that followed people for many years found that those who ate the most fiber had a lower risk for heart disease.

This chapter contains text excerpted from the following sources: Text under the heading "Fit More Fiber into Your Day" is excerpted from "Rough up Your Diet," *NIH News in Health*, National Institutes of Health (NIH), August 2010. Reviewed June 2016; Text under the heading "Fiber and Your Meal" is excerpted from "Fiber and Your Child," © 1995–2016. The Nemours Foundation/KidsHealth®. Reprinted with permission.

The links between fiber and cardiovascular health were so consistent that these studies were used by the Institute of Medicine to develop the Dietary Reference Intakes for fiber.

Experts suggest that men get about 38 grams of fiber a day, and women about 25 grams. Unfortunately, in the United States we take in an average of only 14 grams of fiber each day.

High fiber intake seems to protect against several heart-related problems. "There is evidence that high dietary fiber consumption lowers 'bad' cholesterol concentrations in the blood and reduces the risk for developing coronary artery disease, stroke, and high blood pressure," says Dr. Somdat Mahabir, a nutrition and disease expert with NIH's National Cancer Institute.

Fiber may also lessen the risk for type 2 diabetes, the most common form of diabetes. Fiber in the intestines can slow the absorption of sugar, which helps prevent blood sugar from spiking. "With diabetes, it's good to keep glucose levels from peaking too much," explains Dr. Gertraud Maskarinec of the University of Hawaii.

In a recent NIH-funded study, Maskarinec and her colleagues followed more than 75,000 adults for 14 years. Consistent with other large studies, their research found that diabetes risk was significantly reduced in people who had the highest fiber intake.

"We found that it's mostly the fiber from grains that protects against diabetes," Maskarinec says. However, she notes that while high fiber intake may offer some protection, the best way to reduce your risk of diabetes is to exercise and keep your weight in check.

Weight loss is another area where fiber might help. High-fiber foods generally make you feel fuller for longer. Fiber adds bulk but few calories. "In studies where people are put on different types of diets, those on the high-fiber diets typically eat about 10% fewer calories," says Slavin. Other large studies have found that people with high fiber intake tend to weigh less.

Scientists have also looked into links between fiber and different types of cancer, with mixed results. Much research has focused on colorectal cancer, the second-leading cause of cancer death nationwide. Protection against colorectal cancer is sometimes stronger when scientists look at whole-grain intake rather than just fiber. One NIH-funded study of nearly 500,000 older adults found no relationship between fiber and colorectal cancer risk, but whole-grain intake led to a modest risk reduction.

Different types of fiber might affect your health in different ways. That's why the Nutrition Facts Panels on some foods list 2 categories of fiber: soluble and insoluble. Soluble fiber may help to lower blood sugar and cholesterol. It's found in oat bran, beans, peas, and most fruits. Insoluble fiber is often used to treat or prevent constipation and diverticular disease, which affects the large intestine or colon. Insoluble fiber is found in wheat bran and some vegetables.

Still, experts say the type of fiber you eat is less important than making sure you get enough overall. "In general, people should not be too concerned by the specific type of fiber," says Mahabir. "The focus should be more on eating diets that are rich in whole grains, vegetables and fruits to get the daily fiber requirement."

Whole grains, fruits and vegetables are also packed with vitamins and other nutrients, so experts recommend that you get most of your fiber from these natural sources. "Unfortunately, a lot of people tend to pick low-fiber foods. They go for white bread or white rice. Most of the processed foods—foods that are really convenient—tend to be low in fiber," says Slavin.

For people who have trouble getting in enough fiber from natural sources, store shelves are filled with packaged foods that tout added fiber. These fiber-fortified products include yogurts, ice cream, cereals, snack bars, and juices. They generally contain isolated fibers, such as inulin, polydextrose or maltodextrin. These isolated fibers are included in the product label's list of ingredients.

The health benefits of isolated fibers are still unclear. Research suggests they may not have the same effects as the intact fibers found in whole foods. For instance, there's little evidence that isolated fibers help lower blood cholesterol, and they have differing effects on regularity. On the plus side, some studies suggest that inulin, an isolated fiber from chicory root, might boost the growth of good bacteria in the colon.

The bottom line is that most of us need to fit more fiber into our day, no matter what its source. "It would be great if people would choose more foods that are naturally high in fiber," Slavin says.

Increase your fiber intake gradually, so your body can get used to it. Adding fiber slowly helps you avoid gas, bloating and cramps. Eat a variety of fruits, vegetables, whole grains and nuts to add a mix of different fibers and a wide range of nutrients to your diet. A fiber-rich diet can help your health in many ways.

Fiber and Your Meal

Few kids would say they crave a good fiber-rich meal. Although the thought of fiber might bring gags and groans from kids, many appetizing foods are actually great sources of fiber—from fruits to whole-grain cereals.

Foods with fiber are not just for the senior-citizen crowd. They're beneficial to everyone because they're filling, which helps discourage over-eating—even though fiber itself adds no calories. Along with adequate fluid intake, fiber helps move food through the digestive system and can help relieve and prevent constipation. It also may lower LDL cholesterol ("bad" cholesterol) and help prevent diabetes and heart disease.

Figuring out Fiber

Dietary fiber is found in plant foods like fruits, vegetables, and grains. In packaged foods, the amount of fiber per serving is listed on food labels under total carbohydrates.

Some of the best fiber sources are as follows.

- whole-grain breads and cereals
- apples
- oranges
- bananas
- berries
- prunes
- pears
- green peas
- legumes (dried beans, split peas, lentils, etc.)
- artichokes
- almonds

A high-fiber food has 5 grams or more of fiber per serving; a good source of fiber is one that provides 2.5 to 4.9 grams per serving. Here's how some fiber-friendly foods stack up:

- ½ cup (118 milliliters) of cooked beans (kidney, white, black, pinto, lima) (6.2–9.6 grams of fiber)
- 1 medium baked sweet potato with peel (3.8 grams)
- 1 whole-wheat English muffin (4.4 grams)
- ½ cup (118 milliliters) of cooked green peas (4.4 grams)
- 1 medium pear with skin (5.5 grams)
- ½ cup (118 milliliters) of raspberries (4 grams)
- 1 medium baked potato with skin (3 grams)

- 1/3 cup (79 milliliters) of bran cereal (9.1 grams)
- 1 ounce (28 grams) of almonds (3.5 grams)
- 1 small apple with skin (3.6 grams)
- ¼ cup (59 milliliters) of dried figs (3.7 grams)
- ½ cup (118 milliliters) of edamame (3.8 grams)
- 1 medium orange (3.1 grams)
- 1 medium banana (3.1 grams)
- ½ cup (118 milliliters) canned sauerkraut (3.4 grams)

How Much Should Kids Get?

- Toddlers (1–3 years old) should get 19 grams of fiber each day.
- Kids 4–8 years old should get 25 grams a day.
- Older girls (9–13) and teen girls (14–18) should get 26 grams of fiber a day.
- Older boys (9–13) should get 31 grams and teen boys (14–18) should get 38 grams per day.

Adding Fiber to Your Family's Diet

Here are some creative, fun, and tasty ways to incorporate more fiber-rich foods into your family's diet:

Breakfast

- Make oatmeal (a whole grain) part of morning meals.
- Choose whole-grain cereals that have 3 grams or more fiber per serving.
- Make pancakes with whole-grain (or buckwheat) pancake mix and top with apples, berries or raisins.
- Serve bran or whole grain waffles topped with fruit.
- Offer whole-wheat bagels or English muffins, instead of white toast.
- Top fiber-rich cereal with apples, oranges, berries or bananas. Add almonds to pack even more fiber punch.
- Mix kid-favorite cereals with fiber-rich ones or top with a tablespoon of bran.

Lunch and Dinner

- Make sandwiches with whole-grain breads instead of white.

- Make a fiber-rich sandwich with whole-grain bread, peanut but-ter, and bananas.

- Serve whole-grain rolls with dinner instead of white rolls.

- Use whole-grain pastas instead of white.

- Serve wild or brown rice with meals instead of white rice. Add beans (kidney, black, navy, and pinto) to rice dishes for even more fiber.

- Spice up salads with berries and almonds, chickpeas, artichoke hearts, and beans (kidney, black, navy or pinto).

- Use whole-grain (corn or whole wheat) soft-taco shells or torti-llas to make burritos or wraps. Fill them with eggs and cheese for breakfast; turkey, cheese, lettuce, tomato, and light dressing for lunch; and beans, salsa, taco sauce, and cheese for dinner.

- Add lentils or whole-grain barley to soups.

- Create mini-pizzas by topping whole-wheat English muffins or bagels with pizza sauce, low-fat cheese, mushrooms, and pieces of grilled chicken.

- Add bran to meatloaf or burgers. (But not too much bran or your family might catch on!)

- Serve sweet potatoes with the skins as tasty side dishes. Regu-lar baked potatoes with the skins are good sources of fiber, too.

- Top low-fat hot dogs or veggie dogs with sauerkraut and serve them on whole-wheat hot dog buns.

- Pack fresh fruit or vegetables in school lunches.

Snacks and Treats

- Bake cookies or muffins using whole-wheat flour instead of reg-ular. Or use some whole-wheat and some regular flour, so that the texture of your baked treats won't be drastically different. Add raisins, berries, bananas or chopped or pureed apples to the mix for even more fiber.

- Add bran to baking items such as cookies and muffins.

- Top whole-wheat crackers with peanut butter or low-fat cheese.

- Offer air-popped popcorn—a whole-grain food—as a midday treat or while kids watch TV or movies. (However, only give popcorn to kids over 4 years old because it can be a choking hazard.)

- Top ice cream, frozen yogurt or low-fat yogurt with whole-grain cereal, berries or almonds for some added nutrition and crunch.

- Serve apples topped with peanut butter.

- Make fruit salad with pears, apples, bananas, oranges, and berries. Top with almonds for added crunch. Serve as a side dish with meals or alone as a snack.

- Make low-fat breads, muffins or cookies with canned pumpkin.

- Leave the skins on when serving fruits and veggies as snacks or as part of a meal.

Make gradual changes that will add up to a diet that's higher in fiber over time. And keep offering a variety of foods that are good sources of fiber—fruits like pears and berries; vegetables like spinach and green peas; lentils and kidney, white or black beans; and whole-grain breakfast cereals and breads. Kids will get the fiber they need, and you'll set the tone for a lifetime of healthy eating.

Chapter 8

Fluids and Hydration

Water and Nutrition

Getting enough water every day is important for your health. Healthy people meet their fluid needs by drinking when thirsty and drinking with meals. Most of your fluid needs are met through the water and beverages you drink. However, you can get some fluids through the foods that you eat. For example, broth soups and foods with high water content such as celery, tomatoes or melons can contribute to fluid intake.

Water Helps Your Body

- Keep your temperature normal.

- Lubricate and cushion joints.

- Protect your spinal cord and other sensitive tissues.

- Get rid of wastes through urination, perspiration, and bowel movements.

This chapter contains text excerpted from the following sources: Text under the heading "Water and Nutrition" is excerpted from "Water & Nutrition," Centers for Disease Control and Prevention (CDC), June 3, 2014; Text under the heading "Commercially Bottled Water" is excerpted from "Commercially Bottled Water," Centers for Disease Control and Prevention (CDC), April 7, 2014.

Your Body Needs More Water When You Are:

- In hot climates.

- More physically active.

- Running a fever.

- Having diarrhea or vomiting.

If You Think You Are Not Getting Enough Water, These Tips May Help

- Carry a water bottle for easy access when you are at work of running errands.

- Freeze some freezer safe water bottles. Take one with you for ice-cold water all day long.

- Choose water instead of sugar-sweetened beverages. This can also help with weight management. Substituting water for one 20-ounce sugar sweetened soda will save you about 240 calories. For example, during the school day students should have access to drinking water, giving them a healthy alternative to sugar-sweetened beverages.

- Choose water when eating out. Generally, you will save money and reduce calories.

- Add a wedge of lime or lemon to your water. This can help improve the taste and help you drink more water than you usually do.

Commercially Bottled Water

Americans spend billions of dollars every year on bottled water. People choose bottled water for a variety of reasons including aesthetics (for example, taste), health concerns or as a substitute for other beverages.

If you have questions about bottled water, make sure you are informed about where your bottled water comes from and how it has been treated. The standards for bottled water are set by the U.S. Food and Drug Administration (FDA). The FDA bases its standards on the U.S. Environmental Protection Agency (EPA) standards for tap water.

- Read the label on your bottled water. While there is currently no standardized label for bottled water, this label may tell you about the way the bottled water is treated.

- Check the label for a toll-free number or Webpage address of the company that bottled the water. This may be a source of further information.

Bottled Water and Immunocompromised Individuals

People with compromised immune systems may want to take special precautions with the water they drink. In healthy individuals, the parasite *Cryptosporidium parvum* can cause illness; however, for those with weakened immune systems, it can cause severe illness and possibly death. Look for bottled water treatments that protect against *Cryptosporidium parvum*, which include the following:

- Reverse Osmosis

- Distillation

- Filtration with an absolute 1 micron filter

Fluoride and Bottled Water

Some bottled waters contain fluoride, and some do not. Fluoride can occur naturally in source waters used for bottling or be added. Most bottled waters contain fluoride at levels that are less than optimal for good oral health.

Safety and Regulation

The FDA regulates bottled water under the Federal Food, Drug, and Cosmetic Act and sets standards for bottled water that are based on ones developed by EPA. If these standards are met, water is considered safe for most healthy individuals. The bottled water industry must also follow FDA's Current Good Manufacturing Practices (CGMPs) for processing and bottling drinking water.

Bottled Water Outbreaks

Although bottled water outbreaks are not often reported, they do occur. It is important for bottled water manufacturers, distributors, and consumers to:

- protect and properly treat water before bottling;

- maintain good manufacturing processes;

- protect bottled water during shipping and storage; and

- prevent contamination at the point of use (after purchase by the consumer).

The presence of contaminants in water can lead to adverse health effects, including gastrointestinal illness, reproductive problems, and neurological disorders. Infants, young children, pregnant women, the elderly, and people whose immune systems are compromised because of AIDS, chemotherapy or transplant medications, may be especially susceptible to illness from some contaminants.

The FDA regulates the safety of bottled water. If you suspect an illness resulting from the consumption of bottled water, you should contact your local public health department.

Chapter 9

Vitamins

Chapter Contents

Section 9.1

Vitamin A

This section includes text excerpted from "Vitamin A,"
Office on Dietary Supplements (ODS), National Institutes
of Health (NIH), June 5, 2013.

What Is Vitamin A and What Does It Do?

Vitamin A is a fat-soluble vitamin that is naturally present in many foods. Vitamin A is important for normal vision, the immune system, and reproduction. Vitamin A also helps the heart, lungs, kidneys, and other organs work properly.

There are two different types of vitamin A. The first type, preformed vitamin A, is found in meat, poultry, fish, and dairy products. The second type, provitamin A, is found in fruits, vegetables, and other plant-based products. The most common type of provitamin A in foods and dietary supplements is beta-carotene.

How Much Vitamin A Do I Need?

The amount of vitamin A you need depends on your age and reproductive status. Recommended intakes for vitamin A for people aged 14 years and older range between 700 and 900 micrograms (mcg) of retinol activity equivalents (RAE) per day. Recommended intakes for women who are nursing range between 1,200 and 1,300 RAE. Lower values are recommended for infants and children younger than 14.

However, the vitamin A content of foods and dietary supplements is given on product labels in international units (IU), not mcg RAE. Converting between IU and mcg RAE is not easy. A varied diet with 900 mcg RAE of vitamin A, for example, provides between 3,000 and 36,000 IU of vitamin A depending on the foods consumed.

For adults and children aged 4 years and older, the U.S. Food and Drug Administration (FDA) has established a vitamin A Daily Value (DV) of 5,000 IU from a varied diet of both plant and animal foods. DVs are not recommended intakes; they don't vary by age and sex, for example. But trying to reach 100% of the DV each day, on average, is useful to help you get enough vitamin A.

What Foods Provide Vitamin A?

Vitamin A is found naturally in many foods and is added to some foods, such as milk and cereal. You can get recommended amounts of vitamin A by eating a variety of foods, including the following:

- Beef liver and other organ meats (but these foods are also high in cholesterol, so limit the amount you eat).
- Some types of fish, such as salmon.
- Green leafy vegetables and other green, orange, and yellow vegetables, such as broccoli, carrots, and squash.
- Fruits, including cantaloupe, apricots, and mangos.
- Dairy products, which are among the major sources of vitamin A for Americans.
- Fortified breakfast cereals.

What Kinds of Vitamin A Dietary Supplements Are Available?

Vitamin A is available in dietary supplements, usually in the form of retinyl acetate or retinyl palmitate (preformed vitamin A), beta-carotene (provitamin A) or a combination of preformed and provitamin A. Most multivitamin-mineral supplements contain vitamin A. Dietary supplements that contain only vitamin A are also available.

Am I Getting Enough Vitamin A?

Most people in the United States get enough vitamin A from the foods they eat, and vitamin A deficiency is rare. However, certain groups of people are more likely than others to have trouble getting enough vitamin A:

- Premature infants, who often have low levels of vitamin A in their first year;
- Infants, young children, pregnant women, and breastfeeding women in developing countries; and
- People with cystic fibrosis.

What Happens If I Don't Get Enough Vitamin A?

Vitamin A deficiency is rare in the United States, although it is common in many developing countries. The most common symptom of vitamin A deficiency in young children and pregnant women is an eye condition called xerophthalmia. Xerophthalmia is the inability to see in low light, and it can lead to blindness if it isn't treated.

What Are Some Effects of Vitamin A on Health?

Scientists are studying vitamin A to understand how it affects health. Here are some examples of what this research has shown.

Cancer

People who eat a lot of foods containing beta-carotene might have a lower risk of certain kinds of cancer, such as lung cancer or prostate cancer. But studies to date have not shown that vitamin A or beta-carotene supplements can help prevent cancer or lower the chances of dying from this disease. In fact, studies show that smokers who take high doses of beta-carotene supplements have an increased risk of lung cancer.

Age-Related Macular Degeneration

Age-related macular degeneration (AMD) or the loss of central vision as people age, is one of the most common causes of vision loss in older people. Among people with AMD who are at high risk of developing advanced AMD, a supplement containing antioxidants, zinc, and copper with or without beta-carotene has shown promise for slowing down the rate of vision loss.

Measles

When children with vitamin A deficiency (which is rare in North America) get measles, the disease tends to be more severe. In these children, taking supplements with high doses of vitamin A can shorten the fever and diarrhea caused by measles. These supplements can also lower the risk of death in children with measles who live in developing countries where vitamin A deficiency is common.

Can Vitamin A Be Harmful?

Yes, high intakes of some forms of vitamin A can be harmful.

Getting too much preformed vitamin A (usually from supplements or certain medicines) can cause dizziness, nausea, headaches, coma, and even death. High intakes of preformed vitamin A in pregnant women can also cause birth defects in their babies. Women who might be pregnant should not take high doses of vitamin A supplements.

Consuming high amounts of beta-carotene or other forms of provitamin A can turn the skin yellow-orange, but this condition is harmless. High intakes of beta-carotene do not cause birth defects or the other more serious effects caused by getting too much preformed vitamin A.

The upper limits for preformed vitamin A in IU are listed below. These levels do not apply to people who are taking vitamin A for medical reasons under the care of a doctor. Upper limits for beta-carotene and other forms of provitamin A have not been established.

Table 9.1. Upper Limits for Preformed Vitamin A in International Units (IU)

Life Stage	Upper Limit
Birth to 12 months	2,000 IU
Children 1–3 years	2,000 IU
Children 4–8 years	3,000 IU
Children 9–13 years	5,667 IU
Teens 14–18 years	9,333 IU
Adults 19 years and older	10,000 IU

Section 9.2

The Vitamin B Family

This section contains text excerpted from the following sources: Text under the heading "Thiamin" is excerpted from "Thiamin," Office on Dietary Supplements (ODS), National Institutes of Health (NIH), April 13, 2016; Text under the heading "Riboflavin" is excerpted from "Riboflavin," Office on Dietary Supplements (ODS), National Institutes of Health (NIH), February 17, 2016; Text under the heading "Vitamin B6" is excerpted from "Vitamin B6," Office on Dietary Supplements (ODS), National Institutes of Health (NIH), February 17, 2016; Text under the heading "Vitamin B12" is excerpted from "Vitamin B12 Fact Sheet for Consumers," Office on Dietary Supplements (ODS), National Institutes of Health (NIH), February 17, 2016.

Thiamin

What Is Thiamin and What Does It Do?

Thiamin (also called vitamin B1) helps turn the food you eat into the energy you need. Thiamin is important for the growth, development, and function of the cells in your body.

How Much Thiamin Do I Need?

The amount of thiamin you need depends on your age and sex. Average daily recommended amounts are listed below in milligrams (mg).

Table 9.2. Average Daily Recommended Amount of Thiamin

Life Stage	Recommended Amount
Birth to 6 months	0.2 mg
Infants 7–12 months	0.3 mg
Children 1–3 years	0.5 mg
Children 4–8 years	0.6 mg
Children 9–13 years	0.9 mg
Teen boys 14–18 years	1.2 mg

Table 9.2. Continued

Life Stage	Recommended Amount
Teen girls 14–18 years	1.0 mg
Men	1.2 mg
Women	1.1 mg
Pregnant teens and women	1.4 mg
Breastfeeding teens and women	1.4 mg

What Foods Provide Thiamin?

Thiamin is found naturally in many foods and is added to some fortified foods. You can get recommended amounts of thiamin by eating a variety of foods, including the following:

- Whole grains and fortified bread, cereal, pasta, and rice.

- Meat (especially pork) and fish.

- Legumes (such as black beans and soybeans), seeds, and nuts.

What Kinds of Thiamin Dietary Supplements Are Available?

Thiamin is found in multivitamin/multimineral supplements, in B-complex dietary supplements, and in supplements containing only thiamin. Common forms of thiamin in dietary supplements are thiamin mononitrate and thiamin hydrochloride. Some supplements use a synthetic form of thiamin called benfotiamine.

What Are Some Effects of Thiamin on Health?

Scientists are studying thiamin to better understand how it affects health. Here are some examples of what this research has shown.

Diabetes

People with diabetes often have low levels of thiamin in their blood. Scientists are studying whether thiamin supplements can improve blood sugar levels and glucose tolerance in people with type 2 diabetes. They are also studying whether benfotiamine (a synthetic form of thiamin) supplements can help with nerve damage caused by diabetes.

Heart Failure

Many people with heart failure have low levels of thiamin. Scientists are studying whether thiamin supplements might help people with heart failure.

Alzheimer Disease

Scientists are studying the possibility that thiamin deficiency could affect the dementia of Alzheimer disease. Whether thiamin supplements may help mental function in people with Alzheimer disease needs further study.

Can Thiamin Be Harmful?

Thiamin has not been shown to cause any harm.

Riboflavin

What Is Riboflavin and What Does It Do?

Riboflavin (also called vitamin B2) is important for the growth, development, and function of the cells in your body. It also helps turn the food you eat into the energy you need.

How Much Riboflavin Do I Need?

The amount of riboflavin you need depends on your age and sex. Average daily recommended amounts are listed below in milligrams (mg).

Table 9.3. Average Daily Recommended Amounts of Riboflavin

Life Stage	Recommended Amount
Birth to 6 months	0.3 mg
Infants 7–12 months	0.4 mg
Children 1–3 years	0.5 mg
Children 4–8 years	0.6 mg
Children 9–13 years	0.9 mg
Teen boys 14–18 years	1.3 mg
Teen girls 14–18 years	1.0 mg
Men	1.3 mg
Women	1.1 mg

Table 9.3. Continued

Life Stage	Recommended Amount
Pregnant teens and women	1.4 mg
Breastfeeding teens and women	1.6 mg

What Foods Provide Riboflavin?

Riboflavin is found naturally in some foods and is added to many fortified foods. You can get recommended amounts of riboflavin by eating a variety of foods, including the following:

- Eggs, organ meats (such as kidneys and liver), lean meats, and low-fat milk.

- Green vegetables (such as asparagus, broccoli, and spinach).

- Fortified cereals, bread, and grain products.

What Kinds of Riboflavin Dietary Supplements Are Available?

Riboflavin is found in multivitamin/multimineral supplements, in B-complex dietary supplements, and in supplements containing only riboflavin. Some supplements have much more than the recommended amounts of riboflavin, but your body can't absorb more than about 27 mg at a time.

What Is an Effect of Riboflavin Supplements on Health?

Scientists are studying riboflavin to better understand how it affects health. Here is an example of what this research has shown.

Migraine Headache

Some studies show that riboflavin supplements might help prevent migraine headaches, but other studies do not. Riboflavin supplements usually have very few side effects, so some medical experts recommend trying riboflavin, under the guidance of a healthcare provider, for preventing migraines.

Vitamin B6

What Is Vitamin B6 and What Does It Do?

Vitamin B6 is a vitamin that is naturally present in many foods. The body needs vitamin B6 for more than 100 enzyme reactions involved in metabolism. Vitamin B6 is also involved in brain development during pregnancy and infancy as well as immune function.

How Much Vitamin B6 Do I Need?

The amount of vitamin B6 you need depends on your age. Average daily recommended amounts are listed below in milligrams (mg).

Table 9.4. Average daily recommended amount of Vitamin B6

Life Stage	Recommended Amount
Birth to 6 months	0.1 mg
Infants 7–12 months	0.3 mg
Children 1–3 years	0.5 mg
Children 4–8 years	0.6 mg
Children 9–13 years	1.0 mg
Teens 14–18 years (boys)	1.3 mg
Teens 14–18 years (girls)	1.2 mg
Adults 19–50 years	1.3 mg
Adults 51+ years (men)	1.7 mg
Adults 51+ years (women)	1.5 mg
Pregnant teens and women	1.9 mg
Breastfeeding teens and women	2.0 mg

What Foods Provide Vitamin B6?

Vitamin B6 is found naturally in many foods and is added to other foods. You can get recommended amounts of vitamin B6 by eating a variety of foods, including the following:

- Poultry, fish, and organ meats, all rich in vitamin B6.
- Potatoes and other starchy vegetables, which are some of the major sources of vitamin B6 for Americans.
- Fruit (other than citrus), which are also among the major sources of vitamin B6 for Americans.

What Kinds of Vitamin B6 Dietary Supplements Are Available?

Vitamin B6 is available in dietary supplements, usually in the form of pyridoxine. Most multivitamin-mineral supplements contain vitamin B6. Dietary supplements that contain only vitamin B6 or vitamin B6 with other B vitamins, are also available.

What Are Some Effects of Vitamin B6 on Health?

Scientists are studying vitamin B6 to understand how it affects health. Here are some examples of what this research has shown.

Heart Disease

Some scientists had thought that certain B vitamins (such as folic acid, vitamin B12, and vitamin B6) might reduce heart disease risk by lowering levels of homocysteine, an amino acid in the blood. Although vitamin B supplements do lower blood homocysteine, research shows that they do not actually reduce the risk or severity of heart disease or stroke.

Cancer

People with low levels of vitamin B6 in the blood might have a higher risk of certain kinds of cancer, such as colorectal cancer. But studies to date have not shown that vitamin B6 supplements can help prevent cancer or lower the chances of dying from this disease.

Cognitive Function

Some research indicates that elderly people who have higher blood levels of vitamin B6 have better memory. However, taking vitamin B6 supplements (alone or combined with vitamin B12 and/or folic acid) does not seem to improve cognitive function or mood in healthy people or in people with dementia.

Premenstrual Syndrome

Scientists aren't yet certain about the potential benefits of taking vitamin B6 for premenstrual syndrome (PMS). But some studies show that vitamin B6 supplements could reduce PMS symptoms, including moodiness, irritability, forgetfulness, bloating, and anxiety.

Nausea and Vomiting in Pregnancy

At least half of all women experience nausea, vomiting or both in the first few months of pregnancy. Based on the results of several studies, the American Congress of Obstetricians and Gynecologists

(ACOG) recommends taking vitamin B6 supplements under a doctor's care for nausea and vomiting during pregnancy.

Can Vitamin B6 Be Harmful?

People almost never get too much vitamin B6 from food. But taking high levels of vitamin B6 from supplements for a year or longer can cause severe nerve damage, leading people to lose control of their bodily movements. The symptoms usually stop when they stop taking the supplements. Other symptoms of too much vitamin B6 include painful, unsightly skin patches, extreme sensitivity to sunlight, nausea, and heartburn.

The upper limits for vitamin B6 are listed below. These levels do not apply to people who are taking vitamin B6 for medical reasons under the care of a doctor.

Table 9.5. Upper Limits for Vitamin B6

Life Stage	Upper Limit
Birth to 12 months	Not established
Children 1–3 years	30 mg
Children 4–8 years	40 mg
Children 9–13 years	60 mg
Teens 14–18 years	80 mg
Adults	100 mg

Vitamin B12

What Is Vitamin B12 and What Does It Do?

Vitamin B12 is a nutrient that helps keep the body's nerve and blood cells healthy and helps make DNA, the genetic material in all cells. Vitamin B12 also helps prevent a type of anemia called megaloblastic anemia that makes people tired and weak.

Two steps are required for the body to absorb vitamin B12 from food. First, hydrochloric acid in the stomach separates vitamin B12 from the protein to which vitamin B12 is attached in food. After this, vitamin B12 combines with a protein made by the stomach called intrinsic factor and is absorbed by the body. Some people have pernicious anemia, a condition where they cannot make intrinsic factor. As a result, they have trouble absorbing vitamin B12 from all foods and dietary supplements.

How Much Vitamin B12 Do I Need?

The amount of vitamin B12 you need each day depends on your age. Average daily recommended amounts for different ages are listed below in micrograms (mcg):

Table 9.6. Upper Limits for Vitamin B6

Life Stage	Recommended Amount
Birth to 6 months	0.4 mcg
Infants 7–12 months	0.5 mcg
Children 1–3 years	0.9 mcg
Children 4–8 years	1.2 mcg
Children 9–13 years	1.8 mcg
Teens 14–18 years	2.4 mcg
Adults	2.4 mcg
Pregnant teens and women	2.6 mcg
Breastfeeding teens and women	2.8 mcg

What Foods Provide Vitamin B12?

Vitamin B12 is found naturally in a wide variety of animal foods and is added to some fortified foods. Plant foods have no vitamin B12 unless they are fortified. You can get recommended amounts of vitamin B12 by eating a variety of foods including the following:

- Beef liver and clams, which are the best sources of vitamin B12.

- Fish, meat, poultry, eggs, milk, and other dairy products, which also contain vitamin B12.

- Some breakfast cereals, nutritional yeasts, and other food products that are fortified with vitamin B12. To find out if vitamin B12 has been added to a food product, check the product labels.

What Kinds of Vitamin B12 Dietary Supplements Are Available?

Vitamin B12 is found in almost all multivitamins. Dietary supplements that contain only vitamin B12 or vitamin B12 with nutrients such as folic acid and other B vitamins, are also available. Check the Supplement Facts label to determine the amount of vitamin B12 provided.

Vitamin B12 is also available in sublingual forms (which are dissolved under the tongue). There is no evidence that sublingual forms are better absorbed than pills that are swallowed.

A prescription form of vitamin B12 can be administered as a shot. This is usually used to treat vitamin B12 deficiency. Vitamin B12 is also available as a prescription medication in nasal gel form (for use in the nose).

Am I Getting Enough Vitamin B12?

Most people in the United States get enough vitamin B12 from the foods they eat. But some people have trouble absorbing vitamin B12 from food. As a result, vitamin B12 deficiency affects between 1.5% and 15% of the public. Your doctor can test your vitamin B12 level to see if you have a deficiency.

Certain groups may not get enough vitamin B12 or have trouble absorbing it:

• Many older adults, who do not have enough hydrochloric acid in their stomach to absorb the vitamin B12 naturally present in food. People over 50 should get most of their vitamin B12 from fortified foods or dietary supplements because, in most cases, their bodies can absorb vitamin B12 from these sources.

• People with pernicious anemia whose bodies do not make the intrinsic factor needed to absorb vitamin B12. Doctors usually treat pernicious anemia with vitamin B12 shots, although very high oral doses of vitamin B12 might also be effective.

• People who have had gastrointestinal surgery, such as weight loss surgery or who have digestive disorders, such as celiac disease or Crohn's disease. These conditions can decrease the amount of vitamin B12 that the body can absorb.

• Some people who eat little or no animal foods such as vegetarians and vegans. Only animal foods have vitamin B12 naturally. When pregnant women and women who breastfeed their babies are strict vegetarians or vegans, their babies might also not get enough vitamin B12.

What Happens If I Don't Get Enough Vitamin B12?

Vitamin B12 deficiency causes tiredness, weakness, constipation, loss of appetite, weight loss, and megaloblastic anemia. Nerve problems, such as numbness and tingling in the hands and feet, can also occur. Other symptoms of vitamin B12 deficiency include problems with balance, depression, confusion, dementia, poor memory, and soreness of the mouth or tongue. Vitamin B12 deficiency can damage the nervous system even in people who don't have anemia, so it is important to treat a deficiency as soon as possible.

In infants, signs of a vitamin B12 deficiency include failure to thrive, problems with movement, delays in reaching the typical developmental milestones, and megaloblastic anemia.

Large amounts of folic acid can hide a vitamin B12 deficiency by correcting megaloblastic anemia, a hallmark of vitamin B12 deficiency. But folic acid does not correct the progressive damage to the nervous system that vitamin B12 deficiency also causes. For this reason, healthy adults should not get more than 1,000 mcg of folic acid a day.

What Are Some Effects of Vitamin B12 on Health?

Scientists are studying vitamin B12 to see how it affects health. Here are several examples of what this research has shown.

Heart Disease

Vitamin B12 supplements (along with folic acid and vitamin B6) do not reduce the risk of getting heart disease. Scientists had thought that these vitamins might be helpful because they reduce blood levels of homocysteine, a compound linked to an increased risk of having a heart attack or stroke.

Dementia

As they get older, some people develop dementia. These people often have high levels of homocysteine in the blood. Vitamin B12 (with folic acid and vitamin B6) can lower homocysteine levels, but scientists don't know yet whether these vitamins actually help prevent or treat dementia.

Energy and Athletic Performance

Advertisements often promote vitamin B12 supplements as a way to increase energy or endurance. Except in people with a vitamin B12 deficiency, no evidence shows that vitamin B12 supplements increase energy or improve athletic performance.

Section 9.3

Vitamin C

This section includes text excerpted from "Vitamin C," Office on Dietary Supplements (ODS), National Institutes of Health (NIH), June 24, 2011. Reviewed June 2016.

What Is Vitamin C and What Does It Do?

Vitamin C, also known as ascorbic acid, is a water-soluble nutrient found in some foods. In the body, it acts as an antioxidant, helping to protect cells from the damage caused by free radicals. Free radicals are compounds formed when our bodies convert the food we eat into energy. People are also exposed to free radicals in the environment from cigarette smoke, air pollution, and ultraviolet light from the sun.

The body also needs vitamin C to make collagen, a protein required to help wounds heal. In addition, vitamin C improves the absorption of iron from plant-based foods and helps the immune system work properly to protect the body from disease.

How Much Vitamin C Do I Need?

The amount of vitamin C you need each day depends on your age. Average daily recommended amounts for different ages are listed below in milligrams (mg).

Table 9.7. Average Daily Recommended Amounts of Vitamin C

Life Stage	Recommended Amount
Birth to 6 months	40 mg
Infants 7–12 months	50 mg
Children 1–3 years	15 mg
Children 4–8 years	25 mg
Children 9–13 years	45 mg
Teens 14–18 years (boys)	75 mg
Teens 14–18 years (girls)	65 mg

Table 9.7. continued

Life Stage	Recommended Amount
Adults (men)	90 mg
Adults (women)	75 mg
Pregnant teens	80 mg
Pregnant women	85 mg
Breastfeeding teens	115 mg
Breastfeeding women	120 mg

If you smoke, add 35 mg to the above values to calculate your total daily recommended amount.

What Foods Provide Vitamin C?

Fruits and vegetables are the best sources of vitamin C. You can get recommended amounts of vitamin C by eating a variety of foods including the following:

- Citrus fruits (such as oranges and grapefruit) and their juices, as well as red and green pepper and kiwifruit, which have a lot of vitamin C.

- Other fruits and vegetables—such as broccoli, strawberries, cantaloupe, baked potatoes, and tomatoes—which also have vitamin C.

- Some foods and beverages that are fortified with vitamin C. To find out if vitamin C has been added to a food product, check the product labels.

The vitamin C content of food may be reduced by prolonged storage and by cooking. Steaming or microwaving may lessen cooking losses. Fortunately, many of the best food sources of vitamin C, such as fruits and vegetables, are usually eaten raw.

What Kinds of Vitamin C Dietary Supplements Are Available?

Most multivitamins have vitamin C. Vitamin C is also available alone as a dietary supplement or in combination with other nutrients. The vitamin C in dietary supplements is usually in the form of ascorbic acid, but some supplements have other forms, such as sodium ascorbate, calcium ascorbate, other mineral ascorbates, and ascorbic acid with bioflavonoids. Research has not shown that any form of vitamin C is better than the other forms.

What Are Some Effects of Vitamin C on Health?

Scientists are studying vitamin C to understand how it affects health. Here are several examples of what this research has shown.

Cancer Prevention and Treatment

People with high intakes of vitamin C from fruits and vegetables might have a lower risk of getting many types of cancer, such as lung, breast, and colon cancer. However, taking vitamin C supplements, with or without other antioxidants, doesn't seem to protect people from getting cancer.

It is not clear whether taking high doses of vitamin C is helpful as a treatment for cancer. Vitamin C's effects appear to depend on how it is administered to the patient. Oral doses of vitamin C can't raise blood levels of vitamin C nearly as high as intravenous doses given through injections. A few studies in animals and test tubes indicate that very high blood levels of vitamin C might shrink tumors. But more research is needed to determine whether high-dose intravenous vitamin C helps treat cancer in people.

Vitamin C dietary supplements and other antioxidants might interact with chemotherapy and radiation therapy for cancer. People being treated for cancer should talk with their oncologist before taking vitamin C or other antioxidant supplements, especially in high doses.

Cardiovascular Disease

People who eat lots of fruits and vegetables seem to have a lower risk of cardiovascular disease. Researchers believe that the antioxidant content of these foods might be partly responsible for this association because oxidative damage is a major cause of cardiovascular disease. However, scientists aren't sure whether vitamin C itself, either from food or supplements, helps protect people from cardiovascular disease. It is also not clear whether vitamin C helps prevent cardiovascular disease from getting worse in people who already have it.

Age-Related Macular Degeneration (AMD) and Cataracts

AMD and cataracts are two of the leading causes of vision loss in older people. Researchers do not believe that vitamin C and other antioxidants affect the risk of getting AMD. However, research suggests that vitamin C combined with other nutrients might help slow AMD progression.

In a large study among older people with AMD who were at high risk of developing advanced AMD, those who took a daily dietary supplement with 500mg vitamin C, 80 mg zinc, 400 IU vitamin E, 15 mg beta-carotene, and 2 mg copper for about 6 years had a lower chance of developing advanced AMD. They also had less vision loss than those who did not take the dietary supplement. People who have or are developing the disease might want to talk with their doctor about taking dietary supplements.

The relationship between vitamin C and cataract formation is unclear. Some studies show that people who get more vitamin C from foods have a lower risk of getting cataracts. But further research is needed to clarify this association and to determine whether vitamin C supplements affect the risk of getting cataracts.

The Common Cold

Although vitamin C has long been a popular remedy for the common cold, research shows that for most people, vitamin C supplements do not reduce the risk of getting the common cold. However, people who take vitamin C supplements regularly might have slightly shorter colds or somewhat milder symptoms when they do have a cold. Using vitamin C supplements after cold symptoms start does not appear to be helpful.

Can Vitamin C Be Harmful?

Taking too much vitamin C can cause diarrhea, nausea, and stomach cramps. In people with a condition called hemochromatosis, which causes the body to store too much iron, high doses of vitamin C could worsen iron overload and damage body tissues.

The upper limits for vitamin C are listed below:

Table 9.8. Upper Limits for Vitamin C

Life Stage	Upper Limit
Birth to 12 months	Not established
Children 1–3 years	400 mg
Children 4–8 years	650 mg
Children 9–13 years	1,200 mg
Teens 14–18 years	1,800 mg
Adults	2,000 mg

Section 9.4

Vitamin D

This section includes text excerpted from "Vitamin D Fact Sheet for Consumers," Office on Dietary Supplements (ODS), National Institutes of Health (NIH), February 17, 2016.

What Is Vitamin D and What Does It Do?

Vitamin D is a nutrient found in some foods that is needed for health and to maintain strong bones. It does so by helping the body absorb calcium (one of bone's main building blocks) from food and supplements. People who get too little vitamin D may develop soft, thin, and brittle bones, a condition known as rickets in children and osteomalacia in adults.

Vitamin D is important to the body in many other ways as well. Muscles need it to move, for example, nerves need it to carry messages between the brain and every body part, and the immune system needs vitamin D to fight off invading bacteria and viruses. Together with calcium, vitamin D also helps protect older adults from osteoporosis. Vitamin D is found in cells throughout the body.

How Much Vitamin D Do I Need?

The amount of vitamin D you need each day depends on your age. Average daily recommended amounts from the Food and Nutrition Board (a national group of experts) for different ages are listed below in International Units (IU):

Table 9.9. Average Daily Recommended Amounts of Vitamin D

Life Stage	Recommended Amount
Birth to 12 months	400 IU
Children 1–13 years	600 IU
Teens 14–18 years	600 IU
Adults 19–70 years	600 IU
Adults 71 years and older	800 IU

Table 9.9. continued

Life Stage	Recommended Amount
Pregnant and breastfeeding women and teens	600 IU

What Foods Provide Vitamin D?

Very few foods naturally have vitamin D. Fortified foods provide most of the vitamin D in American diets.

- Fatty fish such as salmon, tuna, and mackerel are among the best sources.

- Beef liver, cheese, and egg yolks provide small amounts.

- Mushrooms provide some vitamin D. In some mushrooms that are newly available in stores, the vitamin D content is being boosted by exposing these mushrooms to ultraviolet light.

- Almost all of the U.S. milk supply is fortified with 400 IU of vitamin D per quart. But foods made from milk, like cheese and ice cream, are usually not fortified.

- Vitamin D is added to many breakfast cereals and to some brands of orange juice, yogurt, margarine, and soy beverages; check the labels.

Can I Get Vitamin D from the Sun?

The body makes vitamin D when skin is directly exposed to the sun, and most people meet at least some of their vitamin D needs this way. Skin exposed to sunshine indoors through a window will not produce vitamin D. Cloudy days, shade, and having dark-colored skin also cut down on the amount of vitamin D the skin makes.

However, despite the importance of the sun to vitamin D synthesis, it is prudent to limit exposure of skin to sunlight in order to lower the risk for skin cancer. When out in the sun for more than a few minutes, wear protective clothing and apply sunscreen with an SPF (sun protection factor) of 8 or more. Tanning beds also cause the skin to make vitamin D, but pose similar risks for skin cancer.

People who avoid the sun or who cover their bodies with sunscreen or clothing should include good sources of vitamin D in their diets or take a supplement. Recommended intakes of vitamin D are set on the assumption of little sun exposure.

What Kinds of Vitamin D Dietary Supplements Are Available?

Vitamin D is found in supplements (and fortified foods) in two different forms: D2 (ergocalciferol) and D3 (cholecalciferol). Both increase vitamin D in the blood.

What Are Some Effects of Vitamin D on Health?

Vitamin D is being studied for its possible connections to several diseases and medical problems, including diabetes, hypertension, and autoimmune conditions such as multiple sclerosis. Two of them discussed below are bone disorders and some types of cancer.

Bone Disorders

As they get older, millions of people (mostly women, but men too) develop or are at risk of, osteoporosis, where bones become fragile and may fracture if one falls. It is one consequence of not getting enough calcium and vitamin D over the long term. Supplements of both vitamin D3 (at 700–800 IU/ day) and calcium (500–1,200 mg/day) have been shown to reduce the risk of bone loss and fractures in elderly people aged 62–85 years. Men and women should talk with their healthcare providers about their needs for vitamin D (and calcium) as part of an overall plan to prevent or treat osteoporosis.

Cancer

Some studies suggest that vitamin D may protect against colon cancer and perhaps even cancers of the prostate and breast. But higher levels of vitamin D in the blood have also been linked to higher rates of pancreatic cancer. At this time, it's too early to say whether low vitamin D status increases cancer risk and whether higher levels protect or even increase risk in some people.

Can Vitamin D Be Harmful?

Yes, when amounts in the blood become too high. Signs of toxicity include nausea, vomiting, poor appetite, constipation, weakness, and weight loss. And by raising blood levels of calcium, too much vitamin D can cause confusion, disorientation, and problems with heart rhythm. Excess vitamin D can also damage the kidneys.

The upper limit for vitamin D is 1,000 to 1,500 IU/day for infants, 2,500 to 3,000 IU/day for children 1–8 years, and 4,000 IU/day for children 9 years and older, adults, and pregnant and breastfeeding teens and women. Vitamin D toxicity almost always occurs from overuse of supplements. Excessive sun exposure doesn't cause vitamin D poisoning because the body limits the amount of this vitamin it produces.

Section 9.5

Vitamin E

This section includes text excerpted from "Vitamin E Fact Sheet for Consumers," Office on Dietary Supplements (ODS), National Institutes of Health (NIH), May 11, 2016.

What Is Vitamin E and What Does It Do?

Vitamin E is a fat-soluble nutrient found in many foods. In the body, it acts as an antioxidant, helping to protect cells from the damage caused by free radicals. Free radicals are compounds formed when our bodies convert the food we eat into energy. People are also exposed to free radicals in the environment from cigarette smoke, air pollution, and ultraviolet light from the sun.

The body also needs vitamin E to boost its immune system so that it can fight off invading bacteria and viruses. It helps to widen blood vessels and keep blood from clotting within them. In addition, cells use vitamin E to interact with each other and to carry out many important functions.

How Much Vitamin E Do I Need?

The amount of vitamin E you need each day depends on your age. Average daily recommended intakes are listed below in milligrams (mg) and in International Units (IU). Package labels list the amount of vitamin E in foods and dietary supplements in IU.

Table 9.10. Average Daily Recommended Intakes of Vitamin E

Life Stage	Recommended Amount
Birth to 6 months	4 mg (6 IU)
Infants 7–12 months	5 mg (7.5 IU)
Children 1–3 years	6 mg (9 IU)
Children 4–8 years	7 mg (10.4 IU)
Children 9–13 years	11 mg (16.4 IU)
Teens 14–18 years	15 mg (22.4 IU)
Adults	15 mg (22.4 IU)
Pregnant teens and women	15 mg (22.4 IU)
Breastfeeding teens and women	19 mg (28.4 IU)

What Foods Provide Vitamin E?

Vitamin E is found naturally in foods and is added to some fortified foods. You can get recommended amounts of vitamin E by eating a variety of foods including the following:

- Vegetable oils like wheat germ, sunflower, and safflower oils are among the best sources of vitamin E. Corn and soybean oils also provide some vitamin E.

- Nuts (such as peanuts, hazelnuts, and, especially, almonds) and seeds (like sunflower seeds) are also among the best sources of vitamin E.

- Green vegetables, such as spinach and broccoli, provide some vitamin E.

- Food companies add vitamin E to some breakfast cereals, fruit juices, margarines and spreads, and other foods. To find out which ones have vitamin E, check the product labels.

What Kinds of Vitamin E Dietary Supplements Are Available?

Vitamin E supplements come in different amounts and forms. Two main things to consider when choosing a vitamin E supplement are:

1. **The amount of vitamin E:** Most once-daily multivitamin mineral supplements provide about 30 IU of vitamin E, whereas vitamin E-only supplements usually contain 100 to 1,000 IU per pill. The doses in vitamin E-only supplements are

much higher than the recommended amounts. Some people take large doses because they believe or hope that doing so will keep them healthy or lower their risk of certain diseases.

2. **The form of vitamin E:** Although vitamin E sounds like a single substance, it is actually the name of eight related compounds in food, including alpha-tocopherol. Each form has a different potency or level of activity in the body.

Vitamin E from natural (food) sources is listed as "d-alpha tocopherol" on food packaging and supplement labels. Synthetic (laboratory-made) vitamin E is listed as "dl-alpha tocopherol." The natural form is more potent. For example, 100 IU of natural vitamin E is equal to about 150 IU of the synthetic form.

Some vitamin E supplements provide other forms of the vitamin, such as gamma-tocopherol, tocotrienols, and mixed tocopherols. Scientists do not know if any of these forms are superior to alpha-tocopherol in supplements.

What Are Some Effects of Vitamin E on Health?

Scientists are studying vitamin E to see how it affects health. Here are several examples of what this research has shown.

Heart Disease

Some studies link higher intakes of vitamin E from supplements to lower chances of developing heart disease. But the best research finds no benefit. People in these studies are randomly assigned to take vitamin E or a placebo (dummy pill with no vitamin E or active ingredients) and they don't know which they are taking. Vitamin E supplements do not seem to prevent heart disease, reduce its severity or affect the risk of death from this disease. Scientists do not know whether high intakes of vitamin E might protect the heart in younger, healthier people who do not have a high risk of heart disease.

Cancer

Most research indicates that vitamin E does not help prevent cancer and may be harmful in some cases. Large doses of vitamin E have not consistently reduced the risk of colon and breast cancer in studies, for example. A large study found that taking vitamin E supplements (400 IU/day) for several years increased the risk of developing prostate cancer in men. Two studies that followed middle-aged men and women for 7 or more years found that extra vitamin E (300–400 IU/day, on average) did not protect them from any form of cancer. However, one study found a link between the use of vitamin E supplements for 10 years or more and a lower risk of death from bladder cancer.

Vitamin E dietary supplements and other antioxidants might interact with chemotherapy and radiation therapy. People undergoing these treatments should talk with their doctor or oncologist before taking vitamin E or other antioxidant supplements, especially in high doses.

Eye Disorders

Age-related macular degeneration (AMD) or the loss of central vision in older people, and cataracts are among the most common causes of vision loss in older people. The results of research on whether vitamin E can help prevent these conditions are inconsistent. Among people with AMD who were at high risk of developing advanced AMD, a supplement containing large doses of vitamin E combined with other antioxidants, zinc, and copper showed promise for slowing down the rate of vision loss.

Mental Function

Several studies have investigated whether vitamin E supplements might help older adults remain mentally alert and active as well as prevent or slow the decline of mental function and Alzheimer disease. So far, the research provides little evidence that taking vitamin E supplements can help healthy people or people with mild mental functioning problems to maintain brain health.

Can Vitamin E Be Harmful?

Eating vitamin E in foods is not risky or harmful. In supplement form, however, high doses of vitamin E might increase the risk of bleeding (by reducing the blood's ability to form clots after a cut or injury) and of serious bleeding in the brain (known as hemorrhagic stroke). Because of this risk, the upper limit for adults is 1,500 IU/day for supplements made from the natural form of vitamin E and 1,100 IU/day for supplements made from synthetic vitamin E. The upper limits for children are lower than those for adults. Some research suggests that taking vitamin E supplements even below these upper limits might cause harm. In one study, for example, men who took 400 IU of vitamin E each day for several years had an increased risk of prostate cancer.

Section 9.6

Vitamin K

This section includes text excerpted from "Vitamin K," Office on Dietary Supplements (ODS), National Institutes of Health (NIH), May April 13, 2016.

What Is Vitamin K and What Does It Do?

Vitamin K is a nutrient that the body needs to stay healthy. It's important for blood clotting and healthy bones and also has other functions in the body. If you are taking a blood thinner such as warfarin (Coumadin®), it's very important to get about the same amount of vitamin K each day.

How Much Vitamin K Do I Need?

The amount of vitamin K you need depends on your age and sex. Average daily recommended amounts are listed below in micrograms (mcg).

Table 9.11. Average Daily Recommended Intakes of Vitamin K

Life Stage	Recommended Amount
Birth to 6 months	2.0 mcg
7–12 months	2.5 mcg
1–3 years	30 mcg
4–8 years	55 mcg
9–13 years	60 mcg
14–18 years	75 mcg
Adult men 19 years and older	120 mcg
Adult women 19 years and older	90 mcg
Pregnant or breastfeeding teens	75 mcg
Pregnant or breastfeeding women	90 mcg

What Foods Provide Vitamin K?

Vitamin K is found naturally in many foods. You can get recommended amounts of vitamin K by eating a variety of foods, including the following:

- Green leafy vegetables, such as spinach, kale, broccoli, and lettuce.

- Vegetable oils.

- Some fruits, such as blueberries and figs.

- Meat, cheese, eggs, and soybeans.

What Kinds of Vitamin K Dietary Supplements Are Available?

Vitamin K is found in multivitamin/multimineral supplements. Vitamin K is also available in supplements of vitamin K alone or of vitamin K with a few other nutrients such as calcium, magnesium, and/or vitamin D. Common forms of vitamin K in dietary supplements are phylloquinone and phytonadione (also called vitamin K1), menaquinone-4, and menaquinone-7 (also called vitamin K2).

What Are Some Effects of Vitamin K on Health?

Scientists are studying vitamin K to understand how it affects our health. Here are some examples of what this research has shown.

Osteoporosis

Vitamin K is important for healthy bones. Some research shows that people who eat more vitamin K-rich foods have stronger bones and are less likely to break a hip than those who eat less of these foods. A few studies have found that taking vitamin K supplements improves bone strength and the chances of breaking a bone, but other studies have not. More research is needed to better understand if vitamin K supplements can help improve bone health and reduce osteoporosis risk.

Coronary Heart Disease

Scientists are studying whether low blood levels of vitamin K increase the risk of heart disease, perhaps by making blood vessels that feed the heart stiffer and narrower.

Can Vitamin K Be Harmful?

Vitamin K has not been shown to cause any harm. However, it can interact with some medications, particularly warfarin (Coumadin®)

Chapter 10

Minerals

Chapter Contents

Section 10.1

Calcium

This section includes text excerpted from "Calcium," Office on Dietary Supplements (ODS), National Institutes of Health (NIH), March 19, 2013.

What Is Calcium and What Does It Do?

Calcium is a mineral found in many foods. The body needs calcium to maintain strong bones and to carry out many important functions. Almost all calcium is stored in bones and teeth, where it supports their structure and hardness.

The body also needs calcium for muscles to move and for nerves to carry messages between the brain and every body part. In addition, calcium is used to help blood vessels move blood throughout the body and to help release hormones and enzymes that affect almost every function in the human body.

How Much Calcium Do I Need?

The amount of calcium you need each day depends on your age. Average daily recommended amounts are listed below in milligrams (mg):

Table 10.1. Average Daily Recommended Amount of Calcium

Life Stage	Recommended Amount
Birth to 6 months	200 mg
Infants 7–12 months	260 mg
Children 1–3 years	700 mg
Children 4–8 years	1,000 mg
Children 9–13 years	1,300 mg
Teens 14–18 years	1,300 mg
Adults 19–50 years	1,000 mg
Adult men 51–70 years	1,000 mg

Table 10.1. Continued

Life Stage	Recommended Amount
Adult women 51–70 years	1,200 mg
Adults 71 years and older	1,200 mg
Pregnant and breastfeeding teens	1,300 mg
Pregnant and breastfeeding adults	1,000 mg

What Foods Provide Calcium?

Calcium is found in many foods. You can get recommended amounts of calcium by eating a variety of foods, including the following:

- Milk, yogurt, and cheese are the main food sources of calcium for the majority of people in the United States.

- Kale, broccoli, and Chinese cabbage are fine vegetable sources of calcium.

- Fish with soft bones that you eat, such as canned sardines and salmon, are fine animal sources of calcium.

- Most grains (such as breads, pastas, and unfortified cereals), while not rich in calcium, add significant amounts of calcium to the diet because people eat them often or in large amounts.

- Calcium is added to some breakfast cereals, fruit juices, soy and rice beverages, and tofu. To find out whether these foods have calcium, check the product labels.

What Kinds of Calcium Dietary Supplements Are Available?

Calcium is found in many multivitamin-mineral supplements, though the amount varies by product. Dietary supplements that contain only calcium or calcium with other nutrients such as vitamin D are also available. Check the Supplement Facts label to determine the amount of calcium provided.

The two main forms of calcium dietary supplements are carbonate and citrate. Calcium carbonate is inexpensive, but is absorbed best when taken with food. Some over-the-counter antacid products, such as Tums® and Rolaids®, contain calcium carbonate. Each pill or chew provides 200–400 mg of calcium. Calcium citrate, a more expensive form of the supplement, is absorbed well on an empty or a full stomach. In addition, people with low levels of stomach acid (a condition more common in people older than 50) absorb calcium citrate more easily than calcium carbonate. Other forms of calcium in supplements and fortified foods include gluconate, lactate, and phosphate.

Calcium absorption is best when a person consumes no more than 500 mg at one time. So a person who takes 1,000 mg/day of calcium from supplements, for example, should split the dose rather than take it all at once.

Calcium supplements may cause gas, bloating, and constipation in some people. If any of these symptoms occur, try spreading out the calcium dose throughout the day, taking the supplement with meals or changing the supplement brand or calcium form you take.

What Are Some Effects of Calcium on Health?

Scientists are studying calcium to understand how it affects health. Here are several examples of what this research has shown:

Bone Health and Osteoporosis

Bones need plenty of calcium and vitamin D throughout childhood and adolescence to reach their peak strength and calcium content by about age 30. After that, bones slowly lose calcium, but people can help reduce these losses by getting recommended amounts of calcium throughout adulthood and by having a healthy, active lifestyle that includes weight-bearing physical activity (such as walking and running).

Osteoporosis is a disease of the bones in older adults (especially women) in which the bones become porous, fragile, and more prone to fracture. Osteoporosis is a serious public health problem for more than 10 million adults over the age of 50 in the United States. Adequate calcium and vitamin D intakes as well as regular exercise are essential to keep bones healthy throughout life.

Taking calcium and vitamin D supplements reduce the risk of breaking a bone and the risk of falling in frail, elderly adults who live in nursing homes and similar facilities. But it's not clear if the supplements help prevent bone fractures and falls in older people who live at home.

Cardiovascular Disease

Whether calcium affects the risk of cardiovascular disease is not clear. Some studies show that getting enough calcium might protect people from heart disease and stroke. But other studies show that some people who consume high amounts of calcium, particularly from supplements, might have an increased risk of heart disease.

High Blood Pressure

Some studies have found that getting recommended intakes of calcium can reduce the risk of developing high blood pressure (hypertension). One large study in particular found that eating a diet high in fat-free and low-fat dairy products, vegetables, and fruits lowered blood pressure.

Cancer

Studies have examined whether calcium supplements or diets high in calcium might lower the risks of developing cancer of the colon or rectum or increase the risk of prostate cancer. The research to date provides no clear answers. Given that cancer develops over many years, longer term studies are needed.

Kidney Stones

Most kidney stones are rich in calcium oxalate. Some studies have found that higher intakes of calcium from dietary supplements are linked to a greater risk of kidney stones, especially among older adults. But calcium from foods does not appear to cause kidney stones. For most people, other factors (such as not drinking enough fluids) probably have a larger effect on the risk of kidney stones than calcium intake.

Weight Loss

Although several studies have shown that getting more calcium helps lower body weight or reduce weight gain over time, most studies have found that calcium—from foods or dietary supplements—has little if any effect on body weight and amount of body fat.

Can Calcium Be Harmful?

Getting too much calcium can cause constipation. It might also interfere with the body's ability to absorb iron and zinc, but this effect is not well established. In adults, too much calcium (from dietary supplements but not food) might increase the risk of kidney stones. Some studies show that people who consume high amounts of calcium might have increased risks of prostate cancer and heart disease, but more research is needed to understand these possible links.

The upper limits for calcium are listed below. Most people do not get amounts above the upper limits from food alone; excess intakes usually come from the use of calcium supplements. Surveys show that some older women in the United States probably get amounts somewhat above the upper limit since the use of calcium supplements is common among these women.

Table 10.2. The Upper Limits for Calcium

Life Stage	Upper Limit
Birth to 6 months	1,000 mg
Infants 7–12 months	1,500 mg
Children 1–8 years	2,500 mg
Children 9–18 years	3,000 mg
Adults 19–50 years	2,500 mg
Adults 51 years and older	2,000 mg
Pregnant and breastfeeding teens	3,000 mg
Pregnant and breastfeeding adults	2,500 mg

Section 10.2

Iron

This section includes text excerpted from "Iron," Office on Dietary Supplements (ODS), National Institutes of Health (NIH), February 17, 2016.

What Is Iron and What Does It Do?

Iron is a mineral that the body needs for growth and development. Your body uses iron to make hemoglobin, a protein in red blood cells that carries oxygen from the lungs to all parts of the body, and myoglobin, a protein that provides oxygen to muscles. Your body also needs iron to make some hormones and connective tissue.

How Much Iron Do I Need?

The amount of iron you need each day depends on your age, your sex, and whether you consume a mostly plant-based diet. Average daily recommended amounts are listed below in milligrams (mg). Vegetarians who do not eat meat, poultry or seafood need almost twice as much iron as listed in the table because the body doesn't absorb nonheme iron in plant foods as well as heme iron in animal foods.

Table 10.3. Average Daily Recommended Amount of Iron

Life Stage	Recommended Amount
Birth to 6 months	0.27 mg
Infants 7–12 months	11 mg
Children 1–3 years	7 mg
Children 4–8 years	10 mg
Children 9–13 years	8 mg
Teens boys 14–18 years	11 mg
Teens girls 14–18 years	15 mg
Adult men 19–50 years	8 mg
Adult women 19–50 years	18 mg
Adults 51 years and older	8 mg
Pregnant teens	27 mg
Pregnant women	27 mg
Breastfeeding teens	10 mg
Breastfeeding women	9 mg

What Foods Provide Iron?

Iron is found naturally in many foods and is added to some fortified food products. You can get recommended amounts of iron by eating a variety of foods, including the following:

- Lean meat, seafood, and poultry.
- Iron-fortified breakfast cereals and breads.
- White beans, lentils, spinach, kidney beans, and peas.
- Nuts and some dried fruits, such as raisins.

Iron in food comes in two forms: heme iron and nonheme iron. Nonheme iron is found in plant foods and iron-fortified food products. Meat, seafood, and poultry have both heme and nonheme iron.

Your body absorbs iron from plant sources better when you eat it with meat, poultry, seafood, and foods that contain vitamin C, like citrus fruits, strawberries, sweet peppers, tomatoes, and broccoli.

What Kinds of Iron Dietary Supplements Are Available?

Iron is available in many multivitamin-mineral supplements and in supplements that contain only iron. Iron in supplements is often in the form of ferrous sulfate, ferrous gluconate, ferric citrate or ferric sulfate. Dietary supplements that contain iron have a statement on the label warning that they should be kept out of the reach of children. Accidental overdose of iron-containing products is a leading cause of fatal poisoning in children under 6.

What Are Some Effects of Iron on Health?

Scientists are studying iron to understand how it affects health. Iron's most important contribution to health is preventing iron deficiency anemia and resulting problems.

Pregnant Women

During pregnancy, the amount of blood in a woman's body increases, so she needs more iron for herself and her growing baby. Getting too little iron during pregnancy increases a woman's risk of iron deficiency anemia and her infant's risk of low birthweight, premature birth, and low levels of iron. Getting too little iron might also harm her infant's brain development.

Women who are pregnant or breastfeeding should take an iron supplement as recommended by an obstetrician or other healthcare provider.

Infants and Toddlers

Iron deficiency anemia in infancy can lead to delayed psychological development, social withdrawal, and less ability to pay attention. By age 6 to 9 months, full-term infants could become iron deficient unless they eat iron-enriched solid foods or drink iron-fortified formula.

Anemia of Chronic Disease

Some chronic diseases—like rheumatoid arthritis, inflammatory bowel disease, and some types of cancer—can interfere with the body's ability to use its stored iron. Taking more iron from foods or supplements usually does not reduce the resulting anemia of chronic disease because iron is diverted from the blood circulation to storage sites. The main therapy for anemia of chronic disease is treatment of the underlying disease.

Can Iron Be Harmful?

Yes, iron can be harmful if you get too much. In healthy people, taking high doses of iron supplements (especially on an empty stomach) can cause an upset stomach, constipation, nausea, abdominal pain, vomiting, and fainting. High doses of iron can also decrease zinc absorption. Extremely high doses of iron (in the hundreds or thousands of mg) can cause organ failure, coma, convulsions, and death. Childproof packaging and warning labels on iron supplements have greatly reduced the number of accidental iron poisonings in children.

Some people have an inherited condition called hemochromatosis that causes toxic levels of iron to build up in their bodies. Without medical treatment, people with hereditary hemochromatosis can develop serious problems like liver cirrhosis, liver cancer, and heart disease. People with this disorder should avoid using iron supplements and vitamin C supplements.

The upper limits for iron from foods and dietary supplements are listed below. A doctor might prescribe more than the upper limit of iron to people who need higher doses for a while to treat iron deficiency.

Table 10.4. The Upper Limits for Iron from Foods and Dietary Supplements

Ages	Upper Limit
Birth to 12 months	40 mg
Children 1–13 years	40 mg
Teens 14–18 years	45 mg
Adults 19+ years	45 mg

Section 10.3

Magnesium

This section includes text excerpted from "Magnesium," Office on Dietary Supplements (ODS), National Institutes of Health (NIH), February 17, 2016.

What Is Magnesium and What Does It Do?

Magnesium is a nutrient that the body needs to stay healthy. Magnesium is important for many processes in the body, including regulating muscle and nerve function, blood sugar levels, and blood pressure and making protein, bone, and DNA.

How Much Magnesium Do I Need?

The amount of magnesium you need depends on your age and sex. Average daily recommended amounts are listed below in milligrams (mg):

Table 10.5. Average Daily Recommended Amount of Magnesium

Life Stage	Recommended Amount
Birth to 6 months	30 mg
Infants 7–12 months	75 mg
Children 1–3 years	80 mg
Children 4–8 years	130 mg
Children 9–13 years	240 mg
Teen boys 14–18 years	410 mg
Teen girls 14–18 years	360 mg
Men	400–420 mg
Women	310–320 mg
Pregnant teens	400 mg
Pregnant women	350–360 mg
Breastfeeding teens	360 mg
Breastfeeding women	310–320 mg

What Foods Provide Magnesium?

Magnesium is found naturally in many foods and is added to some fortified foods. You can get recommended amounts of magnesium by eating a variety of foods, including the following:

- Legumes, nuts, seeds, whole grains, and green leafy vegetables (such as spinach).
- Fortified breakfast cereals and other fortified foods.
- Milk, yogurt, and some other milk products.

What Kinds of Magnesium Dietary Supplements Are Available?

Magnesium is available in multivitamin-mineral supplements and other dietary supplements. Forms of magnesium in dietary supplements that are more easily absorbed by the body are magnesium aspartate, magnesium citrate, magnesium lactate, and magnesium chloride.

Magnesium is also included in some laxatives and some products for treating heartburn and indigestion.

What Are Some Effects of Magnesium on Health?

Scientists are studying magnesium to understand how it affects health. Here are some examples of what this research has shown.

High Blood Pressure and Heart Disease

High blood pressure is a major risk factor for heart disease and stroke. Magnesium supplements might decrease blood pressure, but only by a small amount. Some studies show that people who have more magnesium in their diets have a lower risk of some types of heart disease and stroke. But in many of these studies, it's hard to know how much of the effect was due to magnesium as opposed to other nutrients.

Type 2 Diabetes

People with higher amounts of magnesium in their diets tend to have a lower risk of developing type 2 diabetes. Magnesium helps the body break down sugars and might help reduce the risk of insulin resistance (a condition that leads to diabetes). Scientists are studying whether magnesium supplements might help people who already have type 2 diabetes control their disease.

Osteoporosis

Magnesium is important for healthy bones. People with higher intakes of magnesium have a higher bone mineral density, which is important in reducing the risk of bone fractures and osteoporosis. Getting more magnesium from foods or dietary supplements might help older women improve their bone mineral density.

Migraine Headaches

People who have migraine headaches sometimes have low levels of magnesium in their blood and other tissues. Several small studies found that magnesium supplements can modestly reduce the frequency of migraines. However, people should only take magnesium for this purpose under the care of a healthcare provider.

Can Magnesium Be Harmful?

Magnesium that is naturally present in food is not harmful and does not need to be limited. In healthy people, the kidneys can get rid of any excess in the urine. But magnesium in dietary supplements and medications should not be consumed in amounts above the upper limit, unless recommended by a healthcare provider.

The upper limits for magnesium from dietary supplements and/ or medications are listed below. For many age groups, the upper limit appears to be lower than the recommended amount. This occurs because the recommended amounts include magnesium from all sources—food, dietary supplements and medications. The upper limits include magnesium from only dietary supplements and medications; they do not include magnesium found naturally in food.

Table 10.6. he Upper Limits for Magnesium from Dietary Supplements and/or Medications

Ages	Upper Limit for Magnesium in Dietary Supplements and Medications
Birth to 12 months	Not established
Children 1–3 years	65 mg
Children 4–8 years	110 mg
Children 9–18 years	350 mg
Adults	350 mg

High intakes of magnesium from dietary supplements and medications can cause diarrhea, nausea, and abdominal cramping. Extremely high intakes of magnesium can lead to irregular heartbeat and cardiac arrest.

Section 10.4

Zinc

This section includes text excerpted from "Zinc," Office on Dietary Supplements (ODS), National Institutes of Health (NIH), February 17, 2016.

What Is Zinc and What Does It Do?

Zinc is a nutrient that people need to stay healthy. Zinc is found in cells throughout the body. It helps the immune system fight off invading bacteria and viruses. The body also needs zinc to make proteins and DNA, the genetic material in all cells. During pregnancy, infancy, and childhood, the body needs zinc to grow and develop properly. Zinc also helps wounds heal and is important for proper senses of taste and smell.

How Much Zinc Do I Need?

The amount of zinc you need each day depends on your age. Average daily recommended amounts for different ages are listed below in milligrams (mg):

Table 10.7. Average Daily Recommended Amount of Zinc

Life Stage	Recommended Amount
Birth to 6 months	2 mg
Infants 7–12 months	3 mg
Children 1–3 years	3 mg
Children 4–8 years	5 mg

Table 10.7. Continued

Life Stage	Recommended Amount
Children 9–13 years	8 mg
Teens 14–18 years (boys)	11 mg
Teens 14–18 years (girls)	9 mg
Adults (men)	11 mg
Adults (women)	8 mg
Pregnant teens	12 mg
Pregnant women	11 mg
Breastfeeding teens	13 mg
Breastfeeding women	12 mg

What Foods Provide Zinc?

Zinc is found in a wide variety of foods. You can get recommended amounts of zinc by eating a variety of foods including the following:

- Oysters, which are the best source of zinc.

- Red meat, poultry, seafood such as crab and lobsters, and fortified breakfast cereals, which are also good sources of zinc.

- Beans, nuts, whole grains, and dairy products, which provide some zinc.

What Kinds of Zinc Dietary Supplements Are Available?

Zinc is present in almost all multivitamin/mineral dietary supplements. It is also available alone or combined with calcium, magnesium or other ingredients in dietary supplements. Dietary supplements can have several different forms of zinc including zinc gluconate, zinc sulfate, and zinc acetate. It is not clear whether one form is better than the others.

Zinc is also found in some oral over-the-counter products, including those labeled as homeopathic medications for colds. Use of nasal sprays and gels that contain zinc has been associated with the loss of the sense of smell, in some cases long-lasting or permanent. These safety concerns have not been found to be associated with oral products containing zinc, such as cold lozenges.

Zinc is also present in some denture adhesive creams. Using large amounts of these products, well beyond recommended levels, could lead to excessive zinc intake and copper deficiency. This can cause neurological problems, including numbness and weakness in the arms and legs.

What Are Some Effects of Zinc on Health?

Scientists are studying zinc to learn about its effects on the immune system (the body's defense system against bacteria, viruses, and other foreign invaders). Scientists are also researching possible connections between zinc and the health problems discussed below.

Immune System and Wound Healing

The body's immune system needs zinc to do its job. Older people and children in developing countries who have low levels of zinc might have a higher risk of getting pneumonia and other infections. Zinc also helps the skin stay healthy. Some people who have skin ulcers might benefit from zinc dietary supplements, but only if they have low levels of zinc.

Diarrhea

Children in developing countries often die from diarrhea. Studies show that zinc dietary supplements help reduce the symptoms and duration of diarrhea in these children, many of whom are zinc deficient or otherwise malnourished. The World Health Organization (WHO) and United Nations Children's Emergency Fund (UNICEF) recommend that children with diarrhea take zinc for 10–14 days (20 mg/day or 10 mg/day for infants under 6 months). It is not clear whether zinc dietary supplements can help treat diarrhea in children who get enough zinc, such as most children in the United States.

The Common Cold

Some studies suggest that zinc lozenges or syrup (but not zinc dietary supplements in pill form) help speed recovery from the common cold and reduce its symptoms if taken within 24 hours of coming down with a cold. However, more study is needed to determine the best dose and form of zinc, as well as how long it should be taken before zinc can be recommended as a treatment for the common cold.

Age-Related Macular Degeneration (AMD)

AMD is an eye disease that gradually causes vision loss. Research suggests that zinc might help slow AMD progression. In a large study among older people with AMD who were at high risk of developing advanced AMD, those who took a daily dietary supplement with 80 mg zinc, 500 mg vitamin C, 400 IU vitamin E, 15 mg beta-carotene, and 2 mg copper for about 6 years had a lower chance of developing advanced AMD and less vision loss than those who did not take the dietary supplement. In the same study, people at high risk of the disease who took dietary supplements containing only zinc also had a lower risk of getting advanced AMD than those who did not take zinc dietary supplements. People who have or are developing the disease might want to talk with their doctor about taking dietary supplements.

Can Zinc Be Harmful?

Yes, if you get too much. Signs of too much zinc include nausea, vomiting, loss of appetite, stomach cramps, diarrhea, and headaches. When people take too much zinc for a long time, they sometimes have problems such as low copper levels, lower immunity, and low levels of HDL cholesterol (the "good" cholesterol).

The upper limits for zinc are listed below. These levels do not apply to people who are taking zinc for medical reasons under the care of a doctor:

Table 10.8. The Upper Limits for Zinc

Life Stage	Upper Limit
Birth to 6 months	4 mg
Infants 7–12 months	5 mg
Children 1–3 years	7 mg
Children 4–8 years	12 mg
Children 9–13 years	23 mg
Teens 14–18 years	34 mg
Adults	40 mg

Chapter 11

Food Groups

Chapter Contents

Section 11.1

Vegetables

This section includes text excerpted from "All about the Vegetable Group," ChooseMyPlate.gov, U.S. Department of Agriculture (USDA), March 28, 2016.

What Foods Are in the Vegetable Group?

Any vegetable or 100% vegetable juice counts as a member of the Vegetable Group. Vegetables may be raw or cooked; fresh, frozen, canned or dried/dehydrated; and may be whole, cut-up or mashed.

Based on their nutrient content, vegetables are organized into five subgroups: dark-green vegetables, starchy vegetables, red and orange vegetables, beans and peas, and other vegetables.

How Many Vegetables Are Needed?

The amount of vegetables you need to eat depends on your age, sex, and level of physical activity. Recommended total daily amounts and recommended weekly amounts from each vegetable subgroup are shown in the two tables below.

Table 11.1. Daily Vegetable Table

Daily Recommendation		
Children	2–3 years old	1 cup
	4–8 years old	1 ½ cups
Girls	9–13 years old	2 cups
	14–18 years old	2 ½ cups
Boys	9–13 years old	2 ½ cups
	14–18 years old	3 cups
Women	19–30 years old	2 ½ cups
	31–50 years old	2 ½ cups
	51+ years old	2 cups

Table 11.1. Continued

Men	19–30 years old	3 cups
	31–50 years old	3 cups
	51+ years old	2 ½ cups

*These amounts are appropriate for individuals who get less than 30 minutes per day of moderate physical activity, beyond normal daily activities. Those who are more physically active may be able to consume more while staying within calorie needs.

Vegetable subgroup recommendations are given as amounts to eat WEEKLY. It is not necessary to eat vegetables from each subgroup daily. However, over a week, try to consume the amounts listed from each subgroup as a way to reach your daily intake recommendation.

Table 11.2. Weekly Vegetable Subgroup Table

	Dark green vegetables	Red and orange vegetables	Beans and peas	Starchy vegetables	Other vegetables
	Amount per Week				
Children 2-3 yrs old 4-8 yrs old	½ cup 1 cup	2 ½ cups 3 cups	½ cup ½ cup	2 cups 3 ½ cups	1 ½ cups 2 ½ cups
Girls 9-13 yrs old 14-18 yrs old	1 ½ cups 1 ½ cups	4 cups 5 ½ cups	1 cup 1 ½ cups	4 cups 5 cups	3 ½ cups 4 cups
Boys 9-13 yrs old 14-18 yrs old	1 ½ cups 2 cups	5 ½ cups 6 cups	1 ½ cups 2 cups	5 cups 6 cups	4 cups 5 cups
Women 19-30 yrs old 31-50 yrs old 51+ yrs old	1 ½ cups 1 ½ cups 1 ½ cups	5 ½ cups 5 ½ cups 4 cups	1 ½ cups 1 ½ cups 1 cup	5 cups 5 cups 4 cups	4 cups 4 cups 3 ½ cups

Table 11.2. Continued

	Dark green vegetables	Red and orange vegetables	Beans and peas	Starchy vegetables	Other vegetables
	Amount per Week				
Men **19-30 yrs** **old** **31-50 yrs** **old** **51+ yrs old**	2 cups 2 cups 1 ½ cups	6 cups 6 cups 5 ½ cups	2 cups 2 cups 1 ½ cups	6 cups 6 cups 5 cups	5 cups 5 cups 4 cups

What Counts as a Cup of Vegetables?

In general, 1 cup of raw or cooked vegetables or vegetable juice or 2 cups of raw leafy greens can be considered as 1 cup from the Vegetable Group.

Why Is It Important to Eat Vegetables?

Eating vegetables provides health benefits–people who eat more vegetables and fruits as part of an overall healthy diet are likely to have a reduced risk of some chronic diseases. Vegetables provide nutrients vital for health and maintenance of your body.

Nutrients

- Most vegetables are naturally low in fat and calories. None have cholesterol. (Sauces or seasonings may add fat, calories, and/or cholesterol.)

- Vegetables are important sources of many nutrients, including potassium, dietary fiber, folate (folic acid), vitamin A, and vitamin C.

- Diets rich in potassium may help to maintain healthy blood pressure. Vegetable sources of potassium include sweet potatoes, white potatoes, white beans, tomato products (paste, sauce, and juice), beet greens, soybeans, lima beans, spinach, lentils, and kidney beans.

- Dietary fiber from vegetables, as part of an overall healthy diet, helps reduce blood cholesterol levels and may lower risk of heart disease. Fiber is important for proper bowel function. It helps reduce constipation and diverticulosis. Fiber-containing foods such as vegetables help provide a feeling of fullness with fewer calories.

- Folate (folic acid) helps the body form red blood cells. Women of childbearing age who may become pregnant should consume adequate folate from foods, and in addition 400 mcg of synthetic folic acid from fortified foods or supplements. This reduces the risk of neural tube defects, spina bifida, and anencephaly during fetal development.

- Vitamin A keeps eyes and skin healthy and helps to protect against infections.

- Vitamin C helps heal cuts and wounds and keeps teeth and gums healthy. Vitamin C aids in iron absorption

Health Benefits

- Eating a diet rich in vegetables and fruits as part of an overall healthy diet may reduce risk for heart disease, including heart attack and stroke.

- Eating a diet rich in some vegetables and fruits as part of an overall healthy diet may protect against certain types of cancers.

- Diets rich in foods containing fiber, such as some vegetables and fruits, may reduce the risk of heart disease, obesity, and type 2 diabetes.

- Eating vegetables and fruits rich in potassium as part of an overall healthy diet may lower blood pressure, and may also reduce the risk of developing kidney stones and help to decrease bone loss.

- Eating foods such as vegetables that are lower in calories per cup instead of some other higher-calorie food may be useful in helping to lower calorie intake.

Tips to Help You Eat Vegetables

In General:

- Buy fresh vegetables in season. They cost less and are likely to be at their peak flavor.

- Stock up on frozen vegetables for quick and easy cooking in the microwave.

- Buy vegetables that are easy to prepare. Pick up pre-washed bags of salad greens and add baby carrots or grape tomatoes for a salad in minutes. Buy packages of veggies such as baby carrots or celery sticks for quick snacks.

- Use a microwave to quickly "zap" vegetables. White or sweet potatoes can be baked quickly this way.

- Vary your veggie choices to keep meals interesting.

- Try crunchy vegetables, raw or lightly steamed.

For the Best Nutritional Value:

- Select vegetables with more potassium often, such as sweet potatoes, white potatoes, white beans, tomato products (paste, sauce, and juice), beet greens, soybeans, lima beans, spinach, lentils, and kidney beans.

- Sauces or seasonings can add calories, saturated fat, and sodium to vegetables. Use the Nutrition Facts label to compare the calories and % Daily Value for saturated fat and sodium in plain and seasoned vegetables.

- Prepare more foods from fresh ingredients to lower sodium intake. Most sodium in the food supply comes from packaged or processed foods.

- Buy canned vegetables labeled "reduced sodium," "low sodium," or "no salt added." If you want to add a little salt it will likely be less than the amount in the regular canned product.

At Meals:

- Plan some meals around a vegetable main dish, such as a vegetable stir-fry or soup. Then add other foods to complement it.

- Try a main dish salad for lunch. Go light on the salad dressing.

- Include a green salad with your dinner every night.

- Shred carrots or zucchini into meatloaf, casseroles, quick breads, and muffins.

- Include chopped vegetables in pasta sauce or lasagna.

- Order a veggie pizza with toppings like mushrooms, green peppers, and onions, and ask for extra veggies.

- Use pureed, cooked vegetables such as potatoes to thicken stews, soups, and gravies. These add flavor, nutrients, and texture.

- Grill vegetable kabobs as part of a barbecue meal. Try tomatoes, mushrooms, green peppers, and onions.

Make Vegetables More Appealing:

- Many vegetables taste great with a dip or dressing. Try a low-fat salad dressing with raw broccoli, red and green peppers, celery sticks or cauliflower.

- Add color to salads by adding baby carrots, shredded red cabbage or spinach leaves. Include in-season vegetables for variety through the year.

- Include beans or peas in flavorful mixed dishes, such as chili or minestrone soup.

- Decorate plates or serving dishes with vegetable slices.

- Keep a bowl of cut-up vegetables in a see-through container in the refrigerator. Carrot and celery sticks are traditional, but consider red or green pepper strips, broccoli florets or cucumber slices.

Vegetable Tips for Children:

- Set a good example for children by eating vegetables with meals and as snacks.

- Let children decide on the dinner vegetables or what goes into salads.

- Depending on their age, children can help shop for, clean, peel or cut up vegetables.

- Allow children to pick a new vegetable to try while shopping.

- Use cut-up vegetables as part of afternoon snacks.

- Children often prefer foods served separately. So, rather than mixed vegetables try serving two vegetables separately.

Keep It Safe:

- Rinse vegetables before preparing or eating them. Under clean, running water, rub vegetables briskly with your hands to remove dirt and surface microorganisms. Dry with a clean cloth towel or paper towel after rinsing.

- Keep vegetables separate from raw meat, poultry and seafood while shopping, preparing or storing.

Section 11.2

Fruits

This section includes text excerpted from "All about the Fruit Group," ChooseMyPlate.gov, U.S. Department of Agriculture (USDA), March 28, 2016.

What Foods Are in the Fruit Group?

Any fruit or 100% fruit juice counts as part of the Fruit Group. Fruits may be fresh, canned, frozen or dried, and may be whole, cut-up or pureed.

How Much Fruit Is Needed Daily?

The amount of fruit you need to eat depends on age, sex, and level of physical activity. Recommended daily amounts are shown in the table below.

Table 11.3. Daily Fruit Table

Daily Recommendation*		
Children	2-3 years old	1 cup
	4-8 years old	1 to 1 ½ cups
Girls	9-13 years old	1 ½ cups
	14-18 years old	1 ½ cups
Boys	9-13 years old	1 ½ cups
	14-18 years old	2 cups
Women	19-30 years old	2 cups
	31-50 years old	1 ½ cups
	51+ years old	1 ½ cups

Table 11.3. Continued

Daily Recommendation*		
Men	19-30 years old	2 cups
	31-50 years old	2 cups
	51+ years old	2 cups

These amounts are appropriate for individuals who get less than 30 minutes per day of moderate physical activity, beyond normal daily activities. Those who are more physically active may be able to consume more while staying within calorie needs.

What Counts as a Cup of Fruit?

In general, 1 cup of fruit or 100% fruit juice or ½ cup of dried fruit can be considered as 1 cup from the Fruit Group.

Why Is It Important to Eat Fruit?

Eating fruit provides health benefits—people who eat more fruits and vegetables as part of an overall healthy diet are likely to have a reduced risk of some chronic diseases. Fruits provide nutrients vital for health and maintenance of your body.

Nutrients

- Most fruits are naturally low in fat, sodium, and calories. None have cholesterol.

- Fruits are sources of many essential nutrients that are under consumed, including potassium, dietary fiber, vitamin C, and folate (folic acid).

- Diets rich in potassium may help to maintain healthy blood pressure. Fruit sources of potassium include bananas, prunes and prune juice, dried peaches and apricots, cantaloupe, honeydew melon, and orange juice.

- Dietary fiber from fruits, as part of an overall healthy diet, helps reduce blood cholesterol levels and may lower risk of heart disease. Fiber is important for proper bowel function. It helps reduce constipation and diverticulosis. Fiber-containing foods such as fruits help provide a feeling of fullness with fewer calories. Whole or cut-up fruits are sources of dietary fiber; fruit juices contain little or no fiber.

- Vitamin C is important for growth and repair of all body tissues, helps heal cuts and wounds, and keeps teeth and gums healthy.

- Folate (folic acid) helps the body form red blood cells. Women of childbearing age who may become pregnant should consume adequate folate from foods, and in addition 400 mcg of synthetic folic acid from fortified foods or supplements. This reduces the risk of neural tube defects, spina bifida, and anencephaly during fetal development.

Health Benefits

- Eating a diet rich in vegetables and fruits as part of an overall healthy diet may reduce risk for heart disease, including heart attack and stroke.

- Eating a diet rich in some vegetables and fruits as part of an overall healthy diet may protect against certain types of cancers.

- Diets rich in foods containing fiber, such as some vegetables and fruits, may reduce the risk of heart disease, obesity, and type 2 diabetes.

- Eating vegetables and fruits rich in potassium as part of an overall healthy diet may lower blood pressure, and may also reduce the risk of developing kidney stones and help to decrease bone loss.

- Eating foods such as fruits that are lower in calories per cup instead of some other higher-calorie food may be useful in helping to lower calorie intake.

Tips to Help You Eat Fruits

In General:

- Keep a bowl of whole fruit on the table, counter or in the refrigerator.

- Refrigerate cut-up fruit to store for later.

- Buy fresh fruits in season when they may be less expensive and at their peak flavor.

- Buy fruits that are dried, frozen, and canned (in water or 100% juice) as well as fresh, so that you always have a supply on hand.

- Consider convenience when shopping. Try pre-cut packages of fruit (such as melon or pineapple chunks) for a healthy snack in seconds. Choose packaged fruits that do not have added sugars.

For the Best Nutritional Value:

- Make most of your choices whole or cut-up fruit rather than juice, for the benefits dietary fiber provides.
- Select fruits with more potassium often, such as bananas, prunes and prune juice, dried peaches and apricots, and orange juice.
- When choosing canned fruits, select fruit canned in 100% fruit juice or water rather than syrup.
- Vary your fruit choices. Fruits differ in nutrient content.

At Meals:

- At breakfast, top your cereal with bananas or peaches; add blueberries to pancakes; drink 100% orange or grapefruit juice. Or, mix fresh fruit with plain fat-free or low-fat yogurt.
- At lunch, pack a tangerine, banana or grapes to eat or choose fruits from a salad bar. Individual containers of fruits like peaches or applesauce are easy and convenient.
- At dinner, add crushed pineapple to coleslaw or include orange sections or grapes in a tossed salad.
- Make a Waldorf salad, with apples, celery, walnuts, and a low-calorie salad dressing.
- Try meat dishes that incorporate fruit, such as chicken with apricots or mangoes.
- Add fruit like pineapple or peaches to kabobs as part of a barbecue meal.
- For dessert, have baked apples, pears or a fruit salad.

As Snacks:

- Cut-up fruit makes a great snack. Either cut them yourself or buy pre-cut packages of fruit pieces like pineapples or melons. Or, try whole fresh berries or grapes.
- Dried fruits also make a great snack. They are easy to carry and store well. Because they are dried, ¼ cup is equivalent to ½ cup of other fruits.
- Keep a package of dried fruit in your desk or bag. Some fruits that are available dried include apricots, apples, pineapple,

bananas, cherries, figs, dates, cranberries, blueberries, prunes (dried plums), and raisins (dried grapes).

- As a snack, spread peanut butter on apple slices or top plain fat-free or low-fat yogurt with berries or slices of kiwi fruit.

- Frozen juice bars (100% juice) make healthy alternatives to high-fat snacks.

Make Fruit More Appealing:

- Many fruits taste great with a dip or dressing. Try fat-free or low-fat yogurt as a dip for fruits like strawberries or melons.

- Make a fruit smoothie by blending fat-free or low-fat milk or yogurt with fresh or frozen fruit. Try bananas, peaches, strawberries or other berries.

- Try unsweetened applesauce as a lower calorie substitute for some of the oil when baking cakes.

- Try different textures of fruits. For example, apples are crunchy, bananas are smooth and creamy, and oranges are juicy.

- For fresh fruit salads, mix apples, bananas or pears with acidic fruits like oranges, pineapple or lemon juice to keep them from turning brown.

Fruit Tips for Children:

- Set a good example for children by eating fruit every day with meals or as snacks.

- Offer children a choice of fruits for lunch.

- Depending on their age, children can help shop for, clean, peel or cut up fruits.

- While shopping, allow children to pick out a new fruit to try later at home.

- Decorate plates or serving dishes with fruit slices.

- Top off a bowl of cereal with some berries. Or, make a smiley face with sliced bananas for eyes, raisins for a nose, and an orange slice for a mouth.

- Offer raisins or other dried fruits instead of candy.

- Make fruit kabobs using pineapple chunks, bananas, grapes, and berries.

- Pack a juice box (100% juice) in children's lunches instead of soda or other sugar-sweetened beverages.

- Look for and choose fruit options, such as sliced apples, mixed fruit cup or 100% fruit juice in fast food restaurants.

- Offer fruit pieces and 100% fruit juice to children. There is often little fruit in "fruit-flavored" beverages or chewy fruit snacks.

Keep It Safe:

- Rinse fruits before preparing or eating them. Under clean, running water, rub fruits briskly with your hands to remove dirt and surface microorganisms. Dry with a clean cloth towel or paper towel after rinsing.

- Keep fruits separate from raw meat, poultry and seafood while shopping, preparing or storing.

Section 11.3

Grains

This section includes text excerpted from "All about the Grains Group," ChooseMyPlate.gov, U.S. Department of Agriculture (USDA), March 28, 2016.

What Foods Are in the Grains Group?

Any food made from wheat, rice, oats, cornmeal, barley or another cereal grain is a grain product. Bread, pasta, oatmeal, breakfast cereals, tortillas, and grits are examples of grain products.

Grains are divided into 2 subgroups, Whole Grains and Refined Grains. Whole grains contain the entire grain kernel, the bran, germ, and endosperm. Examples of whole grains include whole-wheat flour, bulgur (cracked wheat), oatmeal, whole cornmeal, and brown rice. Refined grains have been milled, a process that removes the bran and germ. This is done to give grains a finer texture and improve their shelf life, but it also removes dietary fiber, iron, and many B vitamins. *Some examples of refined grain products* are white flour, degermed cornmeal, white bread, and white rice.

Most refined grains are enriched. This means certain B vitamins (thiamin, riboflavin, niacin, folic acid) and iron are added back after processing. Fiber is not added back to enriched grains. Check the ingredient list on refined grain products to make sure that the word "enriched" is included in the grain name. Some food products are made from mixtures of whole grains and refined grains.

How Many Grain Foods Are Needed Daily?

The amount of grains you need to eat depends on your age, sex, and level of physical activity. Recommended daily amounts are listed in this table below. Most Americans consume enough grains, but few are whole grains. **At least half of all the grains eaten should be whole grains.**

Table 11.4. Daily Grain Table

		DAILY RECOMMENDATION*	Daily minimum amount of whole grains
Children	2-3 years old 4-8 years old	3 ounce equivalents 5 ounce equivalents	1 ½ ounce equivalents 2 ½ ounce equivalents
Girls	9-13 years old 14-18 years old	5 ounce equivalents 6 ounce equivalents	3 ounce equivalents 3 ounce equivalents
Boys	9-13 years old 14-18 years old	6 ounce equivalents 8 ounce equivalents	3 ounce equivalents 4 ounce equivalents
Women	19-30 years old 31-50 years old 51+ years old	6 ounce equivalents 6 ounce equivalents 5 ounce equivalents	3 ounce equivalents 3 ounce equivalents 3 ounce equivalents

Table 11.4. Continued

		DAILY RECOMMENDATION*	Daily minimum amount of whole grains
Men	19-30 years old 31-50 years old 51+ years old	8 ounce equivalents 7 ounce equivalents 6 ounce equivalents	4 ounce equivalents 3 ½ ounce equivalents 3 ounce equivalents

*These amounts are appropriate for individuals who get less than 30 minutes per day of moderate physical activity, beyond normal daily activities. Those who are more physically active may be able to consume more while staying within calorie needs.

What Counts as an Ounce-Equivalent of Grains?

In general, 1 slice of bread, 1 cup of ready-to-eat cereal or ½ cup of cooked rice, cooked pasta or cooked cereal can be considered as 1 ounce-equivalent from the Grains Group.

Why Is It Important to Eat Grains, Especially Whole Grains?

Eating grains, especially whole grains, provides health benefits. People who eat whole grains as part of a healthy diet have a reduced risk of some chronic diseases. Grains provide many nutrients that are vital for the health and maintenance of our bodies.

Nutrients

- Grains are important sources of many nutrients, including dietary fiber, several B vitamins (thiamin, riboflavin, niacin, and folate), and minerals (iron, magnesium, and selenium).

- Dietary fiber from whole grains or other foods, may help reduce blood cholesterol levels and may lower risk of heart disease, obesity, and type 2 diabetes. Fiber is important for proper bowel function. It helps reduce constipation and diverticulosis. Fiber-containing foods such as whole grains help provide a feeling of fullness with fewer calories.

- The B vitamins thiamin, riboflavin, and niacin play a key role in metabolism—they help the body release energy from protein, fat, and carbohydrates. B vitamins are also essential for a healthy nervous system. Many refined grains are enriched with these B vitamins.

- Folate (folic acid), another B vitamin, helps the body form red blood cells. Women of childbearing age who may become pregnant should consume adequate folate from foods, and in addition 400 mcg of synthetic folic acid from fortified foods or supplements. This reduces the risk of neural tube defects, spina bifida, and anencephaly during fetal development.

- Iron is used to carry oxygen in the blood. Many teenage girls and women in their childbearing years have iron-deficiency anemia. They should eat foods high in heme-iron (meats) or eat other iron containing foods along with foods rich in vitamin C, which can improve absorption of nonheme iron. Whole and enriched refined grain products are major sources of nonheme iron in American diets.

- Whole grains are sources of magnesium and selenium. Magnesium is a mineral used in building bones and releasing energy from muscles. Selenium protects cells from oxidation. It is also important for a healthy immune system.

Health Benefits

- Consuming whole grains as part of a healthy diet may reduce the risk of heart disease.

- Consuming foods containing fiber, such as whole grains, as part of a healthy diet, may reduce constipation.

- Eating whole grains may help with weight management.

- Eating grain products fortified with folate before and during pregnancy helps prevent neural tube defects during fetal development.

Tips to Help You Eat Whole Grains

At Meals:

- To eat more whole grains, substitute a whole-grain product for a refined product—such as eating whole-wheat bread instead of white bread or brown rice instead of white rice. It's important to substitute the whole-grain product for the refined one, rather than adding the whole-grain product.

- For a change, try brown rice or whole-wheat pasta. Try brown rice stuffing in baked green peppers or tomatoes and whole-wheat macaroni in macaroni and cheese.

- Use whole grains in mixed dishes, such as barley in vegetable soup or stews and bulgur wheat in a casserole or stir-fry.

- Create a whole grain pilaf with a mixture of barley, wild rice, brown rice, broth and spices. For a special touch, stir in toasted nuts or chopped dried fruit.

- Experiment by substituting whole wheat or oat flour for up to half of the flour in pancake, waffle, muffin or other flour-based recipes. They may need a bit more leavening.

- Use whole-grain bread or cracker crumbs in meatloaf.

- Try rolled oats or a crushed, unsweetened whole grain cereal as breading for baked chicken, fish, veal cutlets or eggplant parmesan.

- Try an unsweetened, whole grain ready-to-eat cereal as croutons in salad or in place of crackers with soup.

- Freeze leftover cooked brown rice, bulgur or barley. Heat and serve it later as a quick side dish.

As Snacks:

- Snack on ready-to-eat, whole grain cereals such as toasted oat cereal.

- Add whole-grain flour or oatmeal when making cookies or other baked treats.

- Try 100% whole-grain snack crackers.

- Popcorn, a whole grain, can be a healthy snack if made with little or no added salt and butter.

What to Look for on the Food Label

- Choose foods that name one of the following whole-grain ingredients first on the label's ingredient list:

- **Whole Grain Ingredients**

- Brown rice

- Buckwheat

- Bulgur

- Millet

- Oatmeal

- Popcorn

- Quinoa

- Rolled oats

- Whole-grain barley

- Whole-grain corn

- Whole-grain sorghum

- Whole-grain triticale

- Whole oats

- Whole rye

- Whole wheat

- Wild rice

- Foods labeled with the words "multi-grain," "stone-ground," "100% wheat," "cracked wheat," "seven-grain," or "bran" are usually not whole-grain products.

- Color is not an indication of a whole grain. Bread can be brown because of molasses or other added ingredients. Read the ingredient list to see if it is a whole grain.

- Use the Nutrition Facts label and choose whole grain products with a higher % Daily Value (% DV) for fiber. Many, but not all, whole grain products are good or excellent sources of fiber.

- Read the food label's ingredient list. Look for terms that indicate added sugars (such as sucrose, high-fructose corn syrup, honey, malt syrup, maple syrup, molasses or raw sugar) that add extra calories. Choose foods with fewer added sugars.

- Most sodium in the food supply comes from packaged foods. Similar packaged foods can vary widely in sodium content, including breads. Use the Nutrition Facts label to choose foods with a lower % DV for sodium. Foods with less than 140 mg sodium per serving can be labeled as low sodium foods. Claims such as "low in sodium" or "very low in sodium" on the front of the food label can help you identify foods that contain less salt (or sodium).

Whole Grain Tips for Children

- Set a good example for children by eating whole grains with meals or as snacks.

- Let children select and help prepare a whole grain side dish.

- Teach older children to read the ingredient list on cereals or snack food packages and choose those with whole grains at the top of the list.

Section 11.4

Dairy

This section includes text excerpted from "All about the Dairy Group," ChooseMyPlate.gov, U.S. Department of Agriculture (USDA), March 28, 2016.

What Foods Are Included in the Dairy Group?

All fluid milk products and many foods made from milk are considered part of this food group. Most Dairy Group choices should be fat-free or low-fat. Foods made from milk that retain their calcium content are part of the group. Foods made from milk that have little to no calcium, such as cream cheese, cream, and butter, are not. Calcium-fortified soymilk (soy beverage) is also part of the Dairy Group.

How Much Food from the Dairy Group Is Needed Daily?

The amount of food from the Dairy Group you need to eat depends on age. Recommended daily amounts are shown in the table below.

Table 11.5. Daily Dairy Table

Daily Recommendation					
Children	2-3 years old	2 cups	Women	19-30 years old	3 cups
	4-8 years old	2 ½ cups		31-50 years old	3 cups
Girls	9-13 years old	3 cups		51+ years old	3 cups
	14-18 years old	3 cups	Men	19-30 years old	3 cups
Boys	9-13 years old	3 cups		19-30 years old	3 cups
	14-18 years old	3 cups		19-30 years old	3 cups

What Counts as a Cup in the Dairy Group?

In general, 1 cup of milk, yogurt or soymilk (soy beverage), 1 ½ ounces of natural cheese or 2 ounces of processed cheese can be considered as 1 cup from the Dairy Group.

Selection Tips

- Choose fat-free or low-fat milk, yogurt, and cheese. If you choose milk or yogurt that is not fat-free or cheese that is not low-fat, the fat in the product counts against your maximum limit for "empty calories" (calories from solid fats and added sugars).

- If sweetened milk products are chosen (flavored milk, yogurt, drinkable yogurt, desserts), the added sugars also count against your maximum limit for "empty calories" (calories from solid fats and added sugars).

- For those who are lactose intolerant, smaller portions (such as 4 fluid ounces of milk) may be well tolerated. Lactose-free and lower-lactose products are available. These include lactose-reduced or lactose-free milk, yogurt, and cheese, and calcium-fortified soymilk (soy beverage). Also, enzyme preparations can be added to milk to lower the lactose content.

- Calcium choices for those who do not consume dairy products include: kale leaves

- Calcium-fortified juices, cereals, breads, rice milk or almond milk. Calcium-fortified foods and beverages may not provide the other nutrients found in dairy products. Check the labels.

- Canned fish (sardines, salmon with bones) soybeans and other soy products (tofu made with calcium sulfate, soy yogurt, tempeh), some other beans, and some leafy greens (collard and turnip greens, kale, bok choy). The amount of calcium that can be absorbed from these foods varies.

Nutrients and Health Benefits

Consuming dairy products provides health benefits–especially improved bone health. Foods in the Dairy Group provide nutrients that are vital for health and maintenance of your body. These nutrients include calcium, potassium, vitamin D, and protein.

Nutrients

- Calcium is used for building bones and teeth and in maintaining bone mass. Dairy products are the primary source of calcium in American diets. Diets that provide 3 cups or the equivalent of dairy products per day can improve bone mass.

- Diets rich in potassium may help to maintain healthy blood pressure. Dairy products, especially yogurt, fluid milk, and soymilk (soy beverage), provide potassium.

- Vitamin D functions in the body to maintain proper levels of calcium and phosphorous, thereby helping to build and maintain bones. Milk and soymilk (soy beverage) that are fortified with vitamin D are good sources of this nutrient. Other sources include vitamin D-fortified yogurt and vitamin D-fortified ready-to-eat breakfast cereals.

- Milk products that are consumed in their low-fat or fat-free forms provide little or no solid fat.

Health Benefits

- Intake of dairy products is linked to improved bone health, and may reduce the risk of osteoporosis.

- The intake of dairy products is especially important to bone health during childhood and adolescence, when bone mass is being built.

- Intake of dairy products is also associated with a reduced risk of cardiovascular disease and type 2 diabetes, and with lower blood pressure in adults.

Why Is It Important to Make Fat-Free or Low-Fat Choices from the Dairy Group?

Choosing foods from the Dairy Group that are high in saturated fats and cholesterol can have health implications. Diets high in saturated fats raise "bad" cholesterol levels in the blood. The "bad" cholesterol is called LDL (low-density lipoprotein) cholesterol. High LDL cholesterol, in turn, increases the risk for coronary heart disease. Many cheeses, whole milk, and products made from them are high in saturated fat. To help keep blood cholesterol levels healthy, limit the amount of these foods you eat. In addition, a high intake of fats makes it difficult to avoid consuming more calories than are needed.

Non-Dairy Sources of Calcium

For Those Who Choose Not to Consume Milk Products

Calcium choices for those who do not consume dairy products include:

- Calcium-fortified juices, cereals, breads, rice milk or almond milk.

- Canned fish (sardines, salmon with bones) soybeans and other soy products (tofu made with calcium sulfate, soy yogurt, tempeh), some other beans, and some leafy greens (collard and turnip greens, kale, bok choy). The amount of calcium that can be absorbed from these foods varies.

Tips for Taking Dairy Products

- Include milk or calcium-fortified soymilk (soy beverage) as a beverage at meals. Choose fat-free or low-fat milk.

- If you usually drink whole milk, switch gradually to fat-free milk, to lower saturated fat and calories. Try reduced fat (2%), then low-fat fruits and yogurt (1%), and finally fat-free (skim).

- If you drink cappuccinos or lattes—ask for them with fat-free (skim) milk.

- Add fat-free or low-fat milk instead of water to oatmeal and hot cereals.
- Use fat-free or low-fat milk when making condensed cream soups (such as cream of tomato).
- Have fat-free or low-fat yogurt as a snack.
- Make a dip for fruits or vegetables from yogurt.
- Make fruit-yogurt smoothies in the blender.
- For dessert, make chocolate or butterscotch pudding with fat-free or low-fat milk.
- Top cut-up fruit with flavored yogurt for a quick dessert.
- Top casseroles, soups, stews or vegetables with shredded reduced-fat or low-fat cheese.
- Top a baked potato with fat-free or low-fat yogurt.

Keep It Safe

- Avoid raw (unpasteurized) milk or any products made from unpasteurized milk.
- Chill (refrigerate) perishable food promptly and defrost foods properly. Refrigerate or freeze perishables, prepared food and leftovers as soon as possible. If food has been left at temperatures between 40° and 140° F for more than two hours, discard it, even though it may look and smell good.
- Separate raw, cooked, and ready-to-eat foods.

Section 11.5

Protein Food Group

This section includes text excerpted from "All about the
Protein Foods Group," ChooseMyPlate.gov, U.S. Department
of Agriculture (USDA), March 28, 2016.

What Foods Are in the Protein Foods Group?

All foods made from meat, poultry, seafood, beans and peas, eggs,
processed soy products, nuts, and seeds are considered part of the
Protein Foods Group. Beans and peas are also part of the Vegetable
Group.

Select a variety of protein foods to improve nutrient intake and
health benefits, including at least 8 ounces of cooked seafood per week.
Young children need less, depending on their age and calorie needs.
The advice to consume seafood does not apply to vegetarians. Vegetarian options in the Protein Foods Group include beans and peas,
processed soy products, and nuts and seeds. Meat and poultry choices
should be lean or low-fat.

How Much Food from the Protein Foods Group Is Daily?

The amount of food from the Protein Foods Group you need to eat
depends on age, sex, and level of physical activity. Most Americans eat
enough food from this group, but need to make leaner and more varied
selections of these foods. Recommended daily amounts are shown in
the table below.

Table 11.6. Daily Protein Foods Table

Daily Protein Foods Table		
Daily recommendation*		
Children	2-3 years old 4-8 years old	2 ounce equivalents 4 ounce equivalents
Girls	9-13 years old 14-18 years old	5 ounce equivalents 5 ounce equivalents

Table 11.6. Continued

Daily Protein Foods Table		
Daily recommendation*		
Boys	9-13 years old 14-18 years old	5 ounce equivalents 6 ½ ounce equivalents
Women	19-30 years old 31-50 years old 51+ years old	5 ½ ounce equivalents 5 ounce equivalents 5 ounce equivalents
Men	19-30 years old 31-50 years old 51+ years old	6 ½ ounce equivalents 6 ounce equivalents 5 ½ ounce equivalents

*These amounts are appropriate for individuals who get less than 30 min-
utes per day of moderate physical activity, beyond normal daily activities.
Those who are more physically active may be able to consume more while
staying within calorie needs.*

What Counts as an Ounce-Equivalent in the Protein Foods Group?

In general, 1 ounce of meat, poultry or fish, ¼ cup cooked beans,
1 egg, 1 tablespoon of peanut butter or ½ ounce of nuts or seeds can
be considered as 1 ounce-equivalent from the Protein Foods Group.

Selection Tips

- Choose lean or low-fat meat and poultry. If higher fat choices
  are made, such as regular ground beef (75-80% lean) or chicken
  with skin, the fat counts against your maximum limit for empty
  calories (calories from solid fats or added sugars).

- If solid fat is added in cooking, such as frying chicken in shortening or frying eggs in butter or stick margarine, this also counts
  against your maximum limit for empty calories (calories from
  solid fats and added sugars).

- Select some seafood that is rich in omega-3 fatty acids, such as
  salmon, trout, sardines, anchovies, herring, Pacific oysters, and
  Atlantic and Pacific mackerel.

- Processed meats such as ham, sausage, frankfurters, and luncheon or deli meats have added sodium. Check the Nutrition
  Facts label to help limit sodium intake. Fresh chicken, turkey, and pork that have been enhanced with a salt-containing

solution also have added sodium. Check the product label for statements such as "self-basting" or "contains up to__% of__", which mean that a sodium-containing solution has been added to the product.

- Choose unsalted nuts and seeds to keep sodium intake low.

Why Is It Important to Make Lean or Low-Fat Choices from the Protein Foods Group?

Foods in the meat, poultry, fish, eggs, nuts, and seed group provide nutrients that are vital for health and maintenance of your body. However, choosing foods from this group that are high in saturated fat and cholesterol may have health implications.

The chart below lists specific amounts that count as 1 ounce equivalent in the Protein Foods Group towards your daily recommended intake:

Table 11.7. Protein Foods Group towards Your Daily Recommended Intake

	Amount that counts as 1 ounce equivalent in the Protein Foods Group	**Common portions and ounce equivalents**
Meats	1 ounce cooked lean beef 1 ounce cooked lean pork or ham	1 small steak (eye of round, filet) = 3/12 to 4 ounce equivalents 1 small lean hamburger = 2 to 3 ounce equivalents
Poultry	1 ounce cooked chicken or turkey, without skin 1 sandwich slice of turkey (4 1/2 x 2 1/2 x 1/8")	1 small chicken breast half = 3 ounce equivalents 1/2 Cornish game hen = 4 ounce equivalents
Seafood	1 ounce cooked fish or shell fish	1 can of tuna, drained = 3 to 4 ounce equivalents 1 salmon steak = 4 to 6 ounce equivalents 1 small trout = 3 ounce equivalents
Eggs	1 egg	3 egg whites = 2 ounce equivalents 3 egg yolks = 1 ounce equivalent

Table 11.7. Continued

	Amount that counts as 1 ounce equivalent in the Protein Foods Group	Common portions and ounce equivalents
Beans and peas	1/2 ounce of nuts (12 almonds, 24 pistachios, 7 walnut halves) 1/2 ounce of seeds (pumpkin, sunflower or squash seeds, hulled, roasted) 1 Tablespoon of peanut butter or almond butter	1 ounce of nuts of seeds = 2 ounce equivalents
Beans and peas	1/4 cup of cooked beans (such as black, kidney, pinto or white beans) 1/4 cup of cooked peas (such as chickpeas, cowpeas, lentils or split peas) 1/4 cup of baked beans, refried beans 1/4 cup (about 2 ounces) of tofu 1 ox. tempeh, cooked 1/4 cup roasted soybeans 1 falafel patty (2 1/4", 4 oz) 2 Tablespoons hummus	1 cup split pea soup = 2 ounce equivalents 1 cup lentil soup = 2 ounce equivalents 1 cup bean soup = 2 ounce equivalents 1 soy or bean burger patty = 2 ounce equivalents

Nutrients

- Diets that are high in saturated fats raise "bad" choles-terol levels in the blood. The "bad" cholesterol is called LDL (low-density lipoprotein) cholesterol. High LDL cholesterol, in turn, increases the risk for coronary heart disease. Some food choices in this group are high in saturated fat. These include fatty cuts of beef, pork, and lamb; regular (75% to 85% lean) ground beef; regular sausages, hot dogs, and bacon; some luncheon meats such as regular bologna and salami; and some poultry such as duck. To help keep blood cholesterol levels healthy, limit the amount of these foods you eat.

147

- Diets that are high in cholesterol can raise LDL cholesterol levels in the blood. Cholesterol is only found in foods from animal sources. Some foods from this group are high in cholesterol. These include egg yolks (egg whites are cholesterol-free) and organ meats such as liver and giblets. To help keep blood cholesterol levels healthy, limit the amount of these foods you eat.

- A high intake of fats makes it difficult to avoid consuming more calories than are needed.

Why Is It Important to Eat 8 Ounces of Seafood per Week?

- Seafood contains a range of nutrients, notably the omega-3 fatty acids, EPA, and DHA. Eating about 8 ounces per week of a variety of seafood contributes to the prevention of heart disease. Smaller amounts of seafood are recommended for young children.

- Seafood varieties that are commonly consumed in the United States that are higher in EPA and DHA and lower in mercury include salmon, anchovies, herring, sardines, Pacific oysters, trout, and Atlantic and Pacific mackerel (not king mackerel, which is high in mercury). The health benefits from consuming seafood outweigh the health risk associated with mercury, a heavy metal found in seafood in varying levels.

Health Benefits

- Meat, poultry, fish, dry beans and peas, eggs, nuts, and seeds supply many nutrients. These include protein, B vitamins (niacin, thiamin, riboflavin, and B6), vitamin E, iron, zinc, and magnesium.

- Proteins function as building blocks for bones, muscles, cartilage, skin, and blood. They are also building blocks for enzymes, hormones, and vitamins. Proteins are one of three nutrients that provide calories (the others are fat and carbohydrates).

- B vitamins found in this food group serve a variety of functions in the body. They help the body release energy, play a vital role in the function of the nervous system, aid in the formation of red blood cells, and help build tissues.

- Iron is used to carry oxygen in the blood. Many teenage girls and women in their child-bearing years have iron-deficiency anemia.

They should eat foods high in heme-iron (meats) or eat other non-heme iron containing foods along with a food rich in vitamin C, which can improve absorption of nonheme iron.

- Magnesium is used in building bones and in releasing energy from muscles.

- Zinc is necessary for biochemical reactions and helps the immune system function properly.

- EPA and DHA are omega-3 fatty acids found in varying amounts in seafood. Eating 8 ounces per week of seafood may help reduce the risk for heart disease.

What Are the Benefits of Eating Nuts and Seeds?

Eating peanuts and certain tree nuts (i.e., walnuts, almonds, and pistachios) may reduce the risk of heart disease when consumed as part of a diet that is nutritionally adequate and within calorie needs. Because nuts and seeds are high in calories, eat them in small portions and use them to replace other protein foods, like some meat or poultry, rather than adding them to what you already eat. In addition, choose unsalted nuts and seeds to help reduce sodium intakes.

Vegetarian Choices in the Protein Foods Group

Vegetarians get enough protein from this group as long as the variety and amounts of foods selected are adequate. Protein sources from the Protein Foods Group for vegetarians include eggs (for ovo-vegetarians), beans and peas, nuts, nut butters, and soy products (tofu, tempeh, veggie burgers).

Chapter 12

Phytonutrients and Their Sources

Chapter Contents

Section 12.1

Phytonutrients: An Overview

This section contains text excerpted from the following sources:
Text under the heading "What Are Phytonutrients and Where Are
They Found?" is excerpted from "Phytonutrient FAQs," Agricultural
Research Service (ARS), U.S. Department of Agriculture (USDA),
April 8, 2005. Reviewed June 2016; Text under the heading "How
Plants Protect Us. Unmasking the Secret Power of Phytochemicals"
is excerpted from "How Plants Protect Us Unmasking the Secret
Power of Phytochemicals," Agricultural Research Service
(ARS), U.S. Department of Agriculture (USDA),
March 2008. Reviewed June 2016.

What Are Phytonutrients and Where Are They Found?

The term *"phyto"* originated from a Greek word meaning plant.
Phytonutrients are certain organic components of plants, and these
components are thought to promote human health. Fruits, vegetables,
grains, legumes, nuts, and teas are rich sources of phytonutrients.
Unlike the traditional nutrients (protein, fat, vitamins, minerals),
phytonutrients are not "essential" for life, so some people prefer the
term "phytochemical".

What Are the Major Classes of Phytonutrients?

Some of the Common Classes of Phytonutrients Include:

- Carotenoids

- Flavonoids (Polyphenols) including Isoflavones (Phytoestrogens)

- Inositol Phosphates (Phytates)

- Lignans (Phytoestrogens)

- Isothiocyanates and Indoles

- Phenols and Cyclic Compounds

- Saponins

- Sulfides and Thiols
- Terpenes

About Carotenoids

Of all the phytonutrients, we probably know the most about carotenoids, the red, orange, and yellow pigments in fruits and vegetables. The carotenoids most commonly found in vegetables (and in plasma) are listed below along with common sources of these compounds. Fruits and vegetables that are high in carotenoids appear to protect humans against certain cancers, heart disease, and age related macular degeneration.

Table 12.1. About Carotenoids

Carotenoid	Common Food Source
alpha-carotene	carrots
beta-carotene	leafy green and yellow vegetables (eg broccoli, sweet potato, pumpkin, carrots)
beta-cryptoxanthin	citrus, peaches, apricots
lutein	leafy greens such as kale, spinach, turnip greens
lycopene	tomato products, pink grapefruit, watermelon, guava
zeaxanthin	green vegetables, eggs, citrus

About Polyphenols

Polyphenolic compounds are natural components of a wide variety of plants; they are also known as secondary plant metabolites. Food sources rich in polyphenols include onion, apple, tea, red wine, red grapes, grape juice, strawberries, raspberries, blueberries, cranberries, and certain nuts. The average polyphenol/flavonoid intake in the U.S. has not been determined with precision, in large part, because there is presently no U.S. national food database for these compounds. (U.S. Department of Agriculture(USDA) scientists and their colleagues are in the process of developing a database for foods rich in polyphenols.) It has been estimated that in the Dutch diet a subset of flavonoids (flavonols and flavones) provide 23 mg per day. Earlier estimates of dietary intake that approximated 650 mg per day are generally thought to be too high as the estimate was based on data that were generated by "old" (less specific) methodology. Scientists at the Food Composition Laboratory, Beltsville Human Nutrition Research Center are currently developing new methodology for the accurate measurement of polyphenols in foods.

Polyphenols can be classified as non-flavonoids and flavonoids. The flavonoids quercetin and catechins are the most extensively studied polyphenols relative to absorption and metabolism.

Table 12.2. Non Flavonoids Sources

Non Flavonoids	Sources
ellagic acid	strawberries, blueberries, raspberries
coumarins	

Table 12.3. Flavonoids Sources

Flavonoids	Sources
anthocyanins	fruits
catechins	tea, wine
flavanones	citrus
flavones	fruits and vegetables
flavonols	fruits, vegetables, tea, wine
isoflavones	soybeans

How Do Phytonutrients Protect against Disease?

The following are commonly proposed mechanisms by which phytonutrients may protect human health. More research is needed to firmly establish the mechanisms of action of the various phytochemicals.

Phytonutrients may

- serve as antioxidants;

- enhance immune response;

- enhance cell-to-cell communication;

- alter estrogen metabolism;

- convert to vitamin A (beta-carotene is metabolized to vitamin A);

- cause cancer cells to die (apoptosis);

- repair DNA damage caused by smoking and other toxic exposures; and

- detoxify carcinogens through the activation of the cytocrome P450 and Phase II enzyme systems.

How Plants Protect Us? Unmasking the Secret Power of Phytochemicals

Rosemary, the fragrant herb that enlivens roast chicken and other favorites, and turmeric, the mainstay spice of curry dishes, contain powerful natural compounds that, in test tubes, can kill cells of a childhood cancer. What's more, grapes, strawberries, and other familiar fruits—and some vegetables—also have chemicals that can destroy the cells of this cancer, known as "acute lymphoblastic leukemia."

Death of Leukemia Cells: How Do Phytochemicals Triumph?

For the most part, scientists don't yet have all the details about how phytochemicals bolster healthy cells and battle harmful ones. That's true even for better-known phytochemicals such as the resveratrol in red grapes, blueberries, and some other fruits.

Susan J. Zunino, an Agricultural Research Service molecular biologist, leads the nutrition-focused research that has resulted in these first-ever findings. She's investigating the health-imparting effects of plant chemicals or phytochemicals, using laboratory cultures of both healthy human blood cells and cancerous ones as her models.

Zunino's investigations provide some new clues about how phytochemicals attack cancer cells. She has studied carnosol from rosemary, curcumin from turmeric, resveratrol from grapes, and ellagic acid, kaempferol, and quercetin in strawberries. The work demonstrated the ability of these phytochemicals to kill the acute lymphoblastic leukemia cells and also suggested ways in which the compounds might do that.

For example, Zunino and colleagues showed that the phytochemicals interfere with the orderly operations of mitochondria, the miniature energy-producing power plants inside cells. Without energy, cells die.

Mitochondria exposed to resveratrol and the other phytochemicals became inoperative. But more work is needed to fully understand how the phytochemicals achieved that. And the team wants to know more about the phytochemicals' other modes of action that resulted in the cancer-cell death.

Can Phytochemicals Help Prevent Diabetes?

In related research, Zunino, working with Storms and Charles Stephensen, a physiologist at the Davis research center, determined for the first time that some component of table grapes prevented the progression of type 1 diabetes in mice and increased their survival. That was in contrast to diabetic mice that were not fed grapes.

Scientists provided the fruit in the form of a freeze-dried powder made from table grapes, the kind sold fresh in the produce section of supermarkets. The powder, provided by the California Table Grape Commission, made up 1 percent of the chow fed to some of the mice. That's the human equivalent of about six servings of grapes per day.

Zunino's experiment apparently is the first to show a link between eating grapes and preventing progression of type 1 diabetes. If the results from this study of 30 laboratory mice hold true for humans, the research could offer new options for protection against this chronic autoimmune disease.

According to the National Institutes of Health, an estimated 1 in every 400-600 children and adolescents in the U.S. population has type 1 diabetes.

The researchers don't know which grape compounds provided the protective effect. Similarly, the exact sequence of steps that led to the protection is also not yet proven. But the scientists think that the grape phytochemicals may have prevented unwanted entry of immune cells into the pancreas.

Mice fed the grape powder had fewer immune cells in the pancreas than did the other mice in the experiment. But what's the relation between immune cells in the pancreas and type 1 diabetes?

Immune cells in the pancreas can mistakenly attack specialized cells known as "beta cells." Beta cells produce insulin, which is needed to help regulate the amount of sugar in the bloodstream. If immune cells in the pancreas attack and kill beta cells, the pancreas can run out of beta cells. When that happens, type 1 diabetes can result.

People with type 1 diabetes have to carefully monitor the amounts of sugar-containing foods they eat, including sweet, fresh table grapes. How ironic that this luscious fruit might actually hold a key to preventing the progression of type 1 diabetes. This may be a perplexing riddle of Nature—perhaps one that Zunino's team will soon solve.

Section 12.2

Antioxidants

This section includes text excerpted from "Antioxidants: In Depth," National Center for Complementary and Integrative Health (NCCIH), May 2010. Reviewed June 2016.

Antioxidants are man-made or natural substances that may prevent or delay some types of cell damage. Diets high in vegetables and fruits, which are good sources of antioxidants, have been found to be healthy; however, research has not shown antioxidant supplements to be beneficial in preventing diseases. Examples of antioxidants include vitamins C and E, selenium, and carotenoids, such as beta-carotene, lycopene, lutein, and zeaxanthin. This section provides basic information about antioxidants, summarizes what the science says about antioxidants and health and suggests sources for additional information.

Key Points

- Vegetables and fruits are rich sources of antioxidants. There is good evidence that eating a diet that includes plenty of vegetables and fruits is healthy and official U.S. Government policy urges people to eat more of these foods. Research has shown that people who eat more vegetables and fruits have lower risks of several diseases; however, it is not clear whether these results are related to the amount of antioxidants in vegetables and fruits, to other components of these foods, to other factors in people's diets or to other lifestyle choices.

- Rigorous scientific studies involving more than 100,000 people combined have tested whether antioxidant supplements can help prevent chronic diseases, such as cardiovascular diseases, cancer, and cataracts. In most instances, antioxidants did not reduce the risks of developing these diseases.

- Concerns have not been raised about the safety of antioxidants in food. However, high-dose supplements of antioxidants may be linked to health risks in some cases. Supplementing with high doses of *beta*-carotene may **increase** the risk of lung cancer in smokers. Supplementing with high doses of vitamin E may **increase** risks of prostate cancer and one type of stroke.

- Antioxidant supplements may interact with some medicines.

- Tell all of your healthcare providers about any complementary and integrative health approaches you use. Give them a full picture of what you do to manage your health. This will help ensure coordinated and safe care.

About Free Radicals, Oxidative Stress, and Antioxidants

Free radicals are highly unstable molecules that are naturally formed when you exercise and when your body converts food into energy. Your body can also be exposed to free radicals from a variety of environmental sources, such as cigarette smoke, air pollution, and sunlight. Free radicals can cause "oxidative stress," a process that can trigger cell damage. Oxidative stress is thought to play a role in a variety of diseases including cancer, cardiovascular diseases, diabetes, Alzheimer disease, Parkinson disease, and eye diseases such as cataracts and age-related macular degeneration.

Antioxidant molecules have been shown to counteract oxidative stress in laboratory experiments (for example, in cells or animal studies). However, there is debate as to whether consuming large amounts of antioxidants in supplement form actually benefits health. There is also some concern that consuming antioxidant supplements in excessive doses may be harmful.

Vegetables and fruits are healthy foods and rich sources of antioxidants. Official U.S. Government policy urges people to eat more vegetables and fruits. Concerns have not been raised about the safety of any amounts of antioxidants in food.

Use of Antioxidant Supplements in the United States

An analysis using data from the National Health and Nutrition Examination Survey (NHANES) estimated the amounts of antioxidants adults in the United States get from foods and supplements. Supplements accounted for 54 percent of vitamin C, 64 percent of vitamin E, 14 percent of *alpha*- and *beta*-carotene and 11 percent of selenium intake.

Safety

- High-dose antioxidant supplements may be harmful in some cases. For example, the results of some studies have linked the use of high-dose *beta*-carotene supplements to an increased risk of lung cancer in smokers and use of high-dose vitamin E supplements to increased risks of hemorrhagic stroke (a type of stroke caused by bleeding in the brain) and prostate cancer.

- Like some other dietary supplements, antioxidant supplements may interact with certain medications. For example, vitamin E supplements may increase the risk of bleeding in people who are taking anticoagulant drugs ("blood thinners"). There is conflicting evidence on the effects of taking antioxidant supplements during cancer treatment; some studies suggest that this may be beneficial, but others suggest that it may be harmful. The National Cancer Institute (NCI) recommends that people who are being treated for cancer talk with their healthcare provider before taking supplements.

Why Don't Antioxidant Supplements Work?

Most clinical studies of antioxidant supplements have not found them to provide substantial health benefits. Researchers have suggested several reasons for this, including the following:

- The beneficial health effects of a diet high in vegetables and fruits or other antioxidant-rich foods may actually be caused by other substances present in the same foods, other dietary factors or other lifestyle choices rather than antioxidants.

- The effects of the large doses of antioxidants used in supplementation studies may be different from those of the smaller amounts of antioxidants consumed in foods.

- Differences in the chemical composition of antioxidants in foods versus those in supplements may influence their effects. For example, eight chemical forms of vitamin E are present in foods. Vitamin E supplements, on the other hand, typically include only one of these forms—*alpha*-tocopherol. *Alpha*-tocopherol also has been used in almost all research studies on vitamin E.

- For some diseases, specific antioxidants might be more effective than the ones that have been tested. For example, to prevent eye diseases, antioxidants that are present in the eye, such as lutein, might be more beneficial than those that are not found in the eye, such as *beta*-carotene.

• The relationship between free radicals and health may be more complex than has previously been thought. Under some circumstances, free radicals actually may be beneficial rather than harmful, and removing them may be undesirable.

• The antioxidant supplements may not have been given for a long enough time to prevent chronic diseases, such as cardiovascular diseases or cancer, which develop over decades.

• The participants in the clinical trials discussed above were either members of the general population or people who were at high risk for particular diseases. They were not necessarily under increased oxidative stress. Antioxidants might help to prevent diseases in people who are under increased oxidative stress even if they don't prevent them in other people.

Section 12.3

Carotenoids

This section includes text excerpted from "Fat-Soluble Vitamins and Micronutrients: Vitamins A and E and Carotenoids," Centers for Disease Control and Prevention (CDC), July 30, 2008. Reviewed June 2016.

Carotenoids and Vitamin A

Vitamin A (retinol) and the carotenoids are fat-soluble micronutrients that are found in many foods, including some vegetables, fruits, meats, and animal products. Fish-liver oils, liver, egg yolks, butter, and cream are known for their higher content of vitamin A. At least 700 carotenoids—fat-soluble red and yellow pigments—are found in nature. Americans consume 40–50 of these carotenoids, primarily in fruits and vegetables and smaller amounts in poultry products, including egg yolks and in seafoods. Six major carotenoids are found in human serum: *alpha*-carotene, *beta*-carotene, *beta*-cryptoxanthin, lutein, trans-lycopene and zeaxanthin. Major carotene sources are orange-colored fruits and vegetables such as carrots, pumpkins and mangos. Lutein and zeaxanthin are also found in dark green leafy vegetables, where any orange coloring is overshadowed by chlorophyll. trans-Lycopene is obtained primarily from tomato and tomato products.

Vitamin A, found in foods that come from animal sources, is called preformed vitamin A. Some carotenoids found in colorful fruits and vegetables are called provitamin A; they are metabolized in the body to vitamin A. Among the carotenoids, *beta*-carotene, a retinol dimer, has the most significant provitamin A activity. Because of limitations in the body's ability to absorb and metabolize vitamin A, approximately 12 micrograms (μg) of dietary *beta*-carotene are needed to equal 1 μg of retinol. Other provitamin A carotenoids, such as *alpha*-carotene and *beta* cryptoxanthin, are half as active as *beta*-carotene. The bioconversion of carotenoids to vitamin A is highly variable from person to person.

The absorption of fat-soluble micronutrients from the gastrointestinal tract depends on processes responsible for fat absorption or metabolism. Thus, people with conditions resulting in fat malabsorption (e.g., celiac disease, Crohn disease, pancreatic disorders) can develop vitamin A deficiency over time.

Vitamin A also has interactions with other nutrients. Iron and zinc deficiency can affect vitamin A metabolism and transport of vitamin A stores from the liver to body tissues. The absorption of carotenoids from foods is highly dependent on cooking techniques that break down plant cell walls and release carotenoids and also on the availability of dietary fat to enhance carotenoid uptake. The liver regulates the concentration of vitamin A in the circulation by releasing stored retinyl esters as needed; only when liver reserves are nearly exhausted does serum vitamin A fall into the deficient range. The variation in serum carotenoid concentrations among people in the United States is relatively large, primarily reflecting wide-ranging differences in dietary intake. Inadequate or excessive intake of vitamin A can lead to various disorders.

The U.S. Food and Drug Administration (FDA) recommends that pregnant women obtain vitamin A from foods containing *beta*-carotene.

Carotenoids are considered among the best biological markers for fruit and vegetable intake. The strongest dietary predictors of serum carotenoid concentrations are fruits, carrots and root vegetables (for sources of carotenes) and tomato products (for sources of trans lycopene). Research studies have shown inconsistencies in the relation

161

between carotenoid intake and protection from cancer. Carotenoids in foods, even when consumed over long periods and in large amounts, are not known to produce adverse health effects. However, results of intervention studies of smokers who used 20-30 milligrams (mg) of *beta*-carotene per day showed that this group had more lung cancers than placebo-treated groups.

The American Heart Association advises that antioxidant supplements (such as vitamins E and C and *beta*-carotene) should not be used for primary or secondary prevention of cardiovascular disease. Nevertheless, the American Heart Association recommends consuming food sources of antioxidant nutrients, principally from a variety of plant derived foods such as fruits, vegetables, whole grains and vegetable oils.

The National Academy of Sciences has established dietary-requirement intake values for vitamin A by determining the adequate intake (AI) for infants and the recommended dietary allowance (RDA) for older age groups. The RDA for vitamin A for adults is 900 μg/day of retinol equivalents; for children, the RDA ranges from 300–700 μg/day. For infants (aged 0–12 months), the AI is set at 400–500 μg/day of retinol equivalents. Although no quantitative recommendations are available for the intake of carotenoids, existing recommendations support increased consumption of carotenoid-rich fruits and vegetables. Current public health guidelines advise that people consume 5 to 13 servings of fruits and vegetables a day, depending on caloric need, to ensure adequate nutrient intake.

Clinical laboratories typically use conventional units for serum concentrations of these fat-soluble micronutrients (μg per deciliter [dL]). Conversion factors to international system (SI) units are 1 μg/dL = 0.0349 micromole per liter (μmol/L) for vitamin A. Depending on its molecular weight, each carotenoid has a specific conversion factor.

The diagnosis of vitamin A deficiency is supported by measuring these concentrations in the body. Vitamin A deficiency can be diagnosed in a number of ways. People with serum concentrations of retinol of less than 20 μg/dL are considered vitamin A deficient and those with serum concentrations of less than 10 μg/dL are considered severely deficient. Carotenoid deficiency has no defined serum concentrations.

Section 12.4

Flavonoids

This section includes text excerpted from "USDA's Flavonoid Database: Flavonoids in Fruit," Agricultural Research Service (ARS), U.S. Department of Agriculture (USDA), March 15, 2003. Reviewed June 2016.

Flavonoids are biologically active compounds found in plants that have been associated with decreased risk of some age related and chronic diseases in humans. Food composition data from literature published around the world were evaluated to compile U.S. Department of Agriculture's (USDA) Flavonoid Database. Data are presented for 26 individual flavonoids in five subclasses based on their chemical structure: flavonols, flavones, flavanones, flavan-3-ols, and anthocyanidins. This database can be used to quantify the intake of flavonoids as well as to identify areas where additional research is needed to complete flavonoid profiles for commonly consumed foods.

There are 78 raw and processed fruits and juices in the database. Citrus fruits are the only foods in which flavanones (hesperetin, naringenin, and criodictyol) occur, except for in peppermint. Flavones (apigenin, luteolin) do not occur in significant quantities in fruit. Flavan-3-ols (catechins and epicatechins) are present in apples, cherries and cranberries. Flavonols (quercetin, kaempferol, myricetin, and isorhamnetin) are present only in very small quantities in fruit. Literature data on anthocyanidins (cyanidin, delphinidin, malvidin, pelargonidin, peonidin and petunidin), which are expected to be present in red/purple colored fruit, are available for only blueberries, cherries, elderberries and raspberries. Analytical data have been generated to provide anthocyanidin values for these additional fruits: apples, blackberries, cranberries, red grapefruit, red grapes, plums, strawberries, and watermelon.

Sources

Food sources of flavonoids are vegetables, fruits, nuts, seeds, roots, and beverages like tea and wine. The (U.S. Department of Agriculture)

USDA Database for the Flavonoid Content of Selected Foods contains information on the most prevalent dietary flavonoids. These are organized into five subclasses based on their chemical structure:

- FLAVONOLS: Quercetin, Kaempferol, Myricetin, Isorhamnetin

- FLAVONES: Apigenin, Luteolin FLAVANONES: Hesperetin, Naringenin, Eriodictyol

- FLAVAN-3-OLS: Catechin, Gallocatechin, Epicatechin, Epicatechin 3-gallate, Epigallocatechin, Epigallocatechin 3-gallate, Theaflavin, Theaflavin-3,3'-digallate, Theaflavin-3'-gallate, Theaflavin-3-gallate, Thearubigins

- ANTHOCYANIDINS: Cyanidin, Delphinidin, Malvidin, Pelargonidin, Peonidin, Petunidin

Data on the flavonoid content of fruits was compiled from the scientific literature and evaluated using the Nutrient Data Laboratory data quality evaluation system. Additional samples of commonly consumed fruits were obtained from USDA's National Food and Nutrient Analysis Program (NFANP). Nationwide samples were collected and analyzed by USDA's Food Composition Laboratory (FCL). Below is a summary of the flavonoid content of fruits contained in the database.

- Anthocyanidins are particularly high in blackberries, blueberries, cranberries, cherries, and elderberries. All contain >80 mg/100 g. Elderberries are the highest at 749 mg/100g. Cyanidin is the predominant or only anthocyanidin in most fruits. The only other foods in the database that contain anthocyanidins are wine and red onions.

- Citrus fruits are the only fruits that contain flavanones. The only other food in the database containing flavanones is peppermint, which contains eriodictyol and hesperetin.

- Fruits do not contain flavones, except for small amounts in lemons and pummelo juice.

Section 12.5

Soy Foods: Health Benefits and Risks

This section includes text excerpted from "Soy," National
Center for Complementary and Integrative Health (NCCIH),
April 2012. Reviewed June 2016.

Soy, a plant in the pea family, has been common in Asian diets for
thousands of years. It is found in modern American diets as a food or
food additive. Soybeans, the high-protein seeds of the soy plant, contain isoflavones—compounds similar to the female hormone estrogen.
Traditional or folk uses of soy products include menopausal symptoms,
osteoporosis, memory problems, high blood pressure, high cholesterol
levels, breast cancer, and prostate cancer.

Soy is available in dietary supplements, in forms such as tablets and capsules. Soy supplements may contain isoflavones or soy
protein or both. Soybeans can be cooked and eaten or used to make
tofu, soy milk, and other foods. Also, soy is sometimes used as an
additive in various processed foods, including baked goods, cheese,
and pasta.

What the Science Says

- Research suggests that daily intake of soy protein may
  slightly lower levels of low-density lipoprotein (LDL) ("bad")
  cholesterol.

- Some studies suggest that soy isoflavone supplements may
  reduce hot flashes in women after menopause. However, the
  results have been inconsistent.

- There is not enough scientific evidence to determine whether soy
  supplements are effective for any other health uses.

- National Center for Complementary and Integrative Health
  (NCCIH) supports studies on soy, including its effects in cardiovascular disease and breast cancer and on menopause-related
  symptoms and bone loss.

Side Effects and Cautions

- Soy is considered safe for most people when used as a food or when taken for short periods as a dietary supplement.

- Minor stomach and bowel problems such as nausea, bloating and constipation are possible.

- Allergic reactions such as breathing problems and rash can occur in rare cases.

- The safety of long-term use of soy isoflavones has not been established. Evidence is mixed on whether using isoflavone supplements over time can increase the risk of endometrial hyperplasia (a thickening of the lining of the uterus that can lead to cancer). Studies show no effect of dietary soy on risk for endometrial hyperplasia.

- Soy's possible role in breast cancer risk is uncertain. Until more is known about soy's effect on estrogen levels, women who have or who are at increased risk of developing breast cancer or other hormone-sensitive conditions (such as ovarian or uterine cancer) should be particularly careful about using soy and should discuss it with their healthcare providers.

- Tell all your healthcare providers about any complementary health approaches you use. Give them a full picture of what you do to manage your health. This will help ensure coordinated and safe care.

Part Three

Nutrition through the Life Span

Chapter 13

Feeding Infants and Toddlers

Chapter Contents

Section 13.1

Infants: Breastfeeding and Bottle Feeding

This section includes excerpts from "Breastfeeding vs. Formula
Feeding," © 1995–2016. The Nemours Foundation/
KidsHealth®. Reprinted with permission.

Breastfeeding vs. Formula Feeding

Choosing whether to breastfeed or formula feed their baby is one of
the biggest decisions expectant and new parents will make.

A number of health organizations—including the American Academy of Pediatrics (AAP), the American Medical Association (AMA), and
the World Health Organization (WHO)—recommend breastfeeding as
the best choice for babies. Breastfeeding helps defend against infections,
prevent allergies, and protect against a number of chronic conditions.

The AAP recommends that babies be breastfed exclusively for the
first 6 months. Beyond that, breastfeeding is encouraged until at least
12 months, and longer if both the mother and baby are willing.

Although experts believe breast milk is the best nutritional choice
for infants, breastfeeding may not be possible for all women. For many,
the decision to breastfeed or formula feed is based on their comfort
level, lifestyle, and specific medical situations.

For mothers who are unable to breastfeed or who decide not to,
infant formula is a healthy alternative. Formula provides babies with
the nutrients they need to grow and thrive.

Some mothers worry that if they don't breastfeed, they won't bond
with their baby. But the truth is, loving mothers will always create a
special bond with their children. And feeding—no matter how—is a
great time to strengthen that bond.

The decision to breastfeed or formula feed your baby is a personal
one. Weighing the pros and cons of each method can help you decide
what is best for you and your baby.

All about Breastfeeding

Nursing can be a wonderful experience for both mother and baby.
It provides ideal nourishment and a special bonding experience that
many mothers cherish.

Here are some of the many benefits of breastfeeding:

Fighting infections and other conditions. Breastfed babies have fewer infections and hospitalizations than formula-fed infants. During breastfeeding, antibodies and other germ-fighting factors pass from a mother to her baby and strengthen the immune system. This helps lower a baby's chances of getting many infections such as

- ear infections
- diarrhea
- respiratory infections
- meningitis

Breastfeeding also may protect babies against:

- allergies
- asthma
- diabetes
- obesity
- sudden infant death syndrome (SIDS)

Breastfeeding is particularly beneficial for premature babies.

Nutrition and ease of digestion. Often called the "perfect food" for a human baby's digestive system, breast milk's components—lactose, protein (whey and casein), and fat—are easily digested by a newborn.

As a group, breastfed infants have less difficulty with digestion than do formula-fed infants. Breast milk tends to be more easily digested so that breastfed babies have fewer bouts of diarrhea or constipation.

Breast milk also naturally contains many of the vitamins and minerals that a newborn requires. One exception is vitamin D—the AAP recommends that all breastfed babies begin receiving vitamin D supplements during the first 2 months and continuing until a baby consumes enough vitamin D-fortified formula or milk (after 1 year of age).

The U.S. Food and Drug Administration (FDA) regulates formula companies to ensure they provide all the necessary nutrients (including vitamin D) in their formulas. Still, commercial formulas can't completely match breast milk's exact composition. Why? Because milk is a living substance made by each mother for her individual infant, a process that can't be duplicated in a factory.

Free. Breast milk doesn't cost a cent, while the cost of formula quickly adds up. And unless you're pumping breast milk and giving it to your baby, there's no need for bottles, nipples, and other supplies that can be costly. Since breastfed babies are less likely to be sick, that may mean they make fewer trips to the doctor's office, so fewer co-pays and less money are paid for prescriptions and over-the-counter medicines.

Different tastes. Nursing mothers usually need 500 extra calories per day, which means they should eat a wide variety of well-balanced foods. This introduces breastfed babies to different tastes through their mother's' breast milk, which has different flavors depending on what their mothers have eaten. By tasting the foods of their "culture," breastfed infants more easily accept solid foods.

Convenience. With no last-minute runs to the store for more formula, breast milk is always fresh and available whether you're home or out and about. And when women breastfeed, there's no need to wash bottles and nipples or warm up bottles in the middle of the night.

Smarter babies. Some studies suggest that children who were exclusively breastfed have slightly higher IQs (intelligence quotients) than children who were formula fed.

"Skin-to-skin" contact. Many nursing mothers really enjoy the experience of bonding so closely with their babies. And the skin-to-skin contact can enhance the emotional connection between mother and infant.

Beneficial for mom, too. The ability to totally nourish a baby can help a new mother feel confident in her ability to care for her baby. Breastfeeding also burns calories and helps shrink the uterus, so nursing moms may be able to return to their pre-pregnancy shape and weight quicker. Also, studies show that breastfeeding helps lower the risk of breast cancer, high blood pressure, diabetes, and cardiovascular disease, and also may help decrease the risk of uterine and ovarian cancer.

Breastfeeding Challenges

Breastfeeding can be easy from the get-go for some mothers, but take a while to get used to for others. Moms and babies need plenty of patience to get used to the routine of breastfeeding.

Common concerns of new moms, especially during the first few weeks and months, may include:

Personal comfort. Initially, many moms feel uncomfortable with breastfeeding. But with proper education, support, and practice, most moms overcome this.

Latch-on pain is normal for the first week to ten days, and should last less than a minute with each feeding. But if breastfeeding hurts throughout feedings or if their nipples and/or breasts are sore, it's a good idea for breastfeeding mothers to get help from a lactation consultant or their doctor. Many times, it's just a matter of using the proper technique, but sometimes pain can mean that something else is going on, like an infection.

Time and frequency of feedings. Breastfeeding requires a big time commitment from mothers, especially in the beginning, when babies feed often. A breastfeeding schedule or the need to pump breast milk during the day can make it harder for some moms to work, run errands or travel.

And breastfed babies do need to eat more often than babies who take formula, because breast milk digests faster than formula. This means mom may find herself in demand every 2 or 3 hours (maybe more, maybe less) in the first few weeks.

Diet. Women who are breastfeeding need to be aware of what they eat and drink, since these can be passed to the baby through the breast milk. Just like during pregnancy, breastfeeding women should not eat fish that are high in mercury and limit consumption of lower mercury fish.

If a mom drinks alcohol, a small amount can pass to the baby through breast milk. She should wait at least two hours after a single alcoholic drink to breastfeed to avoid passing any alcohol to the baby. Caffeine intake should be kept to no more than 300 milligrams (about one to three cups of regular coffee) or less per day because it can cause problems like restlessness and irritability in some babies.

Maternal medical conditions, medicines, and breast surgery. Medical conditions such as **HIV or AIDS** or those that involve chemotherapy or treatment with certain medicines can make breastfeeding unsafe. A woman should check with her doctor or a lactation consultant if she's unsure if she should breastfeed with a specific condition. Women should always check with the doctor about the safety of taking medicines while breastfeeding, including over-the-counter and herbal medicines.

Mothers who've had breast surgery, such as a reduction, may have difficulty with their milk supply if their milk ducts have been severed. In this situation, a woman should to talk to her doctor about her concerns and work with a lactation specialist.

All about Formula Feeding

Commercially prepared infant formulas are a nutritious alternative to breast milk, and even contain some vitamins and nutrients that breastfed babies need to get from supplements.

Manufactured under sterile conditions, commercial formulas attempt to duplicate mother's milk using a complex combination of proteins, sugars, fats, and vitamins that aren't possible to create at home. So if you don't breastfeed your baby, it's important to use only commercially prepared formula and not try to make your own.

Besides medical concerns that may prevent breastfeeding, for some women, breastfeeding may be too difficult or stressful. Here are other reasons women may choose to formula feed:

Convenience. Either parent (or another caregiver) can feed the baby a bottle at any time (although this is also true for women who pump their breast milk). This allows mom to share the feeding duties and helps her partner to feel more involved in the crucial feeding process and the bonding that often comes with it.

Flexibility. Once the bottles are made, a formula-feeding mother can leave her baby with a partner or caregiver and know that her little one's feedings are taken care of. There's no need to pump or to schedule work or other obligations and activities around the baby's feeding schedule. And formula-feeding moms don't need to find a private place to nurse in public.

Time and frequency of feedings. Because formula is less digestible than breast milk, formula-fed babies usually need to eat less often than breastfed babies.

Diet. Women who opt to formula feed don't have to worry about the things they eat or drink that could affect their babies.

Formula Feeding Challenges

As with breastfeeding, there are some challenges to consider when deciding whether to formula feed.

Lack of antibodies. None of the antibodies found in breast milk are in manufactured formula. So formula can't provide a baby with the added protection against infection and illness that breast milk does.

Can't match the complexity of breast milk. Manufactured formulas have yet to duplicate the complexity of breast milk, which changes as the baby's needs change.

Planning and organization. Unlike breast milk—which is always available, unlimited, and served at the right temperature—formula feeding your baby requires planning and organization to make sure that you have what you need when you need it. Parents must buy formula and make sure it's always on hand to avoid late-night runs to the store.

And it's important to always have the necessary supplies (like bottles and nipples) clean, easily accessible, and ready to go—otherwise, you will have a very hungry, very fussy baby to answer to. With 8-10 feedings in a 24-hour period, parents can quickly get overwhelmed if they're not prepared and organized.

Expense. Formula can be costly. Powdered formula is the least expensive, followed by concentrated, with ready-to-feed being the most expensive. And specialty formulas (such as soy and hypoallergenic) cost more—sometimes far more—than the basic formulas. During the first year of life, the cost of basic formula can run about $1,500.

Possibility of producing gas and constipation. Formula-fed babies may have more gas and firmer bowel movements than breastfed babies.

Making a Choice

Deciding how you will feed your baby is not an easy decision to make. You'll really only know the right choice for your family once your baby comes.

Many women decide on one method before the birth and then change their minds once their baby is born or in the weeks or months after. And many women decide to breastfeed and supplement with formula because they find that is the best choice for their family and their lifestyle.

While you're weighing the pros and cons, talk to your doctor or lactation consultant. These healthcare providers can give you more information about the options available and help you make the best decision for your family.

Section 13.2

Introducing Solids and Table Foods to Infants

This section contains text excerpted from the following sources: Text
under the heading "Feeding Your 4-to 7-Month-Old," © 1995–2016.
The Nemours Foundation/KidsHealth®. Reprinted with permission;
Text under the heading "Transition to Finger Foods for Your Nine-
Month Old" is excerpted from "Feeding Your 9 Month
Old," Early Childhood Learning and Knowledge Center
(ECLKC), U.S. Department of Health and Human
Services (HHS), November 3, 2014.

Feeding Your 4- to 7-Month-Old

Most babies this age are introduced to solid foods. Experts recommend gradually introducing solid foods when a baby is about 6 months
old, depending on the baby's readiness and nutritional needs.

Be sure to check with your doctor before starting any solid foods.

Is My Baby Ready to Eat Solids?

How can you tell if your baby is ready for solids? Here are a few
hints:

- Is your baby's tongue-thrust reflex gone or diminished? This
  reflex, which prevents infants from choking, also causes them to
  push food out of their mouths.

- Can your baby support his or her own head? To eat solid food, an
  infant needs good head and neck control and should be able to
  sit up.

- Is your baby interested in food? A 6-month-old baby who stares
  and grabs at your food at dinnertime is clearly ready for some
  variety in the food department.

If your doctor gives the go-ahead but your baby seems frustrated or
uninterested as you're introducing solid foods, try waiting a few days
or even weeks before trying again. Since solids are only a supplement
at this point, breastmilk and formula will still meet your baby's basic
nutritional needs.

How to Start Feeding Solids?

When your baby is ready and the doctor has given you the OK to try solid foods, pick a time of day when your baby is not tired or cranky. You want your baby to be a little hungry, but not all-out starving; you might want to let your baby breastfeed a while or provide part of the usual bottle.

Have your baby sit supported in your lap or in an upright infant seat. Infants who sit well, usually around 6 months, can be placed in a high chair with a safety strap.

Most babies' first food is a little iron-fortified infant single-grain cereal mixed with breast milk or formula. Place the spoon near your baby's lips, and let the baby smell and taste. Don't be surprised if this first spoonful is rejected. Wait a minute and try again. Most food offered to your baby at this age will end up on the baby's chin, bib or high-chair tray. Again, this is just an introduction.

Do not add cereal to your baby's bottle unless your doctor instructs you to do so, as this can cause babies to become overweight and doesn't help the baby learn how to eat solid foods.

Once your little one gets the hang of eating cereal off a spoon, it may be time to introduce single-ingredient pureed vegetables, fruit or meat. The order in which foods are introduced doesn't matter but when introducing new foods, go slow. Introduce one food at a time and wait several days before trying something else new. This allows you to identify foods that your baby may be **allergic** to.

Your baby may take a little while to "learn" how to eat solids. During these months you'll still be providing the usual feedings of breastmilk or formula, so don't be concerned if your baby refuses certain foods at first or doesn't seem interested. It may just take some time.

Foods to Avoid

Kids are at higher risk of developing food allergies if one or more close family members have allergies or allergy-related conditions, like food allergies, eczema or asthma. Talk to your doctor about any family history of food allergies.

Possible signs of food allergy or allergic reactions include:

- rash
- bloating or an increase in gassiness
- diarrhea
- vomiting

For more severe allergic reactions, like hives or breathing difficulty, get medical attention right away. If your child has any type of reaction to a food, don't offer that food again until you talk with your doctor.

Also, do not give honey until after a baby's first birthday. Honey may contain certain spores that, while harmless to adults, can cause botulism in babies. And do not give regular cow's milk until your baby is older than 12 months because it does not have the nutrition that infants need.

Tips for Introducing Solids

With the hectic pace of family life, most parents opt for commercially prepared baby foods at first. They come in small, convenient containers, and manufacturers must meet strict safety and nutrition guidelines. Avoid brands with added fillers and sugars.

If you do plan to prepare your own baby foods at home, pureeing them with a food processor or blender, here are some things to keep in mind:

- Protect your baby and the rest of your family from foodborne illness by following the rules for **food safety** (including **washing hands** well and often).

- Try to preserve the nutrients in your baby's food by using cooking methods that retain the most vitamins and minerals. Try steaming or baking fruits and vegetables instead of boiling, which washes away the nutrients.

- Freeze portions that you aren't going to use right away rather than canning them.

- Don't serve home-prepared beets, spinach, green beans, squash or carrots to infants younger than four months old. These can contain high levels of nitrates, which can cause **anemia** in babies. Use jarred varieties of these vegetables instead.

Whether you buy the baby food or make it yourself, remember that texture and consistency are important. At first, babies should have finely pureed single-ingredient foods. (Just applesauce, for example, not apples and pears mixed together).

After you've successfully tried individual foods, it's OK to offer a pureed mix of two foods. When your child is about nine months old, coarser, chunkier textures are going to be tolerated as he or she starts moving to a diet that includes more table foods.

If you use commercially prepared baby food in jars, spoon some of the food into a bowl to feed your baby. Do not feed your baby directly from the jar, because bacteria from the baby's mouth can contaminate the remaining food. If you refrigerate opened jars of baby food, it's best to throw away anything not eaten within a day or two.

Juice can be given after six months of age, which is also a good age to introduce your baby to a cup. Buy one with large handles and a lid (a "sippy cup"), and teach your baby how to handle and drink from it. You might need to try a few different cups to find one that works for your child. Use water at first to avoid messy clean-ups.

Serve only 100% fruit juice, not juice drinks or powdered drink mixes. Do not give juice in a bottle and remember to limit the amount of juice your baby drinks to less than four total ounces (120 ml) a day. Too much juice adds extra calories without the nutrition of breast milk or formula. Drinking too much juice can contribute to **excessive weight gain** and can cause **diarrhea**.

Your goal over the next few months is to introduce a wide variety of foods, including iron-fortified cereals, fruits, vegetables, and pureed meats. If your baby doesn't seem to like a particular food, reintroduce it at later meals. It can take quite a few tries before kids warm up to certain foods.

Transition to Finger Foods for Your Nine-Month Old

- By around nine months, your baby might enjoy many soft, solid foods. This transition to finger foods is an exciting and fun time for parents and babies! However, there are many important things to keep in mind during this time:

  - Soft foods include infant cereal, soft fruits and cooked vegetables, and strained meats.

  - Cut soft foods into small, baby-bite size pieces, no larger than one-half inch, to prevent choking.

  - Your baby does not need much solid food. Start with 1 Tablespoon of each type of food, each time you feed your baby. This will also help you to avoid wasting food.

  - Remember your baby still needs formula and/or breast milk through the first year.

  - Also, continue to offer infant cereal during this time to ensure your baby gets important minerals and vitamins necessary to grow healthy.

- Don't forget to keep offering a variety of foods including fruits and vegetables. Too often during this time healthy foods are replaced by unhealthy snack items like French fries, chips, and other non-nutritious items.

Establishing Meal Time Routines for Your Baby

- Now is a great time to begin enjoying family meals. When possible, include your baby in family mealtime including customs and manners.

- Remember it is important for babies to see you eat healthy foods and use proper table manners.

- Children who eat regularly scheduled meals and snacks are more prepared to learn and less likely to overeat at meals.

- Allow mealtime to end when your baby does not want to eat anymore. You may notice that your baby turns away from the food or cries to tell you he/she is full. This teaches her to listen to her body and know when she is full; a skill that will help her maintain a healthy weight later in life.

Section 13.3

Healthy Nutrition for Toddlers

This section includes excerpts from "Nutrition Guide for Toddlers," © 1995–2016. The Nemours Foundation/ KidsHealth®. Reprinted with permission.

Nutrition through Variety

Growth slows somewhat during the toddler years, but nutrition remains a top priority. It's also a time for parents to shift gears, leaving bottles behind and moving into a new era where kids will eat and drink more independently.

The toddler years are a time of transition, especially between 12-24 months, when they're learning to eat table food and accepting new tastes and textures. Breast milk and formula provided adequate nutrition for your child as an infant, but now it's time for toddlers to start getting what they need through a variety of foods.

How Much Food Do They Need?

Depending on their age, size, and activity level, toddlers need about 1,000-1,400 calories a day. Refer to the chart below to get an idea of how much your child should be eating and what kinds of foods would satisfy the requirements.

Use the chart as a guide, but trust your own judgment and a toddler's cues to tell if he or she is satisfied and getting adequate nutrition. Nutrition is all about averages so don't panic if you don't hit every mark every day—just strive to provide a wide variety of nutrients in your child's diet.

The amounts provided are based on the MyPlate food guide for the average 2-and 3-year-old. For kids between 12 and 24 months, the 2-year-old recommendations can serve as a guide, but during this year toddler diets are still in transition.

Talk with your doctor about specifics for your child. And younger toddlers may not be eating this much—at least at first. When a range of amounts is given, the higher amount applies to kids who are older, bigger or more active and need more calories.

Table 13.1. How Much Food Do We Need?

Food Group	Daily Amount for 2-Year-Olds	Daily Amount for 3-Year-Olds	Help With Servings
Grains	3 ounces, half from whole-grain sources	4-5 ounces, half from whole-grain sources	1 ounce equals: 1 slice of bread, 1 cup of ready-to-eat cereal or ½ cup of cooked rice, cooked pasta or cooked cereal.
Vegetables	1 cup	1½ cups	Use measuring cups to check amounts. Serve veggies that are soft, cut in small pieces, and well cooked to prevent choking.

Table 13.1. Continued

Food Group	Daily Amount for 2-Year-Olds	Daily Amount for 3-Year-Olds	Help With Servings
Fruits	1 cup	1-1½ cups	Use measuring cups to check amounts.
Milk	2 cups	2 cups	1 cup equals: 1 cup of milk or yogurt, 1½ ounces of natural cheese or 2 ounces of processed cheese.
Meat and Beans	2 ounces	3-4 ounces	1 ounce equals: 1 ounce of meat, poultry or fish, ¼ cup cooked dry beans or 1 egg.

Milk Matters

An important part of a toddler's diet, milk provides calcium and vitamin D to help build strong bones. Toddlers should have 700 milligrams of calcium and 600 IU (International Units) of vitamin D (which aids in calcium absorption) a day. This calcium need is met if kids get the recommended two servings of dairy foods every day. But those servings provide less than half of the necessary vitamin D, so doctors often recommend vitamin D supplements. Your doctor will let you know if your toddler needs a supplement.

In general, kids ages 12 to 24 months old should drink whole milk to help provide the dietary fats they need for normal growth and brain development. If overweight or obesity is a concern—or if there is a family history of obesity, high cholesterol or heart disease—talk to your doctor to see if reduced-fat (2%) milk may be given. After age 2, most kids can switch to low-fat (1%) or nonfat milk. Your doctor can help you decide which kind of milk to serve your toddler.

Some kids may reject cow's milk at first because it doesn't taste like the familiar breast milk or formula. If your child is at least 12 months old and having this difficulty, mix whole milk with some formula or breast milk. Gradually adjust the mixture over time so it becomes 100% cow's milk.

Some kids don't like milk or cannot drink or eat dairy products. Explore other calcium sources, such as calcium-fortified soy beverages, calcium-fortified juices, fortified breads and cereals, cooked dried beans, and dark green vegetables like broccoli, bok choy, and kale.

Meeting Iron Requirements

Toddlers should have 7 milligrams of iron each day. After 12 months of age, they're at risk for iron deficiency because they no longer drink iron-fortified formula and may not be eating iron-fortified infant cereal or enough other iron-containing foods to make up the difference.

Cow's milk is low in iron. Drinking a lot of cow's milk also can put a toddler at risk for iron deficiency. Toddlers who drink a lot of cow's milk may be less hungry and less likely to eat iron-rich foods. Milk decreases the absorption of iron and also can irritate the lining of the intestine, causing small amounts of bleeding and the gradual loss of iron in the stool (poop).

Iron deficiency can affect growth and may lead to learning and behavioral problems. And it can lead to anemia (too few red blood cells in the body). Iron is needed to make red blood cells, which carry oxygen throughout the body. Without enough iron and red blood cells, the body's tissues and organs get less oxygen and don't work as well as they should.

To help prevent iron deficiency:

- Limit your child's milk intake to about 16-24 ounces a day (2 to 3 cups).

- Serve more iron-rich foods (meat, poultry, fish, enriched grains, beans, tofu).

- When serving iron-rich meals, include foods that contain vitamin C (like tomatoes, broccoli, oranges, and strawberries), which improve the body's iron absorption.

- Continue serving iron-fortified cereal until your child is 18-24 months old.

Talk to your doctor if you're concerned that your child isn't eating a balanced diet. Many toddlers are checked for iron-deficiency anemia, but never give your child a vitamin or mineral supplement without first discussing it with your doctor.

Chapter 14

Children and Food

Chapter Contents

Section 14.1

Healthy Nutrition for Children

This section includes text excerpted from "Helping Your Child: Tips for Parents," National Institute of Diabetes and Digestive and Kidney Diseases (NIDDK), January 2012. Reviewed June 2016.

How Can I Help My Child Form Healthy Habits?

Parents play a big part in shaping children's habits on eating and physical activity. When parents eat foods that are lower in fat and added sugars and high in fiber, children learn to like these foods as well. If your child does not like a new food right away, don't be upset. Children often need to see a new food many times before they will try it.

Be a Role Model

A powerful example for your child is to be active yourself. You can set a good example by going for a walk or bike ride instead of watching TV, playing a video game or surfing the Internet. Playing ball or jumping rope with your children shows them that being active is fun.

Talk about Being Healthy

Take the time to talk to your children about how a certain food or physical activity may help them. For example, when going for your daily walk, bring your children with you and let them pick the route. Discuss how walking helps you feel better and is a fun way to spend time together. It also offsets calories eaten and inactive time spent in front of TV screens or computers. Use your children's food choices as teaching moments. Speak up when you see unhealthy eating habits. Direct children to healthier options or say, "You can have a little of that, but not too much." Talk to them about why an overly salty or heavily sugared snack is not the best choice. You can also praise your children when they choose a healthy item like fruit or yogurt. Use comments like these:

- "Great choice!"
- "You're giving your body what it needs with that snack!"
- "I like those too."

With physical activity, try upbeat phrases like these to keep your child excited:

- "You run so fast, I can hardly keep up!"
- "You are building a strong, healthy heart!"
- "Let's walk 10 more minutes to make us stronger."

Promote Good Health beyond Your Family

Other adults may play a role in your child's life, too. You can share ideas about healthy habits with them. For instance, many parents work outside the home and need other adults to help with child care. Caregivers like other family members, daycare providers, babysitters or friends may shape your child's eating and activity habits. Talk to your child's caregivers to make sure they offer healthy snacks and meals. Check that caregivers are also providing plenty of active play-time and limiting time with TV or inactive video games.

If your child is in school, you can help promote healthy eating and physical activity in several other ways:

- Find out more about the school's breakfast and lunch programs. Ask for input on menu choices.
- Support physical education and after-school sports at your child's school.
- Take turns with other parents watching your children play outside.

Consider Other Influences

Your children's friends and the media can also affect eating and activity choices. Children may choose to go to fast food places or play video games with their friends instead of playing tag or other active games. TV ads try to persuade children to eat high-fat foods and sugary drinks. You can teach your children to be aware of these pressures. To do so, speak with your children about choices while you watch TV and surf the Internet with them. Talk about how media outlets sell products or values through famous football or basketball players, cartoon figures, and made-up images. Use programs and ads to spark chats about your values. These talks may help your child make healthy choices outside the home.

Healthy Eating

What Should My Child Eat?

Just like adults, children need to eat a wide variety of foods. Every five years, the U.S. Government releases a set of guidelines on healthy eating. The guidelines suggest balancing calories with physical activity. The guidelines also recommend improving eating habits to promote health, reduce the risk of disease, and reduce overweight and obesity. The guidelines encourage Americans ages two years and older to eat a variety of healthy foods. Suggested items include the following:

- Fruits, vegetables, unsalted nuts and seeds, and whole grains.

- Fat-free or low-fat milk and milk products.

- Lean meats, poultry, seafood, beans and peas, soy products, and eggs.

The guidelines also suggest reducing salt (sodium), refined grains, added sugars, and solid fats (like lard, butter, and margarine). Added sugars and solid fats often occur in pizzas, sodas, sugar-sweetened drinks, desserts like cookies or cake, and fast foods. These foods are the main sources of high fat and sugar among children and teens. Another important guideline is to make sure your children eat breakfast to spark the energy they need to focus in school. Not eating breakfast is often linked to overweight and obesity, especially in children and teens.

How Can I Help My Child Eat Better?

Some tips to consider are these:

Use Less Fat, Salt, and Sugar

- Cook with f0ewer solid fats. Use olive or canola oil instead of butter or margarine. Bake or roast instead of frying. You can get a crunchy texture with "oven-frying" recipes that involve little or no oil.

- Choose and prepare foods with less salt. Keep the salt shaker off the table. Have fruits and vegetables on hand for snacks instead of salty snacks like chips.

- Limit the amount of sugar your child eats. Choose cereals with low sugar or with dried fruits as the source of sugar.

- Reshape the plate.

- Make half of what is on your child's plate fruits and vegetables.

- Avoid oversized portions.

Think about the Drink

- Serve water or low-fat or fat-free milk more often as the drink of first choice.

- Reduce the amount of sugar-sweetened sodas and fruit-flavored drinks that your child drinks.

- Offer fresh fruit, which has more fiber than juice, more often than 100% fruit juice.

Healthy Snack Ideas

- Fresh, frozen or canned vegetables or fruit served plain or with low-fat yogurt.

- Pretzels or air-popped popcorn sprinkled with salt-free spice mix.

- Homemade fruit smoothies made with fat-free milk or yogurt and frozen or fresh fruit.

- Dry cereals (with no added sugars) served plain or with low-fat or fat-free milk.

Limit Fast Food

- Order a side fruit bowl or salad instead of fries.

- Ask for sandwiches to be prepared without sauce.

- Order "small." Avoid super-sizing.

Share Food Time as Family Time

- Eat sit-down, family meals together and serve everyone the same thing.

- Involve your children in planning and preparing meals. Children may be more willing to eat the dishes they help prepare.

- Try to limit how much you eat out to control the calories, salt, and fat your children eat. To serve more homemade meals, cook large batches of soup, stew or casseroles and freeze them as a time saver. For handy tips on quick and easy homemade meals.

- Limit eating at home to specific areas such as the kitchen or dining room.

Children of preschool age and younger can easily choke on foods. These foods may be hard to chew, small and round or sticky. Examples are hard vegetables, whole grapes, hard chunks of cheese, raisins, nuts and seeds, and popcorn. Select snacks with care for children in this age group.

Section 14.2

Food Allergies in Children

This section includes text excerpted from "Voluntary Guidelines for Managing Food Allergies in Schools and Early Care and Education Programs," Centers for Disease Control and Prevention (CDC), 2013.

About Food Allergies

A *food allergy* is defined as an adverse health effect arising from a specific immune response that occurs reproducibly on exposure to a given food. The immune response can be severe and life-threatening. Although the immune system normally protects people from germs, in people with food allergies, the immune system mistakenly responds to food as if it were harmful. One way that the immune system causes food allergies is by making a protein antibody called immunoglobulin E (IgE) to the food. The substance in foods that cause this reaction is called the *food allergen*. When exposed to the food allergen, the IgE antibodies alert cells to release powerful substances, such as histamine, that cause symptoms that can affect the respiratory system, gastrointestinal tract, skin or cardiovascular system and lead to a life threatening reaction called *anaphylaxis*.

There are other types of food-related conditions and diseases that range from the frequent problem of digesting lactose in milk, resulting in gas, bloating, and diarrhea, to reactions caused by cereal grains (celiac disease) that can result in severe malabsorption and a variety of other serious health problems. These conditions and diseases may be serious but are not immediately life-threatening.

More than 170 foods are known to cause IgE mediated food allergies. In the United States, the following eight foods or food groups account for 90% of serious allergic reactions: milk, eggs, fish, crustacean shellfish, wheat, soy, peanuts, and tree nuts. Federal law requires food labels in the United States to clearly identify the food allergen source of all foods and ingredients that are (or contain any protein derived from) these common allergens.

The symptoms of allergic reactions to food vary both in type and severity among individuals and even in one individual over time. Symptoms associated with an allergic reaction to food include the following:

- **Mucous Membrane Symptoms:** red watery eyes or swollen lips, tongue or eyes.

- **Skin Symptoms:** itchiness, flushing, rash or hives.

- **Gastrointestinal Symptoms:** nausea, pain, cramping, vomiting, diarrhea or acid reflux.

- **Upper Respiratory Symptoms:** nasal congestion, sneezing, hoarse voice, trouble swallowing, dry staccato cough or numbness around mouth.

- **Lower Respiratory Symptoms:** deep cough, wheezing, shortness of breath or difficulty breathing or chest tightness.

- **Cardiovascular Symptoms:** pale or blue skin color, weak pulse, dizziness or fainting, confusion or shock, hypotension (decrease in blood pressure) or loss of consciousness.

- **Mental or Emotional Symptoms:** sense of "impending doom," irritability, change in alertness, mood change or confusion.

Children sometimes do not exhibit overt and visible symptoms after ingesting an allergen, making early diagnosis difficult. Some children may not be able to communicate their symptoms clearly because of their age or developmental challenges. Complaints such as abdominal pain, itchiness or other discomforts may be the first signs of an allergic reaction.

Signs and symptoms can become evident within a few minutes or up to 1–2 hours after ingestion of the allergen, and rarely, several hours after ingestion. Symptoms of breathing difficulty, voice hoarseness or faintness associated with change in mood or alertness or rapid progression of symptoms that involve a combination of the skin, gastrointestinal tract or cardiovascular symptoms signal a more severe allergic reaction (anaphylaxis) and require immediate attention.

The severity of reactions to food allergens is difficult to predict and varies depending on the child's particular sensitivity to the food and on the type and amount of exposure to the food. Ingesting a food allergen triggers most severe reactions, while inhaling or having skin contact with food allergens generally causes mild reactions. The severity of reaction from food ingestion also can be influenced by the child's age, how quickly the allergen is absorbed (e.g., absorption is faster if food is taken on an empty stomach or ingestion is associated with exercise), and by co-existing health conditions or factors. For example, a person with asthma might be at greater risk of having a more severe anaphylactic reaction. Exercise and certain medications also can increase the harmful effects of certain food allergens.

Allergic Reactions and Anaphylaxis

Anaphylaxis is best described as a severe allergic reaction that is rapid in onset and may cause death. Not all allergic reactions will develop into anaphylaxis. In fact, most are mild and resolve without problems. However, early signs of anaphylaxis can resemble a mild allergic reaction. Unless obvious symptoms—such as throat hoarseness or swelling, persistent wheezing or fainting or low blood pressure—are present, it is not easy to predict whether these initial, mild symptoms will progress to become an anaphylactic reaction that can result in death. Therefore, all children with known or suspected ingestion of a food allergen and the appearance of symptoms consistent with an allergic reaction must be closely monitored and possibly treated for early signs of anaphylaxis.

Characteristics and Risk Factors

Food allergies account for 35%–50% of all cases of anaphylaxis in emergency care settings. Many different food allergens (e.g., milk, egg, fish, shellfish) can cause anaphylaxis. In the United States, fatal or near fatal reactions are most often caused by peanuts (50%–62%) and tree nuts (15%–30%).

Results of studies of fatal allergic reactions to food found that a delay in administering epinephrine was one of the most significant risk factors associated with fatal outcomes. Some population groups, including children with a history of anaphylaxis, are at higher risk of having a severe reaction to food.

Food Allergy Symptoms in Children

Children with food allergies might communicate their symptoms in the following ways:

- It feels like something is poking my tongue.
- My tongue (or mouth) is tingling (or burning).
- My tongue (or mouth) itches.
- My tongue feels like there is hair on it.
- My mouth feels funny.
- There's a frog in my throat; there's something stuck in my throat.
- My tongue feels full (or heavy).
- My lips feel tight.
- It feels like there are bugs in there (to describe itchy ears).
- It (my throat) feels thick.
- It feels like a bump is on the back of my tongue (throat).

Food Allergies and Asthma

One-third of children with food allergies also have asthma, which increases their risk of experiencing a severe or fatal reaction. Data also suggest that children with asthma and food allergies have more visits to hospitals and emergency departments than children who don't have asthma.

Because asthma can pose serious risks to the health of children with food allergies, schools and Early Care and Education (ECE) programs must consider these risks when they develop plans for managing food allergies.

Risk Factors

- Delayed administration of epinephrine.

- Reliance on oral antihistamines alone to treat symptoms.

- Consuming alcohol and the food allergen at the same time.

Groups at Higher Risk

- Adolescents and young adults.

- Children with a known food allergy.

- Children with a prior history of anaphylaxis.

- Children with asthma, particularly those with poorly controlled asthma.

Section 14.3

School Lunches

This section contains text excerpted from the following sources: Text under the heading "How to Make Healthy School Lunches for Your Children?" is excerpted from "How to Make Healthy School Lunches for Your Children," Kids.gov, April 21, 2016; Text under the heading "Keeping "Bag" Lunches Safe" is excerpted from "Back to School," FoodSafety.gov, U.S. Department of Health and Human Services (HHS), May 12, 2016.

How to Make Healthy School Lunches for Your Children?

Being a parent often requires a non-stop juggling routine that begins with morning carpool and ends with bedtime stories. In the rush to get your children to school, it's important not to forget the value of preparing them a healthy lunch.

Switch white bread for whole grain: If sandwiches are a staple in your child's lunch, the easiest way to make a change is to substitute whole grain bread for white. There are many varieties out there to please even the pickiest eater. You can also substitute flour tortillas with wheat ones and white pita with whole grain. Fill them with proteins like turkey slices and cheese. If your child prefers warm food in a thermos, you can fill it with brown rice, whole grain pasta and even oatmeal.

Pack a rainbow: Fruits and vegetables are great sources of nutrition. Make fruits and vegetables more interesting. Pack green and purple grapes or colorful berries, dried apricots, mangos, cut red and orange peppers into strips and send them with a fun dipping sauce like hummus or yogurt and send oranges already peeled and sliced. The prettier the presentation, the higher the chances are your child will reach for it.

Water, water, water: Juice may seem harmless, especially since the labels read things like "packed with fruit." But juice adds a lot of unnecessary sugar and calories to your child's diet. Consider rethinking what they drink and send a bottle of water along with or instead of, the juice box. Not only does drinking water eliminate extra sugar from their diet, but it also keeps children from getting dehydrated throughout the day. Low-fat milk is also a good idea since it provides calcium and protein.

Think about temperature: Would you eat warm yogurt or cold rice? The temperature inside your child's lunchbox is just as important as what is inside. Keep hot foods warm by sending them in a thermos, it helps if you first fill it with boiling water for two minutes to retain some heat. Keep cold items like cheese or hard boiled eggs cool by using ice packs. You can also use a refillable water bottle filled with ice cubes to keep things fresh, plus it will provide drinking water at the same time!

Plan ahead: Making a healthy lunch does take some thought, but the morning rush, when everyone's trying to get out the door, isn't the best time to get creative. Try to make a routine of packing some items the night before. Cutting up fruit, pre-making sandwiches, boiling whole grain pasta are all time-saving steps. Another good habit is to make weekly shopping lists, so you're not stuck searching the cupboard for last-minute—and unhealthy—options.

Keeping "Bag" Lunches Safe

Bacteria that cause foodborne illness, commonly known as food poisoning, grow rapidly at temperatures between 40 and 140 degrees Fahrenheit. In just two hours, these microorganisms can multiply to dangerous levels, which can cause foodborne illness. To make sure lunches and snacks are safe for those you pack for, you should follow the four steps to food safety:

Clean–Separate–Cook–and–Chill

Packing Tips

- If the lunch/snack contains perishable food items like luncheon meats, eggs, cheese or yogurt, make sure to pack it with at least two cold sources. Harmful bacteria multiply rapidly so perishable food transported without an ice source won't stay safe long.

- Frozen juice boxes or water can also be used as freezer packs. Freeze these items overnight and use with at least one other freezer pack. By lunchtime, the liquids should be thawed and ready to drink.

- Pack lunches containing perishable food in an insulated lunch-box or soft-sided lunch bag. Perishable food can be unsafe to eat by lunchtime if packed in a paper bag.

- If packing a hot lunch, like soup, chili or stew, use an insulated container to keep it hot. Fill the container with boiling water, let stand for a few minutes, empty, and then put in the piping hot food. Tell children to keep the insulated container closed until lunchtime to keep the food hot-140 °F or above.

- If packing a child's lunch the night before, parents should leave it in the refrigerator overnight. The meal will stay cold longer because everything will be refrigerator temperature when it is placed in the lunchbox.

- If you're responsible for packing snack for the team, troop or group, keep perishable foods in a cooler with ice or cold packs until snack time. Pack snacks in individual bags or contain-ers, rather than having children share food from one serving dish.

Storage Tips

- If possible, a child's lunch should be stored in a refrigerator or cooler with ice upon arrival. Leave the lid of the lunchbox or bag open in the fridge so that cold air can better circulate and keep the food cold.

Eating and Disposal Tips

- Pack disposable wipes for washing hands before and after eating.

- After lunch, discard all leftover food, used food packaging, and paper bags. Do not reuse packaging because it could contaminate other food and cause foodborne illness.

Chapter 15

Nutrition Information for Teens and Young Adults

Chapter Contents

Section 15.1

Teens and Healthy Eating

This section contains text excerpted from the following sources: Text under the heading "Choose the Foods You Need to Grow: 10 Tips for Teen Guys" is excerpted from "Choose the Foods You Need to Grow," ChooseMyPlate.gov, U.S. Department of Agriculture (USDA), January 2014; Text under the heading "Eat Smart and Be Active as You Grow: 10 Healthy Tips for Teen Girls" is excerpted from "Eat Smart and Be Active as You Grow," ChooseMyPlate.gov, U.S. Department of Agriculture (USDA), January 2014.

Choose the Foods You Need to Grow: Ten Tips for Teen Guys

Feed your growing body by making better food choices today as a teen and as you continue to grow into your twenties. Make time to be physically active every day to help you be fit and healthy as you grow.

1. Get over the Idea of Magic Foods

There are no magic foods to eat for good health. Teen guys need to eat foods such as vegetables, fruits, whole grains, protein foods, and fat-free or low-fat dairy foods. Choose protein foods like unsalted nuts, beans, lean meats, and fish.

2. Always Hungry?

Whole grains that provide fiber can give you a feeling of fullness and provide key nutrients. Choose half your grains as whole grains. Eat whole-wheat breads, pasta, and brown rice instead of white bread, rice or other refined grains. Also, choose vegetables and fruits when you need to "fill-up."

3. Keep Water Handy

Water is a better option than many other drink choices. Keep a water bottle in your backpack and at your desk to satisfy your thirst.

Skip soda, fruit drinks, and energy and sports drinks. They are sugar-sweetened and have few nutrients.

4. Make a List of Favorite Foods

Like green apples more than red apples? Ask your family food shopper to buy quick-to-eat foods for the fridge like mini-carrots, apples oranges, low-fat cheese slices or yogurt. And also try dried fruit; unsalted nuts; whole-grain breads, cereal, and crackers; and popcorn.

5. Start Cooking Often

Get over being hungry by fixing your own snacks and meals. Learn to make vegetable omelets, bean quesadillas or a batch of spaghetti. Prepare your own food so you can make healthier meals and snacks. Microwaving frozen pizzas doesn't count as home cooking.

6. Skip Foods That Can Add Unwanted Pounds

Cut back on calories by limiting fatty meats like ribs, bacon, and hot dogs. Some foods are just occasional treats like pizza, cakes, cookies, candies, and ice cream. Check out the calorie content of sugary drinks by reading the Nutrition Facts label. Many 12-ounce sodas contain 10 teaspoons of sugar.

7. Learn How Much Food You Need

Teen guys may need more food than most adults, teen girls, and little kids. Go to www.SuperTracker.usda.gov. It shows how much food you need based on your age, height, weight, and activity level. It also tracks progress towards fitness goals.

8. Check Nutrition Facts Labels

To grow, your body needs vitamins and minerals. Calcium and vitamin D are especially important for your growing bones. Read Nutrition Facts labels for calcium. Dairy foods provide the minerals your bones need to grow.

9. Strengthen Your Muscles

Work on strengthening and aerobic activities. Work out at least 10 minutes at a time to see a better you. However, you need to get at least 60 minutes of physical activity every day.

10. Fill Your Plate Like Myplate

Go to www.ChooseMyPlate.gov for more easy tips and science-based nutrition from the *Dietary Guidelines for Americans* (www. DietaryGuidelines.gov).

Eat Smart and Be Active as You Grow: Ten Tips for Teen Girls

Young girls, ages 10 to 19, have a lot of changes going on in their bodies. Building healthier habits will help you—now as a growing teen—and later in life. Growing up means you are in charge of foods you eat and the time you spend being physically active every day.

1. Build Strong Bones

A good diet and regular physical activity can build strong bones throughout your life. Choose fat-free or low-fat milk, cheeses, and yogurt to get the vitamin D and calcium your growing bones need. Strengthen your bones three times a week doing activities such as running, gymnastics, and skating.

2. Cut Back on Sweets

Cut back on sugary drinks. Many 12-ounce cans of soda have 10 teaspoons of sugar in them. Drink water when you are thirsty. Sipping water and cutting back on cakes, candies, and sweets helps to maintain a healthy weight.

3. Power up with Whole Grain

Fuel your body with nutrient-packed whole-grain foods. Make sure that at least half your grain foods are whole grains such as brown rice, whole-wheat breads, and popcorn.

4. Choose Vegetables Rich in Color

Brighten your plate with vegetables that are red, orange or dark green. Try acorn squash, cherry tomatoes or sweet potatoes. Spinach and beans also provide vitamins like folate and minerals like potassium that are essential for healthy growth.

5. Check Nutrition Facts Labels for Iron

Read Nutrition Facts labels to find foods containing iron. Most protein foods like meat, poultry, eggs, and beans have iron, and so do fortified breakfast cereals and breads.

6. Be a Healthy Role Model

Encourage your friends to practice healthier habits. Share what you do to work through challenges. Keep your computer and TV time to less than 2 hours a day (unless it's school work).

7. Try Something New

Keep healthy eating fun by picking out new foods you've never tried before like lentils, mango, quinoa or kale.

8. Make Moving Part of Every Event

Being active makes everyone feel good. Aim for 60 minutes of physical activity each day. Move your body often. Dancing, playing active games, walking to school with friends, swimming, and biking are only a few fun ways to be active. Also, try activities that target the muscles in your arms and legs.

9. Include All Food Groups Daily

Use MyPlate as your guide to include all food groups each day.

10. Everyone Has Different Needs

Get nutrition information based on your age, gender, height, weight, and physical activity level. Use SuperTracker to find your calorie level, choose the foods you need, and track progress toward your goals.

Section 15.2

The Importance of Calcium for Bone Development

This section includes text excerpted from "Kids and Their Bones: A Guide for Parents," National Institute of Arthritis and Musculoskeletal and Skin Diseases (NIAMS), March 2015.

Kids and Their Bones

Typically, when parents think about their children's health, they don't think about their bones. But building healthy bones by adopting healthy nutritional and lifestyle habits in childhood is important to help prevent osteoporosis and fractures later in life.

Osteoporosis, the disease that causes bones to become less dense and more prone to fractures, has been called "a pediatric disease with geriatric consequences," because the bone mass attained in childhood and adolescence is an important determinant of lifelong skeletal health. The health habits your kids are forming now can make or literally break, their bones as they age.

Why Is Childhood Such an Important Time for Bone Development?

Bones are the framework for your child's growing body. Bone is living tissue that changes constantly, with bits of old bone being removed and replaced by new bone. You can think of bone as a bank account, where (with your help) your kids make "deposits" and "withdrawals" of bone tissue. During childhood and adolescence, much more bone is deposited than withdrawn as the skeleton grows in both size and density.

For most people, the amount of bone tissue in the skeleton (known as bone mass) peaks by their late twenties. At that point, bones have reached their maximum strength and density. Up to 90 percent of peak bone mass is acquired by age 18 in girls and age 20 in boys, which makes youth the best time for your kids to "invest" in their bone health.

What Is Osteoporosis? Isn't It Something Old People Get?

Osteoporosis is a disease that causes bones to become fragile and break easily. When someone has osteoporosis, it means his/her "bank account" of bone tissue has dropped to a low level. If there is significant bone loss, even sneezing or bending over to tie a shoe can cause a bone in the spine to break. Hips, ribs, and wrist bones also break easily. The fractures from osteoporosis can be painful and disfiguring. There is no cure for the disease.

Osteoporosis is most common in older people but can also occur in young and middle-aged adults. Optimizing peak bone mass and developing lifelong healthy bone behaviors during youth are important ways to help prevent or minimize osteoporosis risk as an adult.

How Can I Help Keep My Kids' Bones Healthy?

The same healthy habits that keep your kids going and growing will also benefit their bones. One of the best ways to encourage healthy habits in your children is to be a good role model yourself. Believe it or not, your kids are watching, and your habits, both good and bad, have a strong influence on theirs.

The two most important lifelong bone health habits to encourage now are proper nutrition and plenty of physical activity.

Eating for healthy bones means getting plenty of foods that are rich in calcium and vitamin D. Most kids do not get enough calcium in their diets to help ensure optimal peak bone mass.

Calcium is found in many foods, but the most common source is milk and other dairy products. Drinking one 8-oz glass of milk provides 300 milligrams (mg) of calcium, which is about one-third of the recommended intake for younger children and about one-fourth of the recommended intake for teens. In addition, milk supplies other minerals and vitamins needed by the body. Table 15.1 lists the calcium content for several high-calcium foods and beverages. Your kids need several servings of these foods each day to meet their need for calcium.

Table 15.1. Selected Food Sources of Calcium

Food	Milligrams (mg) per serving	Percent DV*
Yogurt, plain, low fat, 8 ounces	415	42
Mozzarella, part skim, 1.5 ounces	333	33

Table 15.1. Continued

Food	Milligrams (mg) per serving	Percent DV*
Sardines, canned in oil, with bones, 3 ounces	325	33
Yogurt, fruit, low fat, 8 ounces	313–384	31–38
Cheddar cheese, 1.5 ounces	307	31
Milk, nonfat, 8 ounces**	299	30
Soymilk, calcium-fortified, 8 ounces	299	30
Milk, reduced-fat (2% milk fat), 8 ounces	293	29
Milk, buttermilk, lowfat, 8 ounces	284	28
Milk, whole (3.25% milk fat), 8 ounces	276	28
Orange juice, calcium-fortified, 6 ounces	261	26
Tofu, firm, made with calcium sulfate, ½ cup***	253	25
Salmon, pink, canned, solids with bone, 3 ounces	181	18
Cottage cheese, 1% milk fat, 1 cup	138	14
Tofu, soft, made with calcium sulfate, ½ cup***	138	14
Ready-to-eat cereal, calcium-fortified, 1 cup	100–1,000	10–100
Frozen yogurt, vanilla, soft serve, ½ cup	103	10
Turnip greens, fresh, boiled, ½ cup	99	10
Kale, raw, chopped, 1 cup	100	10
Kale, fresh, cooked, 1 cup	94	9
Ice cream, vanilla, ½ cup	84	8
Chinese cabbage, bok choi, raw, shredded, 1 cup	74	7
Bread, white, 1 slice	73	7
Pudding, chocolate, ready to eat, refrigerated, 4 ounces	55	6

Table 15.1. Continued

Food	Milligrams (mg) per serving	Percent DV*
Tortilla, corn, ready-to-bake/fry, one 6" diameter	46	5
Tortilla, flour, ready-to-bake/fry, one 6" diameter	32	3
Sour cream, reduced fat, cultured, 2 tablespoons	31	3
Bread, whole-wheat, 1 slice	30	3
Broccoli, raw, ½ cup	21	2
Cheese, cream, regular, 1 tablespoon	14	1

DV = Daily Value. The DV for calcium is 1,000 mg for adults and children aged 4 years and older. Foods providing 20% or more of the DV are considered to be high sources of a nutrient, but foods providing lower percentages of the DV also contribute to a healthful diet.
** Calcium content varies slightly by fat content; the more fat, the less calcium the food contains.
*** Calcium content is for tofu processed with a calcium salt. Tofu processed with other salts does not provide significant amounts of calcium.

But My Kids Don't Like Milk

Drinking milk isn't the only way to enjoy its benefits. For example, try making soup and oatmeal or other hot cereals with milk instead of water. Pour milk over cold cereal for breakfast or a snack. Incorporate milk into a fruit smoothie or milkshake. Chocolate milk and cocoa made with milk are also ways to increase the milk in your child's diet.

Sources of calcium also might include an ounce or two of cheese on pizza or a cheeseburger, a cup of calcium-enriched orange juice or a small carton of yogurt. Your kids can also get calcium from dark green, leafy vegetables like kale or bok choy or foods such as broccoli, almonds, tortillas or tofu made with calcium. Many popular foods such as cereals, breads, and juices now have calcium added too. Check the Nutrition Facts label on the package to be sure.

My Teenage Son Loves Milk, but It Seems to Upset His Stomach. Could He Have Lactose Intolerance?

People with lactose intolerance have trouble digesting lactose, the sugar found in milk and dairy foods. Lactose intolerance is not common among infants and young children, but can occur in older children, adolescents, and adults.

Most kids with lactose intolerance are able to digest milk when it is served in small amounts, and combined with other foods like cereal. They may tolerate other dairy products such as cheese or yogurt even if milk is a problem. Lactose-free milk products are now available in most stores, and there are pills and drops you can add to milk and dairy products that make them easier to digest.

Be sure to include plenty of foods with calcium in the meals and snacks you plan for your kids. Almonds, calcium-fortified orange juice, tortillas, fortified cereals, soy beverages, and broccoli with dip are a few great choices. Although it's best to get calcium from food, calcium supplements can also be helpful.

How to Read a Food Label for Calcium?

The food label, called Nutrition Facts, shows you how much one serving of that food contributes to the total amount of calcium, as well as other nutrients, you need every day. This is expressed as a percentage of the daily value (%DV) of calcium that is recommended. For labeling purposes, this is based on the daily calcium recommendation of 1,000 milligrams for people 19 to 50 years old. Since children and teens 9 to 18 years old require more calcium, their %DV target is higher, as indicated below:

Table 15.2

Age	Recommended calcium intake	%DV target
9 to 18	1,300 mg	130%DV
19 to 50	1,000 mg	100%DV

Children and Teens 9 to 18 Years Old Recommended Calcium Intake and %DV Target

Here is an easy rule of thumb for evaluating the calcium content of a food: 20%DV or more is high for calcium. That means it is a high-calcium food and contributes a lot of calcium to the diet. A food with a calcium content of 5%DV or lower contributes little calcium to the diet and is a low source.

If you want to convert the %DV for calcium into milligrams, you can multiply by 10. For example, if a single-serving container of yogurt lists 30%DV for calcium, it contains 300 mg of calcium (30 × 10).

Getting plenty of high-calcium foods every day is important. To meet their calcium needs, children 9 to 18 years old need about four servings of foods with a 30%DV for calcium (300 mg each) or six to seven servings of foods with a 20%DV for calcium (200 mg each) every day. Foods with a lower %DV for calcium are also important to fill gaps and help ensure that your children get all the calcium they need.

My Daughter Is Constantly Dieting. Should I Be Concerned?

Maintaining proper weight is important to overall health, but so is good nutrition. If your daughter is avoiding all milk and dairy products and severely restricting her food intake, she is probably not getting enough calcium. She needs a more balanced diet that includes low-fat milk products and other calcium-rich foods. Calcium supplements may also be helpful to ensure that she gets enough of this essential nutrient.

You should discuss your concerns with your daughter's doctor. If your daughter is one of up to 3 percent of American girls and young women with eating disorders, the problem is even more serious. Eating disorders, especially anorexia nervosa, can lead to missed or irregular menstrual periods or the complete absence of periods, known as amenorrhea. These are signs of low estrogen, a hormone that is essential for developing bone density and reaching peak bone mass. Girls with anorexia nervosa will often have fractures as a first sign of the disease. Furthermore, reduction in estrogen production in adolescence can increase your daughter's risk of osteoporosis and fracture later in life. In severe cases, girls with eating disorders may even develop osteoporosis in their twenties, and they may find the damage to their bones cannot be reversed later in life.

Should I Give My Kids Calcium Supplements?

Experts believe calcium should come from food sources whenever possible. However, if you think your children are not getting adequate calcium from their diet, you may want to consider a calcium supplement.

Section 15.3

Healthy Eating for College Students

This section contains text excerpted from the following sources:
Text under the heading "Be Choosy in the Dining Hall: 10 Tips for
Healthy Eating in the Dining Hall" is excerpted from "Be Choosy
in the Dining Hall," ChooseMyPlate.gov, U.S. Department of
Agriculture (USDA), April 2013; Text under the heading "Healthy
Choices to Keep in Your Dorm Mini-Fridge" is excerpted from
"Mini-Fridge Makeover," ChooseMyPlate.gov, U.S. Department
of Agriculture (USDA), April 2013.

Tips for Healthy Eating in the Dining Hall

Dining halls are full of healthy food options. You just need to
know which foods to put on your tray. Use these tips to plan your food
choices and know which options are best for you.

1. Know What You're Eating

Many dining halls post menus with nutrition information. Look
at the menus ahead of time, so you can be ready to create healthy,
balanced meals when you get there. Having a plan is the first step
in making smarter eating decisions! Visit ChooseMyPlate.gov to find
information and tools like SuperTracker to help you make meal selec-
tion a breeze.

2. Enjoy Your Food, but Eat Less

Everybody loves the all-you-can-eat dining hall! To resist the urge
of eating too much, take smaller portions and use a smaller plate.
Remember you can always go back if you are still hungry.

3. Make Half Your Grains Whole Grains!

Whether you're at the sandwich station or pouring yourself a bowl
of cereal in the morning, make the switch to whole grains like 100%
whole grain-bread and oatmeal.

4. Re-Think Your Drink

Americans drink about 400 calories every day. Consider how often you drink sugary beverages such as sodas, cappuccinos, energy drinks, fruit beverages, sweetened teas, and sports drinks. Drinking water instead of sugary beverages can help you manage your calories.

5. Make Half Your Plate Fruits and Veggies

Fruits and veggies can make your meals more nutritious, colorful, and flavorful. Add to pastas, eggs, pizza, sandwiches, and soups. Try spinach in a wrap or add pineapple to your pizza.

6. Make It Your Own!

Don't feel like you have to choose pre-made plates. Design your own meal! Fresh veggies from the salad bar can be thrown into your omelet for brunch or grab some tofu on your way to the pasta station for lean protein.

7. Slow down on the Sauces

Sauces, gravies, and dressings tend to be high in fat and sodium. Watch out for foods prepared with a lot of oil, butter or topped with heavy condiments, such as mayonnaise. You don't have to do away with sauces and condiments all together; just ask for less or put them on the side. Reducing extras will help you manage your weight.

8. Be on Your Guard at the Salad Bar

Most veggies get the green light but limit foods high in fat and sodium such as olives, bacon bits, fried noodles, croutons, and pasta or potato salads that are made with mayo and oil. Stick to fat-free or low-fat dressings on the side.

9. Make Dessert Special

Save dessert for a Friday night treat or on special occasions. When you can't resist, opt for something healthy, such as a fruit and yogurt parfait.

10. Don't Linger

Dining halls should be just that, where you eat. Although it's great to chat with friends while you eat, avoid staying for long periods of time to reduce your temptation to keep eating.

Healthy Choices to Keep in Your Dorm Mini-Fridge

Stock your dorm-room fridge with a variety of healthy foods. That way, when you need a quick breakfast or study snack, you'll have plenty of options on hand.

1. Low-Fat Cheese

Pair 1 slice cheese with 100% whole-grain bread for an easy snack or munch on a cheese stick for a quick bite between classes. Low-fat cheeses can even be used when making omelets and quesadillas in your dorm microwave!

2. Vegetables

Pre-washed and pre-cut varieties are convenient for quick snacks and meals. Try incorporating green, red, orange, and yellow vegetables into your diet. Pair veggies with your favorite dips, such as carrots with hummus or celery with peanut butter. Add them to omelets and quesadillas.

3. Fruit

Remember that fresh, frozen, dried, and canned fruits all count. Just watch out for varieties with added sugars or syrups. Add a tablespoon of raisins or dried apricots to your morning oatmeal or yogurt and grab an apple for a natural source of energy during a late night study break.

4. Nuts and Nut Butters

These will last longer when stored in the fridge. Try walnuts, almonds, peanuts, hazelnuts, pistachios or cashews. Peanut, butter and almond butter are delicious on apple slices or whole-grain toast.

5. Eggs

Eggs in a dorm room? If you have a refrigerator, yes! Use a microwave safe bowl or mug to scramble eggs for a quick, convenient breakfast or snack. Toss in raw veggies and a tablespoon of cheese for added flavor!

6. Milk and Yogurt

Fat-free (skim) or low-fat milk can be added to oatmeal or whole-grain cereals for a filling, nutritious breakfast. Individual containers of low-fat yogurt or low-fat Greek yogurt are convenient and portable. Mix yogurt with fruit and nuts for an energizing breakfast or top with a few chocolate chips and cinnamon for a healthy dessert.

7. Hummus

Hummus can be paired with almost anything! Enjoy dipping red pepper slices, carrots or other raw veggies into this delicious dip. Spread hummus onto a whole-wheat pita with tomatoes and cucumbers for an easy, nutritious lunch.

8. Salsa

A fresh salsa with tomatoes, jalapenos, cilantro, and onions is a fun and yummy way to incorporate veggies into your diet. Pair low-sodium salsas with a small serving of whole-grain tortilla chips or raw veggies.

9. Use the Nutrition Facts Label

Use the Nutrition Facts label to choose beverages and foods at the store. The label contains information about total sugars, fats, and calories. Reading the Nutrition Facts labels on packaged foods can help you make better choices.

Chapter 16

Nutrition Needs for Women

Chapter Contents

Section 16.1

Nutrition for Pregnancy

This section contains text excerpted from the following sources:
Text beginning with the heading "Nutritional Needs during
Pregnancy" is excerpted from "Nutritional Needs during Pregnancy,"
ChooseMyPlate.gov, U.S. Department of Agriculture (USDA), May
10, 2016; Text beginning with the heading "Pregnancy and Weight
Gain" is excerpted from "Pregnancy Weight Gain Calculator,"
ChooseMyPlate.gov, U.S. Department of Agriculture (USDA), July
2, 2015; Text under the heading "Tips for Pregnant Women" is
excerpted from "Tips for Pregnant Moms," Food and
Nutrition Service (FNS), U.S. Department of Agriculture
(USDA), February 2013.

Nutritional Needs during Pregnancy

When you are pregnant, you have a higher need for some vitamins
and minerals. In each food group, choose foods that have the vitamins
and minerals you need for a healthy pregnancy. Learn more about
choices to make from each food group to provide the vitamins and
minerals you and your baby need.

Vitamin and mineral supplements cannot replace a healthy diet.
Most doctors recommend that pregnant women take a prenatal vitamin
and mineral supplement every day **in addition to** eating a healthy
diet. Taking a supplement ensures that you and your baby get enough
important nutrients like folic acid and iron. But don't overdo it. Taking
extra can be harmful for you and your baby.

Pregnant women and women who may become pregnant should
not drink alcohol. Drinks containing alcohol include beer, wine, liquor,
mixed drinks, malt beverages, etc. Even moderate drinking during
pregnancy can cause behavioral or developmental problems for your
baby. Heavy drinking during pregnancy can result in serious problems
for your baby, including malformation and mental retardation.

Twins, Triplets, and Multiple Births

If you are expecting more than one baby, you should discuss what
and how much to eat with your doctor or healthcare provider. Your

nutrient and calorie needs are higher than those of women carrying one baby. You should also visit your doctor more often than women who are expecting one baby. Women carrying more than one baby need to be monitored more closely.

Pregnancy and Weight Gain

You should gain weight gradually during your pregnancy, with most of the weight gained in the last 3 months. Many doctors suggest women gain weight at the following rate:

- 1 to 4 pounds total during the first 3 months (first trimester).

- 2 to 4 pounds per month during the 4th to 9th months (second and third trimesters).

The total amount of weight you should gain during your pregnancy depends on your weight when you became pregnant. Women whose weight was in the healthy range before becoming pregnant should gain between 25 and 35 pounds while pregnant. The advice is different for those who were overweight or underweight before becoming pregnant.

If you gain too much weight during pregnancy, it can be hard to lose the weight after your baby is born. Most women who gain the suggested amount of weight lose it with the birth of the baby and in the months that follow. Breastfeeding for more than 3 months can also help you lose weight gained during pregnancy. If you gain too little weight during pregnancy, you may have a higher risk for a premature delivery and a low birth weight infant. If you are gaining weight too slowly or too fast, change the amount you are eating:

- If you are gaining weight too fast, cut back on the calories you are currently eating.

- The best way to eat fewer calories is by decreasing the amount of "extras" you are eating.

- "Extras" are added sugars and solid fats in foods like soft drinks, desserts, fried foods, cheese, whole milk, and fatty meats. Look for choices that are low-fat, fat-free, unsweetened or with no-added-sugars.

- Alcohol is also considered an "extra," but you should not drink at all while pregnant.

- If you are not gaining weight or gaining too slowly, you need to eat more calories. You can do this by eating a little more from each food group.

Tips for Pregnant Women

Making healthy food choices along with regular physical activity will help fuel your baby's growth and keep you healthy during pregnancy.

What's on Your Plate?

Before you eat, think about what and how much food goes on your plate or in your cup or bowl. Over the day, include foods from all food groups: vegetables, fruits, whole grains, fat-free or low-fat dairy products, and lean protein foods.

Healthy Food Choices

- **Make half your plate fruits and vegetables.** Choose a variety, including dark-green and red and orange vegetables and beans and peas.

- **Make at least half your grains whole.** Choose whole grains in place of refined grains.

- **Switch to skim or 1% milk.** Choose fat-free or low-fat milk and milk products, such as milk, yogurt, cheese or fortified soy beverages.

- **Vary your protein food choices.** Choose seafood, lean meat and poultry, eggs, beans and peas, soy products, and unsalted nuts and seeds.

- **Use oils to replace solid fats where possible.**

- **Make choices that are low in "empty calories."**

Daily Meal Plan

The Plan shows slightly more amounts of food during the 2nd and 3rd trimesters because you have changing nutritional needs. This is a general Plan. You may need more or less than the Plan.

Table 16.1. Daily Meal Plan for Pregnancy

Food Group	1st Trimester	2nd and 3rd Trimesters	What counts as 1 cup or 1 ounce?
Eat this amount from each group daily			
Vegetables	2½ cups	3 cups	1 cup raw or cooked vegetables or 100% juice 2 cups raw leafy vegetables

Table 16.1. Continued

Food Group	1st Trimester	2nd and 3rd Trimesters	What counts as 1 cup or 1 ounce?
Eat this amount from each group daily			
Fruits	2 cups	2 cups	1 cup fruit or 100% juice ½ cup dried fruit
Grains	6 ounces	8 ounces	1 slice bread 1 ounce ready-to-eat cereal ½ cup cooked pasta, rice or cereal
Dairy	3 cups	3 cups	1 cup milk 8 ounces yogurt 1½ ounces natural cheese 2 ounces processed cheese
Protein Foods	5½ ounces	6½ ounces	1 ounce lean meat, poultry or seafood ¼ cup cooked beans ½ ounce nuts or 1 egg 1 tablespoon peanut butter

If you are not gaining weight or gaining too slowly, you may need to eat a little more from each food group. If you are gaining weight too fast, you may need to cut back by decreasing the amount of "empty calories" you are eating.

Being Physically Active

Unless your doctor advises you not to be physically active, include 2½ hours each week of physical activity such as brisk walking, dancing, gardening or swimming. The activity should be done at least 10 minutes at a time, and preferably spread throughout the week. Avoid activities with a high risk of falling or injury.

Seafood Can Be a Part of a Healthy Diet

Omega-3 fats in seafood have important health benefits for you and your unborn child. Salmon, sardines, and trout are some choices higher in Omega-3 fats.

- Eat 8 to 12 ounces of seafood each week.

- Eat all types of tuna, but limit white (albacore) tuna to 6 ounces each week.

- Do not eat tilefish, shark, swordfish, and king mackerel since they have high levels of mercury.

Section 16.2

Nutrition for Breastfeeding

This section contains text excerpted from the following sources:
Text under the heading "Breastfeeding and Everyday Life" is
excerpted from "Breastfeeding," Office on Women's Health (OWH),
U.S. Department of Health and Human Services (HHS), July 21,
2014; Text under the heading "Weight Loss While Breastfeeding" is
excerpted from "Weight Loss While Breastfeeding," ChooseMyPlate.
gov, U.S. Department of Agriculture (USDA), January 7, 2016; Text
under the heading "Tips for Breastfeeding Women" is excerpted from
"Tips for Breastfeeding Moms," Food and Nutrition Service (FNS),
U.S. Department of Agriculture (USDA), February 2013.

Breastfeeding and Everyday Life

Most breastfeeding moms do not need a special diet, but eating
healthy foods and getting exercise will help make sure you have the
energy you need. Juggling a new baby and a good breastfeeding routine can be stressful. Learning how to keep your stress level as low
as possible can help make the breastfeeding experience a positive one
for you and your baby.

Do I Need to Avoid Certain Foods While Breastfeeding?

Many new mothers wonder if they should be on a special diet while
breastfeeding, but the answer is no. For most breastfeeding moms,
there are no foods you have to avoid. But you may find that some foods
cause stomach upset in your baby. You can try avoiding those foods to
see if your baby feels better, and you can ask your baby's doctor for help.

What Do I Need to Know about Eating Healthy While Breastfeeding?

To eat healthy while breastfeeding, keep these important nutrition
tips in mind:

- Drink plenty of fluids to stay hydrated. A common suggestion is to
  drink a glass of water or other beverage every time you breastfeed.

- Limit drinks with added sugars, such as sodas and fruit drinks.

- Drinking a moderate amount (up to 1 to 2 cups a day) of coffee or other caffeinated beverages does not cause a problem for most breastfeeding babies. But too much caffeine can cause a baby to be fussy or not sleep well.

- In addition to healthy food choices, some breastfeeding women may need a multivitamin and mineral supplement. Talk with your doctor to find out if you need a supplement. Your doctor may recommend that you continue taking your prenatal vitamin while breastfeeding.

Weight Loss While Breastfeeding

Breastfeeding is best for moms and their babies for several reasons. Besides providing nourishment and helping to protect your baby against becoming sick, breastfeeding may help you lose the weight gained in pregnancy. Moderate exercise and eating less can help breastfeeding mothers lose weight.

- A great time to lose weight after pregnancy is while breastfeeding.

- Breastfeeding may make it easier to lose weight because you are using extra calories to feed your infant.

- Women who breastfeed exclusively for more than 3 months tend to lose more weight than those who do not.

- Those who continue breastfeeding beyond 4-6 months may continue to lose weight.

Choose the right amount from each food group. In addition, continue to visit your doctor or healthcare provider while you are breastfeeding. He or she can keep track of your weight and tell you if you are losing weight as you should. If you are losing weight too slowly or too fast, change the amount you are eating.

- If you are **not losing weight** or **losing too slowly**, cut back on the calories you are currently eating.

- The best way to eat fewer calories is by decreasing the amount of "empty calories" you are eating. Empty calories are the calories from added sugars and solid fats, in foods like soft drinks, desserts, fried foods, cheese, whole milk, and fatty meats.

Look for choices that are low-fat, fat-free, unsweetened or with no-added-sugars. They have fewer empty calories. Alcohol is also a source of empty calories.

- If you are **losing weight too fast**, you need to eat more calories. You can do this by eating a little more from each food group. Try adding a healthy snack each day or increasing portion sizes at meals. If you keep losing weight faster than you want to, check with your doctor.

Tips for Breastfeeding Women

Making healthy food choices with regular physical activity will keep you healthy.

Healthy Food Choices

- **Make half your plate fruits and vegetables.** Choose a variety, including dark-green and red and orange vegetables and beans and peas.

- **Make at least half your grains whole.** Choose whole grains in place of refined grains.

- **Switch to skim or 1% milk**. Choose fat-free or low-fat milk and milk products such as milk, yogurt, cheese or fortified soy beverages.

- **Vary your protein food choices.** Choose seafood, lean meat and poultry, eggs, beans and peas, soy products, and unsalted nuts and seeds.

- **Use oils to replace solid fats where possible.**

- **Make choices that are low in "empty calories."**

Daily Meal Plan

The Plan shows different amounts of food depending on how much of your baby's diet is breast milk. Moms who feed only breast milk to their baby need slightly more food. This is a general Plan. You may need more or less than the Plan.

Table 16.2. Daily Meal Plan for Breastfeeding

Food Group	Breastfeeding only	Breastfeeding plus formula	What counts as 1 cup or 1 ounce?
Eat this amount from each group daily			
Vegetables	3 cups	2½ cups	1 cup raw or cooked vegetables or 100% juice 2 cups raw leafy vegetables
Fruits	2 cups	2 cups	1 cup fruit or 100% juice ½ cup dried fruit
Grains	8 ounces	6 ounces	1 slice bread 1 ounce ready-to-eat cereal ½ cup cooked pasta, rice or cereal
Dairy	3 cups	3 cups	1 cup milk 8 ounces yogurt 1½ ounces natural cheese 2 ounces processed cheese
Protein Foods	6½ ounces	5½ ounces	1 ounce lean meat, poultry or seafood ¼ cup cooked beans ½ ounce nuts or 1 egg 1 tablespoon peanut butter

If you are not losing weight you gained in pregnancy, you may need to cut back by decreasing the amount of "empty calories" you are eating

What about Alcohol?

Be very cautious about drinking alcohol, if you choose to drink at all. You may consume a single alcoholic drink if your baby's breastfeeding behavior is well established—no earlier than 3 months old. Then wait at least 4 hours before breastfeeding. Or, you may express breast milk before drinking and feed the expressed milk to your baby later.

Being Physically Active

Unless your doctor advises you not to be physically active, include 2½ hours each week of physical activity such as brisk walking, dancing or swimming. The activity should be done for at least 10 minutes at a time, and preferably spread throughout the week.

Also...

- **Your need for fluids increases while you are breastfeeding.** You may notice that you are thirstier than usual. Drink enough water and other fluids to quench your thirst.

- **Seafood can be part of a healthy diet.** Omega-3 fats in seafood have important health benefits for you and your baby. Salmon, sardines, and trout are some of the choices higher in Omega-3 fats.

- Eat 8 to 12 ounces of seafood each week.

- Eat all types of tuna, but limit white (albacore) tuna to 6 ounces each week.

- Do not eat tilefish, shark, swordfish, and king mackerel since they have high levels of mercury.

Section 16.3

The Importance of Folic Acid for Women of Childbearing Age

This section includes text excerpted from "Get Enough Folic Acid," Office of Disease Prevention and Health Promotion (ODPHP), U.S. Department of Health and Human Services (HHS), March 22, 2016.

Women of childbearing age (typically ages 11 to 49) need an extra 400 to 800 micrograms (mcg) of folic acid every day. Folic acid is found in vitamins and foods like breakfast cereal or bread that have folic acid added.

Why Is Folic Acid Important?

Everyone needs folic acid, but it's especially important for women who are pregnant or who may become pregnant. Folic acid is a vitamin that can prevent birth defects.

Getting enough folic acid is important even when you aren't planning to get pregnant. It's needed during the first few weeks of pregnancy, often before a woman knows she's pregnant.

Talk with Your Doctor about Folic Acid.

If you are pregnant or breastfeeding, your doctor can help you figure out how much folic acid is right for you. You may need more than

400 mcg folic acid if you have a health condition or are taking certain medicines.

How Can I Get Enough Folic Acid?

Getting enough folic acid every day is easy. You can eat foods like breakfast cereal or bread that have folic acid added. Or you can take a vitamin with folic acid.

Look for Breakfast Cereal with Folic Acid.

Check the Nutrition Facts label to see how much folic acid the cereal has. Choose cereal that has 100% DV (Daily Value) of folic acid.

Take a Vitamin with Folic Acid.

You can take a multivitamin or a small pill that has only folic acid. Vitamins and folic acid pills can be found at most pharmacies and grocery stores.

Take Action!

It's easy to get the folic acid you need. Just eat a bowl of cereal with 100% DV of folic acid–or take a vitamin–every day.

Check the Label.

When you are at the grocery store, look for foods with folic acid in them. Choose cereal that has 100% DV of folic acid. Folic acid is also in foods like enriched breads, pastas, and other foods made with grains. Check the Nutrition Facts label. If you buy vitamins, be sure to check the label for folic acid. This label shows a vitamin with 100% DV of folic acid.

Supplement Facts

	Amount Per Serving	% Daily Value
Folic Acid	400 mcg	100%
Vitamin B12	6 mcg	100%
Pantothenic Acid	5 mg	50%
Calcium	450 mg	45%
Iron	18 mg	100%
Magnesium	50 mg	12%
Zinc	15 mg	100%

Figure 16.1. *Supplement Facts*

If You Take a Vitamin, Make It Easy to Remember

- Take it at the same time every day. For example, take it when you brush your teeth in the morning or when you eat breakfast.

- Leave the vitamin bottle somewhere you will notice it every day, like on the kitchen counter.

What about Cost?

Thanks to the Affordable Care Act, the healthcare reform law passed in 2010, health plans must cover folic acid supplements (pills). Depending on your insurance, you may be able to get folic acid supplements at no cost to you. Talk to your insurance company to learn more.

Eat Healthy

Eating healthy means getting plenty of vegetables, fruits, whole grains, and foods with protein. A healthy diet also includes foods with folate (a different type of folic acid).

In addition to eating cereal that has 100% DV of folic acid or taking a vitamin, it's important for women to eat foods with folate, such as:

- Spinach and other leafy greens

- Asparagus

- Oranges and orange juice

- Beans and peas

Section 16.4

Nutrition for Menopause

This section includes text excerpted from "Menopause:
Time for a Change," National Institute on Aging (NIA),
August 2010. Reviewed July 2016.

Staying Healthy

The average woman today has more than one-third of her life ahead of her after menopause. That means the menopausal transition is a good time for lifestyle changes that could help women make the most of the coming years. You've already read some ways to protect or improve your health at this time of life—quitting smoking, exercising daily, and working toward a healthy weight. But, there's even more you can do to stay healthy—other lifestyle changes plus suggestions to help you work with your healthcare providers more effectively.

Good Nutrition

A balanced diet will give you most of the nutrients and calories your body needs to stay healthy. Eat a variety of foods from the five major food groups. Look for foods that have lots of nutrients, like protein and vitamins, but not a lot of calories. These are called nutrient-dense foods. As you grow older, you need fewer calories for energy, but just as many nutrients.

The U.S. Department of Agriculture (USDA) Food Guide is one eating plan suggested by the Federal Government's *Dietary Guidelines for Americans, 2005*. Another eating plan also suggested in the *Dietary Guidelines* is DASH, Dietary Approaches to Stop Hypertension. Contact the National Heart, Lung, and Blood Institute (NHLBI) for more resources about this plan.

The number of calories a woman over age 50 should eat daily depends on how physically active she is. Basically you need:

- 1,600 calories, if your physical activity level is low.

- 1,800 calories, if you are moderately active.

- 2,000-2,200 calories, if you have an active lifestyle.

The more active you are, the more calories you can eat without gaining weight.

Eating the foods recommended in the USDA Food Guide or in DASH will help you get needed nutrients. But, people over 50 have trouble getting enough of some vitamins and minerals through diet alone, including calcium and vitamin D. Just remember that these recommendations include how much of each nutrient you get from food and drinks as well as any supplement you use. Women past menopause who are still having a menstrual cycle because they are using menopausal hormone therapy might need some extra iron over the 8 mg (milligrams) recommended for women over age 50. Iron, important for healthy red blood cells, is found in meat, duck, peas, beans, and fortified bread and grain products.

Women over 50 also need more of two B vitamins. Getting 2.4 mcg (micrograms) of vitamin B12 per day will maintain the health of your blood and nerves. Some foods, such as cereals, are fortified with this vitamin. Vitamin B12 is also found in red meat and, to a lesser extent, fish and poultry. But, up to one-third of older people can no longer absorb natural vitamin B12 from their food. Furthermore, common medicines taken to control the symptoms of GERD (gastroesophageal reflux disease), also known as acid reflux, slow the release of certain stomach acids and, therefore, interfere with the body's absorption of vitamin B12. You might need a supplement if you have GERD.

Another B vitamin, B6, helps your body breakdown proteins and make hemoglobin, a part of red blood cells. Women should have 1.5 mg of vitamin B6 daily. This vitamin is found in fortified cereals, as well as meats, legumes, and eggs.

Don't forget to drink plenty of fluids, especially water. If you drink alcohol, do so in moderation—for a woman, only one drink a day according to the *Dietary Guidelines for Americans*. A drink could be one 12-ounce beer, 5 ounces of wine or 1½ ounces of 80-proof distilled spirits.

U.S. Department of Agriculture (USDA) Food Guide Daily Recommendations for Women Age 50 and Older

Grains—5 to 7 ounces, at least half of which are whole grains.
Vegetables—2 to 3 cups with a variety of colors and types.
Fruits—1½ to 2 cups.
Milk, yogurt, and cheese—3 cups of milk or the equivalent.
Meat, poultry, fish, dry beans, eggs, and nuts—5 to 6 ounces of lean meat, poultry or fish or the equivalent.

Chapter 17

Nutrition for Older Persons

Chapter Contents

Section 17.1

Healthy Eating for Adults 50 and Over

This section contains text excerpted from the following sources: Text in this section begins with excerpts from "Eating Well as You Get Older: Benefits of Eating Well," NIHSeniorHealth, National Institute on Aging (NIA), March 2016; Text under the heading "How Much Should I Eat?" is excerpted from "Healthy Eating after 50," National Institute on Aging (NIA), March 2015.

Eating well is vital for everyone at all ages. Whatever your age, your daily food choices can make an important difference in your health and in how you look and feel.

Eating Well Promotes Health

Eating a well-planned, balanced mix of foods every day has many health benefits. For instance, eating well may reduce the risk of heart disease, stroke, type 2 diabetes, bone loss, some kinds of cancer, and anemia. If you already have one or more of these chronic diseases, eating well, and being physically active may help you better manage them. Healthy eating may also help you reduce high blood pressure, lower high cholesterol, and manage diabetes.

Eating well gives you the nutrients needed to keep your muscles, bones, organs, and other parts of your body healthy throughout your life. These nutrients include vitamins, minerals, protein, carbohydrates, fats, and water.

Eating Well Promotes Energy

Eating well helps keep up your energy level, too. By consuming enough calories—a way to measure the energy you get from food—you give your body the fuel it needs throughout the day. The number of calories needed depends on how old you are, whether you're a man or woman, your height and weight, and how active you are.

Food Choices Can Affect Weight

Consuming the right number of calories for your level of physical activity helps you control your weight, too. Extra weight is a concern for older adults because it can increase the risk for diseases such as type 2 diabetes and heart disease and can increase joint problems. Eating more calories than your body needs for your activity level will lead to extra pounds.

If you become less physically active as you age, you will probably need fewer calories to stay at the same weight. Choosing mostly nutrient-dense foods—foods which have a lot of nutrients but relatively few calories—can give you the nutrients you need while keeping down calorie intake.

Food Choices Affect Digestion

Your food choices also affect your digestion. For instance, not getting enough fiber or fluids may cause constipation. Eating more whole-grain foods with fiber, fruits and vegetables or drinking more water may help with constipation.

Make One Change at a Time

Eating well isn't just a "diet" or "program" that's here today and gone tomorrow. It is part of a healthy lifestyle that you can adopt now and stay with in the years to come.

To eat healthier, you can begin by taking small steps, making one change at a time. For instance, you might

- take the salt shaker off your table. Decreasing your salt intake slowly will allow you to adjust.

- switch to whole-grain bread, seafood or more vegetables and fruits when you shop.

These changes may be easier than you think. They're possible even if you need help with shopping or cooking or if you have a limited budget.

Checking with Your Doctor

If you have a specific medical condition, be sure to check with your doctor or registered dietitian about foods you should include or avoid.

You Can Start Today

Whatever your age, you can start making positive lifestyle changes today. Eating well can help you stay healthy and independent—and look and feel good—in the years to come.

How Much Should I Eat?

How much you should eat depends on how active you are. If you eat more calories than your body uses, you gain weight. What are calories? Calories are a way to count how much energy is in food. The energy you get from food helps you do the things you need to do each day. Try to choose foods that have a lot of the nutrients you need, but not many calories.

Just counting calories is not enough for making smart choices. Think about this: a medium banana, 1 cup of flaked cereal, 1-1/2 cups of cooked spinach, 1 tablespoon of peanut butter or 1 cup of 1% milk all have roughly the same number of calories. But, the foods are different in many ways. Some have more of the nutrients you might need than others do. For example, milk gives you more calcium than a banana, and peanut butter gives you more protein than cereal. Some foods can make you feel fuller than others.

Here's a tip: In the U.S. Department of Agriculture (USDA) Food Patterns, eating the smallest amount suggested for each food group gives you about 1,600 calories. The largest amount has 2,800 calories.

How Much Is on My Plate?

How does the food on your plate compare to how much you should be eating? Here are some ways to see how the food on your plate measures up to how much you should be eating:

- deck of cards = 3 ounces of meat or poultry
- ½ baseball = ½ cup of fruit, rice, pasta or ice cream
- baseball = 1 cup of salad greens
- 4 dice = 1-1/2 ounces of cheese
- tip of your first finger = 1 teaspoon of butter or margarine
- ping pong ball = 2 tablespoons of peanut butter
- fist = 1 cup of flaked cereal or a baked potato
- compact disc or DVD = 1 pancake or tortilla

Having Problems with Food?

Does your favorite chicken dish taste different? As you grow older, your sense of taste and smell may change. Foods may seem to have lost flavor.

Also, medicines may change how food tastes. They can also make you feel less hungry. Talk to your doctor about whether there is a different medicine you could use. Try extra spices or herbs on your foods to add flavor.

Maybe some of the foods you used to eat no longer agree with you. For example, some people become *lactose intolerant*. They have symptoms like stomach pain, gas or diarrhea after eating or drinking something with milk in it, like ice cream. Most can eat small amounts of such food or can try yogurt, buttermilk or hard cheese. Lactose-free foods are available now also. Your doctor can test to see if you are lactose intolerant.

Is it harder to chew your food? Maybe your dentures need to fit better or your gums are sore. If so, a dentist can help you. Until then, you might want to eat softer foods that are easier to chew.

Do I Need to Drink Water?

With age, you may lose some of your sense of thirst. Drink plenty of liquids like water, juice, milk, and soup. Don't wait until you feel thirsty. Try to add liquids throughout the day. You could try soup for a snack or drink a glass of water before exercising or working in the yard. Don't forget to take sips of water, milk or juice during a meal.

What about Fiber?

Fiber is found in foods from plants—fruits, vegetables, beans, nuts, seeds, and whole grains. Eating more fiber might prevent stomach or intestine problems, like **constipation**. It might also help lower cholesterol, as well as blood sugar.

It is better to get fiber from food than dietary supplements. Start adding fiber slowly. That will help avoid unwanted gas. Here are some tips for adding fiber:

- Eat cooked dry beans, peas, and lentils often.
- Leave skins on your fruit and vegetables if possible.
- Choose whole fruit over fruit juice.
- Eat whole-grain breads and cereals.

Drink plenty of liquids to help fiber move through your intestines.

Should I Cut Back on Salt?

The usual way people get sodium is by eating salt. The body needs sodium, but too much can make blood pressure go up in some people.

Most fresh foods contain some sodium, especially those high in protein. Salt is added to many canned and prepared foods.

People tend to eat more salt than they need. If you are 51 or older, about 2/3 of a teaspoon of table salt—1,500 milligrams (mg) sodium—is all you need each day. That includes all the sodium in your food and drink, not just the salt you add. Try to avoid adding salt during cooking or at the table. Talk to your doctor before using salt substitutes. Some contain sodium. And most have potassium which some people also need to limit. Eat fewer salty snacks and processed foods. Look for the word sodium, not salt, on the Nutrition Facts panel. Choose foods labeled "low-sodium." Often, the amount of sodium in the same kind of food can vary greatly between brands.

Here's a tip: Spices, herbs, and lemon juice can add flavor to your food, so you won't miss the salt.

What about Fat?

Fat in your diet comes from two places—the fat already in food and the fat added when you cook. Fat gives you energy and helps your body use certain vitamins, but it is high in calories. To lower the fat in your diet:

- Choose cuts of meat, fish or poultry (with the skin removed) with less fat.
- Trim off any extra fat before cooking.
- Use low-fat dairy products and salad dressings.
- Use non-stick pots and pans, and cook without added fat.
- Choose an unsaturated or mono saturated vegetable oil for cooking—check the label.
- Don't fry foods. Instead, broil, roast, bake, stir-fry, steam, microwave or boil them.

Keeping Food Safe

Older people must take extra care to keep their food safe to eat. You are less able to fight off infections, and some foods could make you very sick. Talk to your doctor or a registered dietitian, a nutrition specialist, about foods to avoid.

Handle raw food with care. Keep it apart from foods that are already cooked or won't be cooked. Use hot soapy water to wash your hands, tools, and work surfaces as you cook.

Don't depend on sniffing or tasting food to tell what is bad. Try putting dates on foods in your fridge. Check the "use by" date on foods. If in doubt, toss it out.

Here's a tip: Make sure food gets into the refrigerator no more than 2 hours after it is cooked.

Can I Afford to Eat Right?

If your budget is limited, it might take some planning to be able to pay for the foods you should eat. Here are some suggestions. First, buy only the foods you need. A shopping list will help with that. Buy only as much food as you will use. Here are some other ways to keep your food costs down:

- Plain (generic) labels or store brands often cost less than name brands.
- Plan your meals around food that is on sale.
- Divide leftovers into small servings, label and date, and freeze to use within a few months.

Federal Government programs are available to help people with low incomes buy groceries. To learn more about these programs or find your Area Agency on Aging, contact the Eldercare Locator.

Section 17.2

Food Safety for Older Adults

This section contains text excerpted from the following sources:
Text in this section begins with excerpts from "Food Safety for Older
Adults," FoodSafety.gov, U.S. Department of Health and Human
Services (HHS), June 8, 2015; Text under the heading "Food Safety
for Home Delivered Meals" is excerpted from "Food Safety for Home
Delivered Meals," FoodSafety.gov, U.S. Department of Health and
Human Services (HHS), June 2, 2015.

Adults 65 and older are at a higher risk for hospitalization and
death from foodborne illness. For example, older adults residing in
nursing homes are ten times more likely to die from bacterial gastroenteritis than the general population. As data shows, food safety is
particularly important for adults 65 and older.

This increased risk of foodborne illness is because our organs and
body systems go through changes as we age. These changes include:

- The gastrointestinal tract holds on to food for a longer period of
  time, allowing bacteria to grow.

- The liver and kidneys may not properly rid our bodies of foreign
  bacteria and toxins.

- The stomach may not produce enough acid. The acidity helps to
  reduce the number of bacteria in our intestinal tract. Without
  proper amounts of acid, there is an increased risk of bacterial
  growth.

- Underlying chronic conditions, such as diabetes and cancer, may
  also increase a person's risk of foodborne illness.

What You Can Do

Learn about safety tips for those at increased risk of foodborne
illness. Older adults should always follow the four steps:

Clean: Wash hands and surfaces often.

Separate: Separate raw meat and poultry from ready-to-eat foods.

Cook: Cook food to the right temperatures.

Chill: Chill raw meat and poultry as well as cooked leftovers promptly (within 2 hours).

Food Safety for Home Delivered Meals

Many people receive home delivered meals from churches, social organizations, senior assistance groups or healthcare organizations. Hot or cold ready-prepared meals are perishable and can cause illness when mishandled. Proper handling is essential to ensure the food is safe to eat.

The "Danger Zone"

Leaving food out too long at room temperature can cause bacteria to grow to dangerous levels that can cause illness.

Bacteria grow most rapidly in the range of temperatures between 40 °F and 140 °F, doubling in number in as little as 20 minutes. This range of temperatures is often called the "Danger Zone." Perishable foods left at room temperature for more than two hours should be discarded. If temperatures are above 90 °F perishable foods should not be left out longer than one hour. Discard food after one hour if the temperature is above 90 °F.

Refrigerate delivered meals if you don't plan to eat them immediately. You can reheat them when you are ready to eat. Follow these steps to refrigerate delivered meals:

- Store food in a refrigerator at 40 °F or below.

- Divide food or cut into smaller portions.

- Use shallow containers to store food.

- Remove any stuffing from whole cooked poultry before refrigerating.

Foods delivered cold should be eaten within 2 hours or refrigerated or frozen for eating at another time.

Table 17.1. Refrigerator Storage at 40 °F or Below

Cooked meat or poultry	3 to 4 days
Pizza	3 to 4 days
Luncheon meats	3 to 5 days
Egg, tuna, and macaroni salads	3 to 5 days

Table 17.2. Freezer Storage at 0 °F or Below

Cooked meat or poultry	2 to 6 months
Pizza	1 to 2 months
Luncheon meats	1 to 2 months

Reheating

You may wish to reheat your meal, whether it was purchased hot and then refrigerated or purchased cold initially.

- Reheat food to 165 °F using a food thermometer. Bring soup or gravy to a rolling boil.

- If using a microwave oven to reheat food, cover food and rotate the dish so that food heats evenly. This prevents any "cold spots" from harboring bacteria. Allow standing time. Consult your owner's manual for complete instructions. Heat food until it reaches at least 165 °F throughout.

Section 17.3

Common Eating and Cooking Problems for Older Adults

This section includes text excerpted from "Common Questions," National Institute on Aging (NIA), October 1, 2011. Reviewed June 2016.

Tired of Cooking or Eating Alone?

Maybe you are tired of planning and cooking dinners every night. Have you considered some potluck meals? If everyone brings one part of the meal, cooking is a lot easier, and there might be leftovers to share. Or try cooking with a friend to make a meal you can enjoy together. Also look into having some meals at a nearby senior center, community center or religious facility. Not only will you enjoy a free or low-cost meal, but you will have some company while you eat.

Problems Chewing Food?

Do you avoid some foods because they are hard to chew? People who have problems with their **teeth or dentures** often avoid eating meat, fruits or vegetables and might miss out on **important nutrients.** If you are having trouble chewing, see your dentist to check for problems. If you wear dentures, the dentist can check how they fit.

Sometimes Hard to Swallow Your Food?

If food seems to get stuck in your throat, it might be that less saliva in your mouth is making it hard for you to swallow your food. Drinking plenty of liquids with your meal might help. Talk to your doctor about what might be causing your **dry mouth** and the problem swallowing.

Food Tastes Different?

Are foods not as tasty as they used to be? It might not be the cook's fault! Maybe your **sense of taste, smell** or both has changed. Growing older can cause your senses to change, but so can a variety of other things such as dental problems or medication side effects. Taste and smell are important for healthy appetite and eating.

Feeling Sad and Don't Want to Eat?

Feeling blue now and then is normal, but if you continue to feel sad, ask your doctor for help. Being unhappy can cause a loss of appetite. Help might be available. For example, you might need to talk with someone trained to work with people who are depressed.

Just Not Hungry?

Maybe you are not sad, but just can't eat very much. Changes to your body as you age can cause some people to feel full sooner than they did when younger. Or lack of appetite might be the side effect of a medicine you are taking—your doctor might be able to suggest a different drug.

Try being more **physically active.** In addition to all the other benefits of exercise and physical activity, it may make you hungrier.

If you aren't hungry because food just isn't appealing, there are ways to make it more interesting. Make sure your foods are seasoned well, but **not with extra salt.** Try using lemon juice, vinegar or herbs to boost the flavor of your food.

Vary the shape, color, and texture of foods you eat. When you go **shopping,** look for a new vegetable, fruit or seafood you haven't tried before or one you haven't eaten in a while. Sometimes grocery stores have recipe cards near items. Or ask the produce staff or meat or seafood department staff for suggestions about preparing the new food. Find recipes online. Type the name of a food and the word "recipes" into a search window to look for ideas.

Foods that are overcooked tend to have less flavor. Try cooking or steaming your vegetables for a shorter time, and see if that gives them a crunch that will help spark your interest.

Trouble Getting Enough Calories?

If you aren't eating enough, add snacks throughout the day to help you get more nutrients and calories. Snacks can be healthy—for example, raw vegetables with a low-fat dip or hummus, low-fat cheese, and whole-grain crackers or a piece of fruit. Unsalted nuts or nut butters are nutrient-dense snacks that give you added protein. You could try putting shredded low-fat cheese on your soup or popcorn or sprinkling nuts or wheat germ on yogurt or cereal.

If you are eating so little that you are losing weight but don't need to, your doctor might suggest protein and energy supplements. Sometimes these help undernourished people gain a little weight. If so, they should be used as snacks between meals or after dinner, not in place of a meal and not right before one. Ask your doctor how to choose a supplement.

Physical Problems Making It Hard to Eat?

Sometimes illnesses like Parkinson disease, stroke or arthritis can make it harder for you to cook or feed yourself. Your doctor might recommend an occupational therapist. He or she might suggest rearranging things in your kitchen, make a custom splint for your hand or give you special exercises to strengthen your muscles. Devices like special utensils and plates might make mealtime easier or help with food preparation.

Can Foods and Medicines Interact?

Medicines can change how food tastes, make your mouth dry or take away your appetite. In turn, some foods can change how certain medicines work. You might have heard that grapefruit juice is a common culprit when used with any of several drugs. Chocolate, licorice, and alcohol are some of the others. Whenever your doctor prescribes a new drug for you, be sure to ask about any food/drug interactions.

Lactose Intolerant?

Some older people believe they are lactose intolerant because they have uncomfortable stomach and intestinal symptoms when they have **dairy products.** Your doctor can do tests to learn whether or not you do indeed need to limit or avoid dairy foods when you eat. If so, **talk to your healthcare practitioner** about how to meet your calcium and vitamin D needs. Even lactose-intolerant people might be able to have small amounts of milk when taken with food. There are non-dairy food sources of calcium, lactose-free milk and milk products, calcium- and vitamin D-fortified foods, and supplements.

Weight Issues Adding to Frailty?

Older people who don't get enough of the right nutrients can be too thin or too heavy. Some may be too thin because they don't get enough food. But others might be overweight partly because they get too much of the wrong types of foods. Keeping track of what you are eating could help you see which foods you should eat less of, more of or not at all.

Obesity is a growing problem in the United States, and the number of older people who are overweight or obese is also increasing. But frailty is also a problem, and not just in thin people. As you grow older, you can lose muscle strength, but you also get more fat tissue. This can make you frail, and in time, you might have problems getting around and taking care of yourself. Being overweight puts you more at risk for frailty and disability.

But, just losing weight is not necessarily the answer. That's because sometimes when older people lose weight, they lose even more muscle than they already have lost. That puts them at greater risk for becoming frail and **falling.** They also might lose **bone strength** and be at more risk for a broken bone after a fall. Exercise helps you keep muscle and bone. Also, for some people, a few extra pounds late in life can act as a safety net should they get a serious illness that limits how much they can eat for a while.

Part Four

Lifestyle and Nutrition

Chapter 18

Nutrition Statistics in America

Chapter Contents

Section 18.1

Attitudes toward Nutrition and Health

This section includes text excerpted from "American Adults Are
Choosing Healthier Foods, Consuming Healthier Diets," U.S.
Department of Agriculture (USDA), January 16, 2014.

American adults are eating better, making better use of available
nutrition information, and consuming fewer calories coming from fat
and saturated fat, consuming less cholesterol and eating more fiber,
according to a report from the U.S. Department of Agriculture's Economic Research Service (ERS).

The study underscores the importance of robust efforts undertaken
since 2009 to improve food choices and diet quality and ensure that
all Americans have access to healthy food and science-based nutrition
education and advice.

"The United States Government is working hard to empower the
American public to make smart choices every day at school, at home
and in their communities," said Agriculture Secretary Tom Vilsack.
"We have made significant progress, but our work is not done. We will
continue to invest in critical programs that expand the availability of
healthy, safe, affordable food for all Americans."

The researchers found that use of nutrition information, including
the Nutrition Facts Panel found on most food packages, increased in
recent years. Forty-two percent of working age adults and 57 percent
of older adults reported using the Nutrition Facts Panel most or all
of the time when making food choices. When asked about nutrition
information in restaurants, 76 percent of working-age adults reported
that they would use the information if it were available.

"We are pleased to hear that this study finds improvements in several key areas of the American diet," said Michael R. Taylor, deputy
commissioner for foods and veterinary medicine at the U.S. Food and
Drug Administration. "FDA will soon propose an updated Nutrition
Facts label designed to provide information that will make it even
easier for people to make healthy choices."

Reduced consumption of food away from home (such as food from
restaurants and fast food) accounted for 20 percent of the improvements

246

in diet quality. A recent study found that during the recession of 2007-2009, U.S. household overall food expenditures declined approximately 5 percent, mostly due to a 12.9 percent decline in spending on food away from home. Calories consumed through food away from home dropped by 127 calories per day, and the average person ate three fewer meals and 1.5 fewer snacks per month away from home. Eating at home more often was also associated with more frequent family meals.

The report also indicates changing attitudes toward food and nutrition. Compared with 2007, the percentage of working-age adults who believed they have the ability to change their body weight increased by three percentage points in 2010. During the same time period, the report shows there was little change in the importance that price played when making choices at the grocery store, but working-age adults placed increased importance on nutrition when choosing items to purchase.

"When individuals believe that their actions directly affect their body weight, they might be more inclined to make healthier food choices," said study author Jessica Todd, Ph.D., of the Economic Research Service.

The researcher used individual dietary intake data for working-age adults from the National Health and Nutrition Examination Survey (NHANES), which collects detailed individual and household information on a wide range of health-related topics through questionnaires, physical exams and lab work, in two-year segments. The survey is designed to be nationally representative, with a sample composed of 9,839 individuals. Overall, daily caloric intake declined by 78 calories per day between 2005 and 2010. There were overall declines in calories from total fat (3.3 percent), saturated fat (5.9 percent), and intake of cholesterol (7.9 percent). Overall fiber intake increased by 1.2 grams per day (7.5 percent).

This research was conducted by the Economic Research Service, which is a primary source of economic information and research at USDA.

Expanding the availability of healthy food to all Americans, while providing science-based nutrition information and advice, is a key focus of USDA's nutrition assistance programs and the Federal Government. USDA is focused on strategies that empower families to make healthy food choices, including:

- USDA's MyPlate symbol and the resources at ChooseMyPlate provide quick, easy reference tools to facilitate healthy eating on a budget for parents, teachers, healthcare professionals, and communities. The site includes shopping strategies and meal planning advice to help families serve more nutritious meals affordably through its 10-Tips Nutrition Series and the Thrifty Food Plan.

- USDA's SuperTracker, a free online planning and tracking tool, helps more than three million Americans improve food choices, maintain a healthy weight, and track physical activity on a daily basis.

- America's students now have healthier and more nutritious school meals due to improved nutrition standards implemented as a result of the historic Healthy, Hunger-Free Kids Act of 2010. USDA recently announced Smart Snacks in Schools, which sets healthy guidelines for all foods and beverages sold in school to ensure that students will be offered only healthier food options during the school day.

- USDA expanded eligibility for $4 million in grants to improve access to fresh produce and healthy foods for SNAP shoppers at America's farmers markets. By increasing the number of farmers markets that are able to accept SNAP benefits, USDA is encouraging SNAP recipients to use their benefits to purchase and prepare healthy foods for their families.

- Through USDA's Know Your Farmer, Know Your Food, the department has worked to increase access to nutritious food through the development of strong local and regional food systems. The number of farmers markets increased by more than 67 percent in the last four years and there are now more than 220 regional food hubs in operation around the country.

Section 18.2

Hunger and Food Security

This section contains text excerpted from the following sources: Text
beginning with the heading "What Is Food Security?" is excerpted
from "Food Security in the U.S.," Economic Research Service (ERS),
U.S. Department of Agriculture (USDA), September 8, 2015; Text
under the heading "Household Food Security in the United States
in 2014" is excerpted from "Household Food Security in the United
States in 2014," Economic Research Service (ERS), U.S. Department
of Agriculture (USDA), September 2015.

What Is Food Security?

Food security for a household means access by all members at all
times to enough food for an active, healthy life. Food security includes
at a minimum:

- The ready availability of nutritionally adequate and safe foods.

- Assured ability to acquire acceptable foods in socially acceptable
  ways (that is, without resorting to emergency food supplies,
  scavenging, stealing or other coping strategies).

... and Food Insecurity?

Food insecurity is limited or uncertain availability of nutritionally adequate and safe foods or limited or uncertain ability to acquire
acceptable foods in socially acceptable ways.

(Definitions are from the Life Sciences Research Office, S.A. Ander-
sen, ed., "Core Indicators of Nutritional State for Difficult to Sample
Populations," The Journal of Nutrition 120:1557S-1600S, 1990.)

Does USDA Measure Hunger?

U.S. Department of Agriculture (USDA) does not have a measure of
hunger or the number of hungry people. Prior to 2006, USDA described
households with very low food security as "food insecure with hunger"
and characterized them as households in which one or more people

were hungry at times during the year because they could not afford enough food. "Hunger" in that description referred to "the uneasy or painful sensation caused by lack of food."

In 2006, USDA introduced the new description "very low food security" to replace "food insecurity with hunger," recognizing more explicitly that, although hunger is related to food insecurity, it is a different phenomenon. Food insecurity is a household-level economic and social condition of limited access to food, while hunger is an individual-level physiological condition that may result from food insecurity.

Information about the incidence of hunger is of considerable interest and potential value for policy and program design. But providing precise and useful information about hunger is hampered by lack of a consistent meaning of the word. "Hunger" is understood variously by different people to refer to conditions across a broad range of severity, from rather mild food insecurity to prolonged clinical undernutrition.

USDA sought guidance from the Committee on National Statistics (CNSTAT) of the National Academies on the use of the word "hunger" in connection with food insecurity. The independent panel of experts convened by CNSTAT concluded that in official statistics, resource-constrained hunger (i.e., physiological hunger resulting from food insecurity)"...should refer to a potential consequence of food insecurity that, because of prolonged, involuntary lack of food, results in discomfort, illness, weakness or pain that goes beyond the usual uneasy sensation."

Validated methods have not yet been developed to measure resource-constrained hunger in this sense, in the context of U.S. conditions. Such measurement would require collection of more detailed and extensive information on physiological experiences of individual household members than could be accomplished effectively in the context of USDA's annual household food security survey.

USDA's measurement of food insecurity, then, provides some information about the economic and social contexts that may lead to hunger but does not assess the extent to which hunger actually ensues.

How Are Food Security and Insecurity Measured?

The food security status of each household lies somewhere along a continuum extending from high food security to very low food security. This continuum is divided into four ranges, characterized as follows:

1. **High food security**—Households had no problems or anxiety about, consistently accessing adequate food.

2. **Marginal food security**—Households had problems at times or anxiety about, accessing adequate food, but the quality, variety, and quantity of their food intake were not substantially reduced.

3. **Low food security**—Households reduced the quality, variety, and desirability of their diets, but the quantity of food intake and normal eating patterns were not substantially disrupted.

4. **Very low food security**—At times during the year, eating patterns of one or more household members were disrupted and food intake reduced because the household lacked money and other resources for food.

For most reporting purposes, USDA describes households with high or marginal food security as food secure and those with low or very low food security as food insecure.

Placement on this continuum is determined by the household's responses to a series of questions about behaviors and experiences associated with difficulty in meeting food needs. The questions cover a wide range of severity of food insecurity.

How Many Households Are Interviewed in the National Food Security Surveys?

USDA's food security statistics are based on a national food security survey conducted as an annual supplement to the monthly Current Population Survey (CPS). The CPS is a nationally representative survey conducted by the Census Bureau for the Bureau of Labor Statistics. The CPS provides data for the Nation's monthly unemployment statistics and annual income and poverty statistics.

In December of each year, after completing the labor force interview, about 45,000 households respond to the food security questions and to questions about food spending and about the use of Federal and community food assistance programs. The households interviewed in the CPS are selected to be representative of all civilian households at State and national levels.

Household Food Security in the United States in 2014

Most U.S. households have consistent, dependable access to enough food for active, healthy living—they are food secure. But a minority of American households experience food insecurity at times during the year, meaning that their access to adequate food is limited by a lack of money and other resources. USDA's food and nutrition assistance programs increase food security by providing low-income households access to food, a healthful diet, and nutrition education.

USDA also monitors the extent and severity of food insecurity in U.S. households through an annual, nationally representative survey sponsored and analyzed by USDA's Economic Research Service (ERS). Reliable monitoring of food security contributes to the effective operation of the Federal food assistance programs, as well as that of private food assistance programs and other government initiatives aimed at reducing food insecurity.

What Did the Study Find?

The estimated percentage of U.S. households that were food insecure remained essentially unchanged from 2013 to 2014; however, food insecurity was down from a high of 14.9 percent in 2011. The percentage of households with food insecurity in the severe range—described as very low food security—was unchanged.

- In 2014, 86.0 percent of U.S. households were food secure throughout the year. The remaining 14.0 percent (17.4 million households) were food insecure. Food-insecure households (those with low and very low food security) had difficulty at some time during the year providing enough food for all their members due to a lack of resources. The changes from 2013 (14.3 percent) and 2012 (14.5 percent) to 2014 were not statistically significant; however, the cumulative decline from 14.9 percent in 2011 was statistically significant.

- In 2014, 5.6 percent of U.S. households (6.9 million households) had very low food security, unchanged from 5.6 percent in 2013. In this more severe range of food insecurity, the food intake of some household members was reduced and normal eating patterns were disrupted at times during the year due to limited resources.

- Children were food insecure at times during the year in 9.4 percent of U.S. households with children (3.7 million households), essentially unchanged from 9.9 percent in 2013. These households were unable at times during the year to provide adequate, nutritious food for their children.

- While children are usually shielded from the disrupted eating patterns and reduced food intake that characterize very low food security, both children and adults experienced instances of very low food security in 1.1 percent of households with children (422,000 households) in 2014. The changes from both 2013 and 2012 were not statistically significant.

- For households with incomes near or below the Federal poverty line, households with children headed by single women or single men, women living alone, and Black- and Hispanic-headed households, the rates of food insecurity were substantially higher than the national average. In addition, the food insecurity rate was highest in rural areas, moderate in large cities, and lowest in suburban and exurban areas around large cities.

- The prevalence of food insecurity varied considerably from State to State. Estimated prevalence of food insecurity in 2012-14 ranged from 8.4 percent in North Dakota to 22.0 percent in Mississippi; estimated prevalence rates of very low food security ranged from 2.9 percent in North Dakota to 8.1 percent in Arkansas. (Data for 3 years were combined to provide more reliable State-level statistics.)

- The typical (median) food-secure household spent 26 percent more for food than the typical food-insecure household of the same size and composition, including food purchased with Supplemental Nutrition Assistance Program (SNAP) benefits (formerly the Food Stamp Program).

- Sixty-one percent of food-insecure households in the survey reported that in the previous month, they had participated in one or more of the three largest Federal food and nutrition assistance programs (SNAP; Special Supplemental Nutrition Program for Women, Infants, and Children (WIC); and National School Lunch Program).

Chapter 19

Smart Food Shopping

Chapter Contents

Section 19.1

Making Healthy Food Choices

This section includes text excerpted from "Tips for Eating Right," National Heart, Lung, and Blood Institute (NHLBI), February 13, 2013.

Tips for Eating Right

Small steps can help your family get on the road to maintaining a healthy weight. Choose a different tip each week for you and your family to try. See if you or they can add to the list. Here are a few:

Change Your Shopping Habits

- Eat before grocery shopping.
- Make a grocery list before you shop.
- Choose a checkout line without a candy display.
- Buy and try serving a new fruit or vegetable (ever had jicama, fava beans, plantain, bokchoy, starfruit or papaya?).

Watch Your Portion Size

- Share an entree with someone.
- If entrees are large, choose an appetizer or side dish.
- Don't serve seconds.
- Share dessert or choose fruit instead.
- Eat sweet foods in small amounts. To reduce temptation, don't keep sweets at home.
- Cut or share high-calorie foods like cheese and chocolate into small pieces and only eat a few pieces.
- Eat off smaller plates.
- Skip buffets.

Change the Way You Prepare Food

- Cut back on added fats and/or oils in cooking or spreads.
- Grill, steam or bake instead of frying.
- Make foods flavorful with herbs, spices, and low-fat seasonings.
- Use fat-free or low-fat sour cream, mayo, sauces, dressings, and condiments.
- Serve several whole-grain foods every day.
- Top off cereal with sliced apples or bananas.

Change Your Eating Habits

- Keep to a regular eating schedule.
- Eat together as a family most days of the week.
- Eat before you get too hungry.
- Make sure every family member eats breakfast every day.
- Drink water before a meal.
- Stop eating when you're full.
- Don't eat late at night.
- Try a green salad instead of fries.
- Ask for salad dressing "on the side."
- Chew slowly every time you eat and remind others to enjoy every bite.
- Serve water or low-fat milk at meals, instead of soda or other sugary drinks.
- Pay attention to flavors and textures.
- Instead of eating out, bring a healthy, low-calorie lunch to work and pack a healthy "brown bag" for your kids.
- Provide fruits and vegetables for snacks.
- Ask your sweetie to bring you fruit or flowers instead of chocolate.

Section 19.2

Stretch Your Food Dollar

This section contains text excerpted from the following sources:
Text in this section begins with excerpts from "Save More at
the Grocery Store," ChooseMyPlate.gov, U.S. Department of
Agriculture (USDA), September 1, 2015; Text under the heading
"Smart Shopping for Veggies and Fruits" is excerpted from
"Smart Shopping for Veggies and Fruits: 10 Tips for Affordable
Vegetables and Fruits," ChooseMyPlate.gov, U.S. Department of
Agriculture (USDA), October 2012. Reviewed June 2016.

Using coupons and looking for the best price are great ways to save money at the grocery store. Knowing how to find them is the first step to cutting costs on food.

1. **Find deals right under your nose**

   Look for coupons with your receipt, as peel-offs on items, and on signs along aisle shelves.

2. **Search for coupons**

   Many stores still send ads and coupons for promotion, so don't overlook that so-called "junk mail." You can also do a Web search for "coupons." Go through your coupons at least once a month and toss out any expired ones.

3. **Look for savings in the newspaper**

   Brand name coupons are found as inserts in the paper every Sunday—except on holiday weekends. Some stores will double the value of brand name coupons on certain days.

4. **Join your store's loyalty program**

   Signup is usually free and you can receive savings and electronic coupons when you provide your email address.

5. **Buy when foods are on sale**

   Maximize your savings by using coupons on sale items. You may find huge deals such as "buy one get one free."

6. **Find out if the store will match competitors' coupons**

   Many stores will accept coupons, as long as they are for the same item. Check with the customer service desk for further details.

7. **Stay organized so coupons are easy to find**

   Sort your coupons either by item or in alphabetical order. Develop a system that's easiest for you and make finding coupons quick and hassle-free. Ideas for coupon storage include 3-ring binders, accordion-style organizers or plain envelopes.

8. **Find a coupon buddy**

   Swap coupons you won't use with a friend. You can get rid of clutter and discover additional discounts.

9. **Compare brands**

   Store brands can be less expensive than some of the name brand foods. Compare the items to find better prices.

10. **Stick to the list**

    Make a shopping list for all the items you need. Keep a running list on your phone, on the refrigerator or in a wallet. When you're in the store, do your best to buy only the items on your list.

Smart Shopping for Veggies and Fruits

It is possible to fit vegetables and fruits into any budget. Making nutritious choices does not have to hurt your wallet. Getting enough of these foods promotes health and can reduce your risk of certain diseases. There are many low-cost ways to meet your fruit and vegetable needs.

- **Celebrate the season**

  Use fresh vegetables and fruits that are in season. They are easy to get, have more flavor, and are usually less expensive. Your local farmer's market is a great source of seasonal produce.

- **Try canned or frozen**

  Compare the price and the number of servings from fresh, canned, and frozen forms of the same veggie or fruit. Canned and frozen items may be less expensive than fresh. For canned items, choose fruit canned in 100% fruit juice and vegetables with "low sodium" or "no salt added" on the label.

- **Buy small amounts frequently**

  Some fresh vegetables and fruits don't last long. Buy small amounts more often to ensure you can eat the foods without throwing any away.

- **Buy in bulk when items are on sale**

  For fresh vegetables or fruits you use often, a large size bag is the better buy. Canned or frozen fruits or vegetables can be bought in large quantities when they are on sale, since they last much longer.

- **Store brands = savings**

  Opt for store brands when possible. You will get the same or similar product for a cheaper price. If your grocery store has a membership card, sign up for even more savings.

- **Keep it simple**

  Buy vegetables and fruits in their simplest form. Pre-cut, pre-washed, ready-to-eat, and processed foods are convenient, but often cost much more than when purchased in their basic forms.

- **Plant your own**

  Start a garden—in the yard or a pot on the deck—for fresh, inexpensive, flavorful additions to meals. Herbs, cucumbers, peppers or tomatoes are good options for beginners. Browse through a local library or online for more information on starting a garden.

- **Plan and cook smart**

  Prepare and freeze vegetable soups, stews or other dishes in advance. This saves time and money. Add leftover vegetables to casseroles or blend them to make soup. Overripe fruit is great for smoothies or baking.

Chapter 20

The Health Benefits of Eating Breakfast

Why Is Breakfast the Most Important Meal of the Day?

Almost everyone is familiar with the idea that breakfast is the most important meal of the day, but the reasons behind that idea may not be so well known. For most people, the time between yesterday's evening meal and this morning's breakfast is the longest period of time that the body goes without food each day. This means that breakfast has a physical effect on the body that is different than any other meal. Eating breakfast within two hours of waking helps the body's metabolism to operate more efficiently, provides a burst of energy to begin the day's activities, helps to curb appetite throughout the day, and can aid in weight management.

Eating a healthy breakfast that contains a variety of foods such as whole grains, dairy, cereal, and fruit makes a difference in the way the body processes blood sugar levels. Sometimes called the "second-meal effect," breakfast kick-starts the metabolism and makes it easier for the body to absorb nutrients and regulate blood sugar throughout the rest of the day. Without breakfast, the body experiences prolonged fasting that triggers a spike in hunger-related hormones, which in turn leads to fluctuating blood sugar levels throughout the day. These fluctuations can cause people to feel tired, irritable, and unable to concentrate on tasks. People who eat a healthy breakfast every day tend to maintain better diets overall and weigh less than people who don't eat breakfast. This is because when the metabolism gets moving with breakfast, the body begins to burn more calories converting food to energy.

Breakfast is especially important for school-aged children. Eating breakfast boosts brain function, enhances memory, and improves concentration, attention span, reasoning, creativity, and learning abilities. Eating a healthy breakfast every day has also been linked to improved academic performance. Children who eat breakfast tend to be more active, have fewer health problems, and fewer absences from school. As with adults, children who eat breakfast also tend to consume fewer calories later in the day. Those who skip breakfast are more likely to overeat during lunch due to excessive hunger.

What Is a Healthy Breakfast?

A healthy breakfast that provides the most physical and mental benefits includes whole grains, dairy, cereal, and fruit, and a balance of carbohydrates, protein, and fiber. Carbohydrates from whole grain bread, muffins, cereals, fruits, and vegetables provide immediate energy that is processed quickly by the body. Longer-term energy from protein in dairy products, lean meats, eggs, nuts, and beans is accessed by the body after the carbohydrates. The fiber in whole-grain breads, waffles, cereals, bran, fruits, vegetables, nuts, and beans helps people feel full longer and discourages overeating. A healthy breakfast is not limited to traditional breakfast foods. As long as a nutritional balance is achieved, breakfast can include leftovers from the previous night's dinner, sandwiches or vegetables and nuts.

Some ideas for a healthy breakfast include:

- Fruit and yogurt
- Fruit and whole-grain cereal with milk
- Whole-grain muffins, pancakes, or waffles with fruit and milk
- Egg omelet with vegetables
- Mixed nuts and dried fruit
- Hard-cooked eggs with whole-wheat bread
- Oatmeal with fruit, nuts, or spices and milk
- Whole-grain toast with peanut butter and fruit and milk

- Cucumbers and hummus with whole-wheat bread or crackers
- Lean turkey with tomato on whole-wheat bread
- Cheese with whole-wheat bread or crackers
- Cheese pizza

Some traditional breakfast items are best avoided, at least on a daily basis. Donuts, pastries, toaster pastries, and certain breakfast bars contain as much fat, sugar, and calories as a regular candy bar. Sugary cereals can be mixed with regular whole-grain cereals to add flavor and fun without the poor nutritional profile of a whole bowl of sugared cereal.

Breakfast Planning

Many people skip breakfast because they don't have time to prepare and eat a meal every morning. A healthy breakfast doesn't have to be complicated or time-consuming, and breakfast can even be planned and prepared the previous night. Rising just ten minutes earlier than usual can provide enough time for everyone to enjoy a bowl of cereal or oatmeal before heading out for the day. Breakfast can be streamlined by stocking the pantry and refrigerator with grab-and-go options such as whole fruit, yogurt parfaits, and individual containers of whole-grain cereals or snack mixes. Peanut butter and whole wheat sandwiches made the night before are another good option.

References

1. Gavin, Mary L, MD. "Breakfast Basics," July 2015.

2. "Why Eating the Right Breakfast is So Important," *Consumer Reports*. August 26, 2015.

3. "Healthy Breakfasts for Kids," U.S. Food and Drug Administration. August 13, 2015.

4. Agan, Cathy, and Terri Crawford. "Smart Choices: Nutrition News for Seniors," Louisiana State University Agricultural Center. n.d.

5. "Why is Breakfast Important?" Agriculture and Horticulture Development Board. 2016

6. Bar-Dayan, Alisa. "The Important of a Healthy Breakfast," April 19, 2010.

Chapter 21

Healthy Eating at Home

Chapter Contents

Section 21.1

The Importance of Family Meals

This section includes excerpts from "Family Meals," © 1995–2016.
The Nemours Foundation/KidsHealth®. Reprinted with permission.

Family Meals

Family meals are making a comeback. And that's good news for a couple of reasons:

- Shared family meals are more likely to be nutritious.

- Kids who eat regularly with their families are less likely to snack on unhealthy foods and more likely to eat fruits, vegetables, and whole grains.

- Teens who take part in regular family meals are less likely to smoke, drink alcohol or use marijuana and other drugs, and are more likely to have healthier diets as adults, studies have shown.

Beyond health and nutrition, family meals provide a valuable opportunity to reconnect. This becomes even more important as kids get older.

Making Family Meals Happen

It can be a big challenge to find the time to plan, prepare, and share family meals, then be relaxed enough to enjoy them.

Try these three steps to schedule family meals and make them enjoyable for everyone who pulls up a chair.

1. Plan

To plan more family meals, look over the calendar to choose a time when everyone can be there.

Figure out what's getting in the way of more family meals—busy schedules, no supplies in the house, no time to cook. Ask for the family's help and ideas on how these roadblocks can be removed. For instance, figure out a way to get groceries purchased for a family meal. Or if time to cook is the problem, try doing some prep work on weekends or even completely preparing a dish ahead of time and putting it in the freezer.

2. Prepare

Once you have all your supplies on hand, involve the kids in preparations. Recruiting younger kids can mean a little extra work, but it's often worth it. Simple tasks such as putting plates on the table, tossing the salad, pouring a beverage, folding the napkins or being a "taster" are appropriate jobs for preschoolers and school-age kids.

Older kids may be able to pitch in even more, such as getting ingredients, washing produce, mixing and stirring, and serving. If you have teens around, consider assigning them a night to cook, with you as the helper.

If kids help out, set a good example by saying please and thanks for their help. Being upbeat and pleasant as you prepare the meal can rub off on your kids. If you're grumbling about the task at hand, chances are they will too. But if the atmosphere is light, you're showing them how the family can work together and enjoy the fruits of its labor.

3. Enjoy

Even if you're thinking of all you must accomplish after dinner's done (doing dishes, making lunches, etc.), try not to focus on that during dinner. Make your time at the table pleasant and a chance for everyone to decompress from the day and enjoy being together as a family.

They may be starving, but have your kids wait until everyone is seated before digging in. Create a moment of calm before the meal begins, so the cook can shift gears. It also presents a chance to say grace, thank the cook, wish everyone a good meal or to raise a glass of milk and toast each other. You're setting the mood and modeling good manners and patience.

Family meals are a good time to teach civilized behavior that kids also can use at restaurants and others' houses, so establish rules about staying seated, passing items instead of grabbing them, putting napkins on laps, and not talking with your mouth full.

You can gently remind when they break the rules, but try to keep tension and discipline at a minimum during mealtime. The focus should remain on making your kids feel loved, connected, and part of the family.

Keep the interactions positive and let the conversation flow. Ask your kids about their days and tell them about yours. Give everyone a chance to talk.

Need some conversation starters? Here are a few:

- If you could have any food for dinner tomorrow night, what would it be?

- Who can guess how many potatoes I used to make that bowl of mashed potatoes?

- What's the most delicious food on the table?

- If you opened a restaurant, what kind would it be?

- Who's the best cook you know? (We hope they say it's you!)

Section 21.2

Healthy Eating Tips for Vegetarians

This section includes text excerpted from "Healthy Eating for Vegetarians," ChooseMyPlate.gov, U.S. Department of Agriculture (USDA), November 13, 2015.

A vegetarian eating pattern can be a healthy option. The key is to consume a variety of foods and the right amount of foods to meet your calorie and nutrient needs.

1. **Think about protein**

    Your protein needs can easily be met by eating a variety of plant foods. Sources of protein for vegetarians include beans and peas, nuts, and soy products (such as tofu, tempeh). Lac-to-ovo vegetarians also get protein from eggs and dairy foods.

2. **Bone up on sources of calcium**

    Calcium is used for building bones and teeth. Some vegetar-ians consume dairy products, which are excellent sources of calcium. Other sources of calcium for vegetarians include cal-cium-fortified soymilk (soy beverage), tofu made with calcium sulfate, calcium-fortified breakfast cereals and orange juice, and some dark-green leafy vegetables (collard, turnip, and mustard greens; and bok choy).

3. Make simple changes

Many popular main dishes are or can be vegetarian—such as pasta primavera, pasta with marinara or pesto sauce, veggie pizza, vegetable lasagna, tofu-vegetable stir-fry, and bean burritos

4. Enjoy a cookout

For barbecues, try veggie or soy burgers, soy hot dogs, marinated tofu or tempeh, and fruit kabobs. Grilled veggies are great, too!

5. Include beans and peas

Because of their high nutrient content, consuming beans and peas is recommended for everyone, vegetarians and nonvegetarians alike. Enjoy some vegetarian chili, three bean salad or split pea soup. Make a hummus filled pita sandwich.

6. Try different veggie versions

A variety of vegetarian products look—and may taste—like their non-vegetarian counterparts but are usually lower in saturated fat and contain no cholesterol. For breakfast, try soy-based sausage patties or links. For dinner, rather than hamburgers, try bean burgers or falafel (chickpea patties).

7. Make some small changes at restaurants

Most restaurants can make vegetarian modifications to menu items by substituting meatless sauces or non meat items, such as tofu and beans for meat, and adding vegetables or pasta in place of meat. Ask about available vegetarian options.

8. Nuts make great snacks

Choose unsalted nuts as a snack and use them in salads or main dishes. Add almonds, walnuts or pecans instead of cheese or meat to a green salad.

9. Get your vitamin B12

Vitamin B12 is naturally found only in animal products. Vegetarians should choose fortified foods such as cereals or soy products or take a vitamin B12 supplement if they do not consume any animal products. Check the Nutrition Facts label for vitamin B12 in fortified products.

10. Find a vegetarian pattern for you

Check the *Dietary Guidelines for Americans* for vegetarian (and vegan) adaptations of the U.S. Department of Agriculture (USDA) food patterns at 12 calorie levels.

Section 21.3

Healthy Cooking and Snacking

This section includes text excerpted from "Healthy Cooking and Snacking," National Heart, Lung, and Blood Institute (NHLBI), February 13, 2013.

Food doesn't have to be high in fat to be good. Get the **whole family** to help slice, dice, and chop, and learn how to cut fat and calories in some foods. You'd be surprised how easy heart healthy cooking and snacking can be.

Healthy Family Snacks

Try these tips for quick and easy snacks:

- Toss sliced apples, berries, bananas or whole-grain cereal on top of fat-free or low-fat yogurt.

- Put a slice of fat-free or low-fat cheese on top of whole-grain crackers.

- Make a whole-wheat pita pocket with hummus, lettuce, tomato, and cucumber.

- Pop some fat-free or low-fat popcorn.

- Microwave or toast a soft whole grain tortilla with fat-free or low-fat cheese and sliced peppers and mushrooms to make a mini-burrito or quesadilla.

- Drink fat-free or low-fat chocolate milk (blend it with a banana or strawberries and some ice for a smoothie).

Healthy Cooking Tips

Make a few changes in the kitchen and you'll be eating healthy in no time.

Tips for Reducing Fat

- Instead of frying, try baking, broiling, boiling or microwaving.
- Choose fat-free or low-fat milk products, salad dressings, and mayonnaise.
- Add salsa on a baked potato instead of butter or sour cream.
- Remove skin from poultry (like chicken or turkey) and do not eat it.
- Cool soups and gravies and skim off fat before reheating them.

Tips for Reducing Sugar

- Serve fruit instead of cookies or ice cream for dessert.
- Eat fruits canned in their own juice rather than syrup.
- Reduce sugar in recipes by 1/4 to 1/3. If a recipe says 1 cup, use 2/3 cup.
- To enhance the flavor when sugar is reduced, add vanilla, cinnamon or nutmeg.

Healthy Baking and Cooking Substitutes

Cut the fat and sugar in your meals by using these substitutes.

Table 21.1. Healthy Baking and Cooking Substitutes

Instead of:	Substitute:
1 cup cream	1 cup evaporated fat-free milk
1 cup butter, margarine or oil	1/2 cup apple butter or applesauce
1 egg	2 egg whites or 1/4 cup egg substitute
Pastry dough	Graham cracker crumb crust
Butter, margarine or vegetable oil for sautéing	Cooking spray, chicken broth or a small amount of olive oil
Bacon	Lean turkey bacon
Ground beef	Extra lean ground beef or ground turkey breast

Table 21.1. Continued

Instead of:	Substitute:
Sour cream	Fat-free sour cream
1 cup chocolate chips	1/4-1/2 cup mini chocolate chips
1 cup sugar	3/4 cup sugar (this works with nearly everything except yeast breads)
1 cup mayonnaise	1 cup fat-free or reduced-fat mayonnaise
1 cup whole milk	1 cup fat-free milk
1 cup cream cheese	1/2 cup ricotta cheese pureed with 1/2 cup fat-free cream cheese
Oil and vinegar dressing with 3 parts oil to 1 part vinegar	1 part olive oil + 1 part vinegar (preferably a flavored vinegar, such as balsamic) + 1 part orange juice
Unsweetened baking chocolate (1 ounce)	3 tablespoons unsweetened cocoa powder + 1 tablespoon vegetable oil or margarine

Chapter 22

Healthy Use of Dietary Supplements

Chapter Contents

273

Section 22.1

Dietary Supplements: What You Need to Know

This section includes text excerpted from "Dietary Supplements: What You Need to Know," U.S. Food and Drug Administration (FDA), June 1, 2016.

You've heard about them, may have used them, and may have even recommended them to friends or family. While some dietary supplements are well understood and established, others need further study.

Before making decisions about whether to take a supplement, talk to your healthcare provider. They can help you achieve a balance between the foods and nutrients you personally need.

What Are Dietary Supplements?

Dietary supplements include such ingredients as vitamins, minerals, herbs, amino acids, and enzymes. Dietary supplements are marketed in forms such as tablets, capsules, softgels, gelcaps, powders, and liquids.

What Are the Benefits of Dietary Supplements?

Some supplements can help assure that you get enough of the vital substances the body needs to function; others may help reduce the risk of disease. But supplements should not replace complete meals which are necessary for a healthful diet–so, be sure you eat a variety of foods as well.

Unlike drugs, **supplements are not intended to treat, diagnose, prevent or cure diseases**. That means supplements should not make claims, such as "reduces pain" or "treats heart disease." Claims like these can only legitimately be made for drugs, not dietary supplements.

Are There Any Risks in Taking Supplements?

Yes. Many supplements contain active ingredients that have strong biological effects in the body. This could make them unsafe in some situations and hurt or complicate your health. For example, the following actions could lead to harmful–even life-threatening–consequences.

- Combining supplements
- Using supplements with medicines (whether prescription or over-the-counter)
- Substituting supplements for prescription medicines
- Taking too much of some supplements, such as vitamin A, vitamin D or iron Some supplements can also have unwanted effects *before, during, and after surgery*. So, be sure to inform your healthcare provider, including your pharmacist about any supplements you are taking

Some Common Dietary Supplements

- Calcium
- Echinacea
- Fish Oil
- Ginseng
- Glucosamine
- Chondroitin Sulphate

- Garlic
- Vitamin D
- St. John Wort
- Saw Palmetto
- Ginkgo
- Green Tea

How Can I Find out More about the Dietary Supplement I'm Taking?

Dietary supplement labels must include name and location information for the manufacturer or distributor.

If you want to know more about the product that you are taking, check with the manufacturer or distributor about:

- Information to support the claims of the product
- Information on the safety and effectiveness of the ingredients in the product

How Can I Be a Smart Supplement Shopper?

Be a savvy supplement user. Here's how:

- When searching for supplements on the internet, use noncommercial sites (e.g., NIH, FDA, USDA) rather than doing blind searches

- Watch out for false statements like "works better than [a prescription drug]," "totally safe," or has "no side effects"

- Be aware that the term *natural* doesn't always means safe

- Ask your healthcare provider for help in distinguishing between reliable and questionable information

- Always remember–safety first!

Report Problems to FDA

Notify FDA if the use of a dietary supplement caused you or a family member to have a serious reaction or illness (even if you are not certain that the product was the cause or you did not visit a doctor or clinic).
Follow these steps:

1. Stop using the product

2. Contact your healthcare provider to find out how to take care of the problem

3. Report problems to FDA in either of these ways:

   i. Contact the Consumer Complaint Coordinator in your area

   ii. File a safety report online through the Safety Reporting Portal

Section 22.2

Safety Tips for Dietary Supplement Users

This section includes text excerpted from "Tips for Dietary Supplement Users," U.S. Food and Drug Administration (FDA), April 4, 2014.

Making Informed Decisions and Evaluating Information

U.S. Food and Drug Administration (FDA), as well as health professionals and their organizations, receive many inquiries each year from consumers seeking health-related information, especially about dietary supplements. Clearly, people choosing to supplement their diets with herbals, vitamins, minerals or other substances want to know more about the products they choose so that they can make informed decisions about them. The choice to use a dietary supplement can be a wise decision that provides health benefits. However, under certain circumstances, these products may be unnecessary for good health or they may even create unexpected risks.

Given the abundance and conflicting nature of information now available about dietary supplements, you may need help to sort the reliable information from the questionable. Below are tips and resources that will help you be a savvy dietary supplement user.

Basic Points to Consider

- **Do I need to think about my total diet?**

  Yes. Dietary supplements are intended to supplement the diets of some people, but not to replace the balance of the variety of foods important to a healthy diet. While you need enough nutrients, too much of some nutrients can cause problems. You can find information on the functions and potential benefits of vitamins and minerals, as well as upper safe limits for nutrients at the National Academy of Sciences Website disclaimer icon.

- **Should I check with my doctor or healthcare provider before using a supplement?**

  This is a good idea, especially for certain population groups. Dietary supplements may not be risk-free under certain circumstances. If you are pregnant, nursing a baby or have a chronic medical condition, such as, diabetes, hypertension or heart disease, be sure to consult your doctor or pharmacist before purchasing or taking any supplement. While vitamin and mineral supplements are widely used and generally considered safe for children, you may wish to check with your doctor or pharmacist before giving these or any other dietary supplements to your child. If you plan to use a dietary supplement in place of drugs or in combination with any drug, tell your healthcare provider first. Many supplements contain active ingredients that have strong biological effects and their safety is not always assured in all users. If you have certain health conditions and take these products, you may be placing yourself at risk.

- **Some supplements may interact with prescription and over-the-counter (OTC) medicines.**

Taking a combination of supplements or using these products together with medications (whether prescription or OTC drugs) could under certain circumstances produce adverse effects, some of which could be life-threatening. Be alert to advisories about these products, whether taken alone or in combination. For example: Coumadin (a prescription medicine), ginkgo biloba (an herbal supplement), aspirin (an OTC drug) and vitamin E (a vitamin supplement) can each thin the blood, and taking any of these products together can increase the potential for internal bleeding. Combining St. John's Wort with certain HIV drugs significantly reduces their effectiveness. St. John's Wort may also reduce the effectiveness of prescription drugs for heart disease, depression, seizures, certain cancers or oral contraceptives.

- **Some supplements can have unwanted effects during surgery:**

  It is important to fully inform your doctor about the vitamins, minerals, herbals or any other supplements you are taking, especially before elective surgery. You may be asked to stop taking these products at least 2-3 weeks ahead of the procedure to avoid potentially dangerous supplement/drug interactions—such as changes in heart rate, blood pressure and increased bleeding-that could adversely affect the outcome of your surgery.

- **Adverse effects from the use of dietary supplements should be reported to MedWatch:**

  You, your healthcare provider or anyone may directly to FDA if you believe it is related to the use of any dietary supplement product, by calling FDA at 1-800-FDA-1088, by fax at 1-800-FDA-0178 or reporting report a serious adverse event or illness on-line. FDA would like to know whenever you think a product caused you a serious problem, even if you are not sure that the product was the cause, and even if you do not visit a doctor or clinic.

- **Who is responsible for ensuring the safety and efficacy of dietary supplements?**

  Under the law, manufacturers of dietary supplements are responsible for making sure their products are safe before they go to market. They are also responsible for determining that the claims on their labels are accurate and truthful. Dietary supplement products are not reviewed by the government before they are marketed, but FDA has the responsibility to take action against any unsafe dietary supplement product that reaches the market. If FDA can prove that claims on marketed dietary supplement products are false and misleading, the agency may take action also against products with such claims.

Tips on Searching the Web for Information on Dietary Supplements

When searching on the Web, try using directory sites of respected organizations, rather than doing blind searches with a search engine. Ask yourself the following questions:

- **Who operates the site?**

  Is the site run by the government, a university or a reputable medical or health-related association (e.g., American Medical Association, American Diabetes Association, American Heart Association, National Institutes of Health, National Academies of Science or U.S. Food and Drug Administration)? Is the information written or reviewed by qualified health professionals, experts in the field, academia, government or the medical community?

- **What is the purpose of the site?**

  Is the purpose of the site to objectively educate the public or just to sell a product? Be aware of practitioners or organizations whose main interest is in marketing products, either directly or through sites with which they are linked. Commercial sites should clearly distinguish scientific information from advertisements. Most nonprofit and government sites contain no advertising; and access to the site and materials offered are usually free

- **What is the source of the information and does it have any references?**

  Has the study been reviewed by recognized scientific experts and published in reputable peer-reviewed scientific journals, like the New England Journal of Medicine? Does the information say "some studies show..." or does it state where the study is listed so that you can check the authenticity of the references? For example, can the study be found in the National Library of Medicine's database of literature citations (PubMed)

- **Is the information current?**

  Check the date when the material was posted or updated. Often new research or other findings are not reflected in old material, e.g., side effects or interactions with other products or new evidence that might have changed earlier thinking. Ideally, health and medical sites should be updated frequently

- **How reliable is the Internet or e-mail solicitations?**

  While the Internet is a rich source of health information, it is also an easy vehicle for spreading myths, hoaxes and rumors about alleged news, studies, products or findings. To avoid falling prey to such hoaxes, be skeptical and watch out for overly emphatic language with UPPERCASE LETTERS and lots of exclamation points!!!! Beware of such phrases such as: "This is not a hoax" or "Send this to everyone you know."

More Tips and To-Do's

- Ask yourself: Does it sound too good to be true?

  Do the claims for the product seem exaggerated or unrealistic? Are there simplistic conclusions being drawn from a complex study to sell a product? While the Web can be a valuable source of accurate, reliable information, it also has a wealth of misinformation that may not be obvious. Learn to distinguish hype from evidence-based science. Nonsensical lingo can sound very convincing. Also, be skeptical about anecdotal information from persons who have no formal training in nutrition or botanicals or from personal testimonials (e.g. from store employees, friends or online chat rooms and message boards) about incredible benefits or results obtained from using a product. Question these people on their training and knowledge in nutrition or medicine.

- Think twice about chasing the latest headline

  Sound health advice is generally based on a body of research, not a single study. Be wary of results claiming a "quick fix" that depart from previous research and scientific beliefs. Keep in mind science does not proceed by dramatic breakthroughs, but by taking many small steps, slowly building towards a consensus. Furthermore, news stories, about the latest scientific study, especially those on TV or radio, are often too brief to include important details that may apply to you or allow you to make an informed decision

- Check your assumptions about the following:

- #1 Questionable Assumption

  "Even if a product may not help me, it at least won't hurt me."
  It's best not to assume that this will always be true. When consumed in high enough amounts, for a long enough time or in
  combination with certain other substances, all chemicals can be
  toxic, including nutrients, plant components, and other biologically active ingredients

- #2 Questionable Assumption

  "When I see the term 'natural,' it means that a product is healthful and safe." Consumers can be misled if they assume this
  term assures wholesomeness or that these food-like substances
  necessarily have milder effects, which makes them safer to use
  than drugs. The term "natural" on labels is not well defined and
  is sometimes used ambiguously to imply unsubstantiated benefits or safety. For example, many weight-loss products claim to
  be "natural" or "herbal" but this doesn't necessarily make them
  safe. Their ingredients may interact with drugs or may be dangerous for people with certain medical conditions

- #3 Questionable Assumption

  "A product is safe when there is no cautionary information on
  the product label." Dietary supplement manufacturers may not
  necessarily include warnings about potential adverse effects on
  the labels of their products. If consumers want to know about
  the safety of a specific dietary supplement, they should contact
  the manufacturer of that brand directly. It is the manufacturer's
  responsibility to determine that the supplement it produces or
  distributes is safe and that there is substantiated evidence that
  the label claims are truthful and not misleading

- #4 Questionable Assumption

  "A recall of a harmful product guarantees that all such harmful products will be immediately and completely removed from
  the marketplace." A product recall of a dietary supplement is
  voluntary and while many manufacturers do their best, a recall
  does not necessarily remove all harmful products from the
  marketplace

Contact the manufacturer for more information about the specific
product that you are purchasing.

If you cannot tell whether the product you are purchasing meets the same standards as those used in the research studies you read about, check with the manufacturer or distributor.

Section 22.3

An Introduction to Probiotics

This section contains text excerpted from the following sources: Text in this section begins with excerpts from "Are Probiotics Good for Your Health?" National Center for Complementary and Integrative Health (NCCIH), August 27, 2013; Text under the heading "What the Science Says about the Effectiveness of Probiotics" is excerpted from "Probiotics: In Depth," National Center for Complementary and Integrative Health (NCCIH), July 2015.

Probiotics are gaining in popularity in the United States, and chances are you've heard about them as "good bacteria" or seen them advertised in your supermarket's yogurt aisle. But what are probiotics, and do they have any real health benefits?

Probiotics are live microorganisms—bacteria, for example—that are either the same or similar to microorganisms found naturally in our bodies. Although we tend to think of bacteria as harmful "germs," many bacteria actually help the body function properly. Probiotics are available as dietary supplements and in dairy foods, and our research tells us that probiotics are among the top five natural products used for children. It is important to note that the U.S. Food and Drug Administration (FDA) has not approved any health claims for probiotics; however, there is some evidence that probiotics may be helpful for conditions such as acute diarrhea, antibiotic-associated diarrhea, and possibly atopic eczema.

What the Science Says about the Effectiveness of Probiotics

Researchers have studied probiotics to find out whether they might help prevent or treat a variety of health problems, including:

- Digestive disorders such as diarrhea caused by infections, antibiotic-associated diarrhea, irritable bowel syndrome, and inflammatory bowel disease

- Allergic disorders such as atopic dermatitis (eczema) and allergic rhinitis (hay fever)

- Tooth decay, periodontal disease, and other oral health problems

- Colic in infants

- Liver disease

- The common cold

- Prevention of necrotizing enterocolitis in very low birth weight infants

There's preliminary evidence that some probiotics are helpful in preventing diarrhea caused by infections and antibiotics and in improving symptoms of irritable bowel syndrome, but more needs to be learned. We still don't know which probiotics are helpful and which are not. We also don't know how much of the probiotic people would have to take or who most likely benefit from taking probiotics would. Even for the conditions that have been studied the most, researchers are still working toward finding the answers to these questions.

Probiotics are not all alike. For example, if a specific kind of *Lactobacillus* helps prevent an illness, that doesn't necessarily mean that another kind of Lactobacillus would have the same effect or that any of the *Bifidobacterium* probiotics would do the same thing.

Although some probiotics have shown promise in research studies, strong scientific evidence to support specific uses of probiotics for most health conditions is lacking. The U.S. Food and Drug Administration (FDA) has not approved any probiotics for preventing or treating any health problem. Some experts have cautioned that the rapid growth in marketing and use of probiotics may have outpaced scientific research for many of their proposed uses and benefits.

How Might Probiotics Work?

Many probiotics are sold as dietary supplements, which do not require FDA approval before they are marketed. Dietary supplement labels may make claims about how the product affects the structure or function of the body without FDA approval, but they cannot make health claims (claims that the product reduces the risk of a disease) without the FDA's consent. If a probiotic is marketed as a drug for specific treatment of a disease or disorder in the future, it will be required to meet more stringent requirements. It must be proven safe and effective for its intended use through clinical trials and be approved by the FDA before it can be sold.

What the Science Says about the Safety and Side Effects of Probiotics

Whether probiotics are likely to be safe for you depends on the state of your health.

- In people who are generally healthy, probiotics have a good safety record. Side effects, if they occur at all, usually consist only of mild digestive symptoms such as gas

- On the other hand, there have been reports linking probiotics to severe side effects, such as dangerous infections, in people with serious underlying medical problems

- The people who are most at risk of severe side effects include critically ill patients, those who have had surgery, very sick infants, and people with weakened immune systems

Even for healthy people, there are uncertainties about the safety of probiotics. Because many research studies on probiotics haven't looked closely at safety, there isn't enough information right now to answer some safety questions. Most of our knowledge about safety comes from studies of *Lactobacillus* and *Bifidobacterium*; less is known about other probiotics. Information on the long-term safety of probiotics is limited, and safety may differ from one type of probiotic to another. For example, even though a National Center for Complementary and Integrative Health (NCCIH)-funded study showed that a particular kind of *Lactobacillus* appears safe in healthy adults age 65 and older, this does not mean that all probiotics would necessarily be safe for people in this age group.

Quality Concerns about Probiotic Products

NCCIH-Funded Research

NCCIH is sponsoring a variety of research projects related to probiotics:

- Whether a specific probiotic is helpful for irritable bowel syndrome

- The mechanisms by which certain probiotics may enhance the response to vaccines

- How prebiotics influence probiotic bacteria

- Whether a yogurt beverage can be used as a way of giving probiotics to children.

Section 22.4

FDA's Role in Regulating Dietary Supplements

This section includes text excerpted from "Questions and Answers on Dietary Supplements," U.S. Food and Drug Administration (FDA), January 2016.

What Is a Dietary Supplement?

Congress defined the term "dietary supplement" in the Dietary Supplement Health and Education Act (DSHEA) of 1994. A dietary supplement is a product taken by mouth that contains a "dietary ingredient" intended to supplement the diet. The "dietary ingredients" in these products may include: vitamins, minerals, herbs or other botanicals, amino acids, and substances such as enzymes, organ tissues, glandulars, and metabolites. Dietary supplements can also be extracts or concentrates, and may be found in many forms such as tablets, capsules, softgels, gelcaps, liquids or powders. They can also be in other forms, such as a bar, but if they are, information on their label must not represent the product as a conventional food or a sole item of a meal or diet. Whatever their form may be, DSHEA places dietary supplements in a special category under the general umbrella of "foods," not drugs, and requires that every supplement be labeled a dietary supplement.

What Is a "New Dietary Ingredient" in a Dietary Supplement?

The Dietary Supplement Health and Education Act (DSHEA) of 1994 defined both of the terms "dietary ingredient" and "new dietary ingredient" as components of dietary supplements. In order for an ingredient of a dietary supplement to be a "dietary ingredient," it must be one or any combination of the following substances:

- a vitamin

- a mineral

- an herb or other botanical

- an amino acid

- a dietary substance for use by man to supplement the diet by increasing the total dietary intake (e.g., enzymes or tissues from organs or glands) or

- a concentrate, metabolite, constituent or extract

A "new dietary ingredient" is one that meets the above definition for a "dietary ingredient" and was not sold in the U.S. in a dietary supplement before October 15, 1994.

What Is FDA's Role in Regulating Dietary Supplements Versus the Manufacturer's Responsibility for Marketing Them?

In October 1994, the Dietary Supplement Health and Education Act (DSHEA) was signed into law by President Clinton. Before this time, dietary supplements were subject to the same regulatory requirements as were other foods. This new law, which amended the Federal Food, Drug, and Cosmetic Act, created a new regulatory framework for the safety and labeling of dietary supplements. Under DSHEA, a firm is responsible for determining that the dietary supplements it manufactures or distributes are safe and that any representations or claims made about them are substantiated by adequate evidence to show that they are not false or misleading. This means that dietary supplements do not need approval from FDA before they are marketed.

Except in the case of a new dietary ingredient, where pre-market review for safety data and other information is required by law, a firm does not have to provide FDA with the evidence it relies on to substantiate safety or effectiveness before or after it markets its products.

Also, manufacturers need to register themselves pursuant to the Bioterrorism Act with FDA before producing or selling supplements. In June, 2007, FDA published comprehensive regulations for Current Good Manufacturing Practices for those who manufacture, package or hold dietary supplement products. These regulations focus on practices that ensure the identity, purity, quality, strength and composition of dietary supplements.

What Information Must the Manufacturer Disclose on the Label of a Dietary Supplement?

FDA regulations require that certain information appear on dietary supplement labels. Information that must be on a dietary supplement label includes: a descriptive name of the product stating that it is a "supplement;" the name and place of business of the manufacturer, packer or distributor; a complete list of ingredients; and the net contents of the product. In addition, each dietary supplement (except for some small volume products or those produced by eligible small businesses) must have nutrition labeling in the form of a "Supplement Facts" panel. This label must identify each dietary ingredient contained in the product.

Must All Ingredients Be Declared on the Label of a Dietary Supplement?

Yes, ingredients not listed on the "Supplement Facts" panel must be listed in the "other ingredient" statement beneath the panel. The types of ingredients listed there could include the source of dietary ingredients, if not identified in the "Supplement Facts" panel (e.g., rose hips as the source of vitamin C), other food ingredients (e.g., water and sugar), and technical additives or processing aids (e.g., gelatin, starch, colors, stabilizers, preservatives, and flavors).

Is It Legal to Market a Dietary Supplement Product as a Treatment or Cure for a Specific Disease or Condition?

No, a product sold as a dietary supplement and promoted on its label or in labeling* as a treatment, prevention or cure for a specific disease or condition would be considered an unapproved—and thus illegal—drug. To maintain the product's status as a dietary supplement, the label and labeling must be consistent with the provisions in the Dietary Supplement Health and Education Act (DSHEA) of 1994.

Labeling refers to the label as well as accompanying material that is used by a manufacturer to promote and market a specific product.

Who Validates Claims and What Kinds of Claims Can Be Made on Dietary Supplement Labels?

FDA receives many consumer inquiries about the validity of claims for dietary supplements, including product labels, advertisements, media, and printed materials. The responsibility for ensuring the validity of these claims rests with the manufacturer, FDA, and, in the case of advertising, with the Federal Trade Commission. By law, manufacturers may make three types of claims for their dietary supplement products: health claims, structure/function claims, and nutrient content claims. Some of these claims describe: the link between a food substance and disease or a health-related condition; the intended benefits of using the product; or the amount of a nutrient or dietary substance in a product. Different requirements generally apply to each type of claim, and are described in more detail.

Why Do Some Supplements Have Wording (a Disclaimer) That Says: "This Statement Has Not Been Evaluated by the FDA. This Product Is Not Intended to Diagnose, Treat, Cure or Prevent Any Disease"?

This statement or "disclaimer" is required by law (DSHEA) when a manufacturer makes a structure/function claim on a dietary supplement label. In general, these claims describe the role of a nutrient or dietary ingredient intended to affect the structure or function of the body. The manufacturer is responsible for ensuring the accuracy and truthfulness of these claims; they are not approved by FDA. For this reason, the law says that if a dietary supplement label includes such a claim, it must state in a "disclaimer" that FDA has not evaluated this claim. The disclaimer must also state that this product is not intended to "diagnose, treat, cure or prevent any disease," because only a drug can legally make such a claim.

How Are Advertisements for Dietary Supplements Regulated?

The Federal Trade Commission (FTC) regulates advertising, including infomercials, for dietary supplements and most other products sold to consumers. FDA works closely with FTC in this area, but FTC's work is directed by different laws. Advertising and promotional material received in the mail are also regulated under different laws and are subject to regulation by the U.S. Postal Inspection Service.

How Do I, My healthcare Provider or Any Informed Individual Report a Problem or Illness Caused by a Dietary Supplement to FDA?

If you think you have suffered a serious harmful effect or illness from a dietary supplement, the first thing you should do is contact or see your healthcare provider immediately. Then, you or your healthcare provider can report this by submitting a report through the Safety Reporting Portal. If you do not have access to the internet, you may submit a report by calling FDA's MedWatch hotline at 1-800-FDA-1088.

Chapter 23

Organic Food

Chapter Contents

Section 23.1

The Market for Organic Food

This section includes text excerpted from "Organic Agriculture,"
Economic Research Service (ERS), U.S. Department of Agriculture
(USDA), May 7, 2014.

Consumer demand for organically produced goods continues to show double-digit growth, providing market incentives for U.S. farmers across a broad range of products. Organic products are now available in nearly 20,000 natural food stores and nearly 3 out of 4 conventional grocery stores. Organic sales account for over 4 percent of total U.S. food sales, according to recent industry statistics.

- Organic food is sold to consumers through three main venues in the United States—conventional grocery stores, natural food stores, and direct-to-consumer markets.

- A typical organic consumer is difficult to pinpoint, but new research continues to shed light on consumer attitudes and purchasing behavior.

- Organic price premiums continue to remain high in many markets as the demand for organic products expands.

Organic Sales Widen in All Food Categories

U.S. Department of Agriculture (USDA) does not have official statistics on U.S. organic retail sales, but information is available from industry sources. U.S. sales of organic products were an estimated $28.4 billion in 2012—over 4 percent of total food sales—and will reach an estimated $35 billion in 2014, according to the *Nutrition Business Journal.*

Fresh fruits and vegetables have been the top selling category of organically grown food since the organic food industry started retailing products over 3 decades ago, and they are still outselling other food categories, according to the *Nutrition Business Journal.* Produce accounted for 43 percent of U.S. organic food sales in 2012, followed by dairy (15 percent), packaged/prepared foods (11 percent), beverages

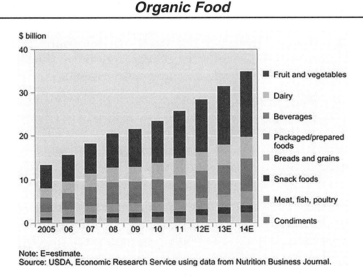

$ billion

Note: E=estimate.
Source: USDA, Economic Research Service using data from Nutrition Business Journal.

Figure 23.1. *U.S. Organic Food Sales by Category, 2005-14E*

(11 percent), bread/grains (9 percent), snack foods (5 percent), meat/fish/poultry (3 percent), and condiments (3 percent).

Most organic sales (93 percent) take place through conventional and natural food supermarkets and chains, according to the Organic Trade Association (OTA). OTA estimates the remaining 7 percent of U.S. organic food sales occur through farmers' markets, food service, and marketing channels other than retail stores. One of the most striking differences between conventional and organic food marketing is the use of direct markets—Cornell University estimates that only about 1.6 percent of U.S. fresh produce sales are through direct sales. The number of farmers' markets in the United States has grown steadily from 1,755 markets in 1994, when USDA began to track them, to over 8,144 in 2013. Participating farmers are responding to heightened demand for locally grown organic product.

A USDA survey of market managers found that demand for organic products was strong or moderate in most of the farmers' markets surveyed around the country, and that managers felt more organic farmers were needed to meet consumer demand in many States.

Organic Price Premiums Remain High

Over the last decade, USDA's Agricultural Marketing Service (AMS) has expanded wholesale price reporting for organic fruits and vegetables, and added new price reports on organic grains, poultry and eggs, and sales volume for milk. Prices for organic products continue to be higher than for their conventional counterparts.

- *AMS Market News* publishes organic prices for fruit and vegetable crops in a number of terminal markets where prices are collected, including Atlanta and San Francisco. See ERS (Economic Research Service) data on organic farmgate and wholesale prices for a comparison of organic and conventional prices from 1999 to 2013.

- *Market News* began reporting organic poultry prices in the weekly Organic Poultry and Egg report in January 2004. The report tracks prices paid to poultry or egg companies by the first receiver (such as a retailer, distributor or manufacturer).

- In January 2006, AMS began reporting sales (in volume) of organic fluid milk products in monthly milk marketing order reports.

- In January 2007, AMS began biweekly regional price reporting on organic grains, and now publishes single national grain and feedstuffs report available through the Market News website.

At the retail level, organic produce and milk, the two top organic food sales categories, receive significant price premiums over conventionally grown products.

ERS analyzed organic prices for 18 fruits and 19 vegetables using 2005 data on produce purchases, and found that the organic premium as a share of the corresponding conventional price was less than 30 percent for over two-thirds of the items. The premium for only one item—blueberries—exceeded 100 percent. In contrast, in 2006, organic price premiums for a half-gallon container of milk ranged from 60 percent for private-label organic milk above branded conventional milk to 109 percent for branded organic milk above private-label conventional milk.

Organic Consumers Are Increasingly Mainstream

Numerous studies have been conducted on the buying habits and demographics of consumers of organic foods. Results have varied depending on the type of survey, sample size, and geographic coverage. However, a few general themes have emerged.

Consumers prefer organically produced food because of their concerns regarding health, the environment, and animal welfare, and they show a willingness to pay the price premiums established in the marketplace.

Organic products have shifted from being a lifestyle choice for a small share of consumers to being consumed at least occasionally by a majority of Americans. National surveys conducted by the Hartman Group and Food Marketing Institute during the early 2000s found that two-thirds of surveyed shoppers bought organically grown foods.

Section 23.2

Understanding Organic Labeling

This section includes text excerpted from "Labeling Organic Products," Agricultural Marketing Service (AMS), U.S. Department of Agriculture (USDA), October 2012. Reviewed June 2016.

Organic products have strict production and labeling requirements. Unless noted below, organic products must meet the following requirements:

- Produced without excluded methods (e.g., genetic engineering), ionizing radiation or sewage sludge.

- Produced per the National List of Allowed and Prohibited Substances (National List).

- Overseen by a U.S. Department of Agriculture (USDA) National Organic Program authorized certifying agent, following all USDA organic regulations.

Overall, if you make a product and want to claim that it or its ingredients are organic, your final product probably needs to be certified. If you are not certified, you must not make any organic claim on the principal display panel or use the USDA organic seal anywhere on the package. You may only, on the information panel, identify the certified organic ingredients as organic and the percentage of organic ingredients.

- **Principal Display Panel:** portion of the package most likely to be seen by customers at the time of purchase.

- **Information Panel:** includes ingredient statement (list of ingredients contained in a product, from highest to lowest percentage of final product) and other product information.

Your certifying agent will review and approve each of your product labels to ensure compliance.

100 Percent Organic

Raw or processed agricultural products in the "100 percent organic" category:

- Must meet these criteria:

  - All ingredients must be certified organic.

  - Any processing aids must be organic.

  - Product labels must state the name of the certifying agent on the information panel.

- May include USDA organic seal and/or 100 percent organic claim.

- Must identify organic ingredients (e.g., organic dill) or via asterisk or other mark.

Organic

Raw or processed agricultural products in the "organic" category:

- Must meet these criteria:

  - All agricultural ingredients must be certified organic, except where specified on National List.

  - Non-organic ingredients allowed per National List may be used, up to a combined total of five percent of non-organic content (excluding salt and water).

  - Product labels must state the name of the certifying agent on the information panel.

- May include USDA organic seal and/or organic claim.

- Must identify organic ingredients (e.g., organic dill) or via asterisk or other mark.

"Made With" Organic

Multi-ingredient agricultural products in the "made with" category:

- Must meet these criteria:
  - At least 70 percent of the product must be certified organic ingredients (excluding salt and water).
  - Any remaining agricultural products are not required to be organically produced but must be produced without excluded methods.
  - Non-agricultural products must be specifically allowed on the National List.
  - Product labels must state the name of the certifying agent on the information panel.
- May state "made with organic (insert up to three ingredients or ingredient categories)." Must not include USDA organic seal anywhere, represent finished product as organic or state "made with organic ingredients."
- Must identify organic ingredients (e.g., organic dill) or via asterisk or other mark.

Specific Organic Ingredients

Multi-ingredient products with less than 70 percent certified organic content (excluding salt and water) don't need to be certified. Any non-certified product:

- Must not include USDA organic seal anywhere or the word "organic" on principal display panel.
- May only list certified organic ingredients as organic in the ingredient list and the percentage of organic ingredients. Remaining ingredients are not required to follow the USDA organic regulations.

Based on the label, IF the product contains at least 70 percent certified organic content (excluding salt and water) AND is overseen by a certifying agent, your muffin mix would qualify for the "made with" organic labeling category. To qualify for the "organic" category and use the USDA organic seal, your blueberries and cinnamon would also need to be certified organic.

Alcohol: In addition to the USDA organic requirements, alcoholic beverages must meet the Alcohol and Tobacco Tax and Trade Bureau (TTB) regulations, including sulfite labeling requirements. Any use of added sulfites means that the wine is only eligible for the "made with" labeling category and may not use the USDA organic seal.

Please note that sulfites may only be added to wine "made with" organic grapes; wine labeled as "made with" other organic fruit (e.g., apples) may not contain added sulfites. Organic alcohol labels must be reviewed by an organic certifying agent and the TTB.

Chapter 24

Healthy Eating Out

Chapter Contents

Section 24.1

Tips for Eating Out

This section contains text excerpted from documents published
by two public domain sources. Text under the heading marked
1 is excerpted from "Tips for Eating Out," National Heart,
Lung, and Blood Institute (NHLBI), December 2013; Text
under the heading marked 2 is excerpted from "Eating Foods
Away from Home," ChooseMyPlate.gov, U.S. Department of
Agriculture (USDA), June 2015.

Eating Foods Away from Home[1]

Restaurants, convenience and grocery stores or fast-food places
offer a variety of options when eating out. But larger portions and too
many extras can make it difficult to stay within your calorie needs.
Think about ways to make healthier choices when eating food away
from home.

General Tips[2]

- Let the restaurant know your dietary needs, so they can suggest
  ways to meet your needs, if possible.

- Instead of buffets, order healthy choices from the menu.

- On the day you are planning to eat out, eat foods with less
  sodium in your other meals and snacks. Many meals at restaurants are high in sodium.

- Ask that no salt be added to your meal.

- When eating Asian food, use light soy sauce to season the food.

For Main Dishes

- Choose rotisserie-style chicken rather than fried chicken.
  Always remove the skin.

- Order pizza with vegetable toppings, such as peppers, mushrooms or onions. Ask for half the usual amount of cheese.

- Choose grilled, steamed or baked fish instead of deep-fried fish.
- Leave off all butter, gravy, and sauces.
- Make sure the restaurant does not use monosodium glutamate (MSG) in the dishes. MSG is high in sodium!

For Side Dishes

- Choose a baked potato over french fries.
- Share a small order of french fries instead of eating a large order by yourself.
- Use low-calorie, low-fat salad dressing. Ask that it be served on the side, and use less
- Order a green vegetable or salad instead of two or more starches.
- Ask for low-fat cheese and lowfat sour cream.

10 Tips for Eating Out[1]

1. **Consider your drink**

   Choose water, fat-free or low-fat milk, unsweetened tea, and other drinks without added sugars to complement your meal.

2. **Savor a salad**

   Start your meal with a salad packed with vegetables to help you feel satisfied sooner. Ask for dressing on the side and use a small amount of it.

3. **Share a main dish**

   Divide a main entree between family and friends. Ask for small plates for everyone at the table.

4. **Select from the sides**

   Order a side dish or an appetizer-sized portion instead of a regular entree. They're usually served on smaller plates and in smaller amounts.

5. **Pack your snack**

   Pack fruit, sliced vegetables, low-fat string cheese or unsalted nuts to eat during road trips or long commutes. No need to stop for other food when these snacks are ready-to-eat.

6. **Fill your plate with vegetables and fruit**

   Stir-fries, kabobs or vegetarian options are usually filled with vegetables. Order options without creamy sauces or heavy gravies. Select fruits for dessert.

7. **Compare the calories, fat, and sodium**

   Many menus now include nutrition information. Look for items that are lower in calories, saturated fat, and sodium. Check with your server if you don't see them on the menu

8. **Pass on the buffet**

   Have an item from the menu and avoid the "all-you-can-eat" buffet. Steamed, grilled or broiled dishes have fewer calories than foods that are fried in oil or cooked in butter.

9. **Get your whole grains**

   Request 100% whole-wheat breads, rolls, and pasta when choosing sandwiches, burgers or main dishes.

10. **Quit the "clean your plate club"**

    When you've eaten enough food, leave the rest. Take leftovers home in a container and chill in the refrigerator right away.

Section 24.2

Making Healthy Fast Food Choices

This section contains text excerpted from the following sources: Text beginning with the heading "Food Away from Home" is excerpted from "Food Consumption and Demand," Economic Research Service (ERS), U.S. Department of Agriculture (USDA), October 29, 2014; Text under the heading "Fast-Food Alternatives" is excerpted from "Fast-Food Alternatives," U.S. Department of Veterans Affairs (VA), March 23, 2016; Text under the heading "Eating Healthy at Restaurants" is excerpted from "Eating Healthy at Restaurants," Office on Women's Health (OWH), U.S. Department of Health and Human Services (HHS), January 13, 2014.

Food Away from Home

Consumption of food prepared away from home plays an increasingly large role in the American diet. In 1970, 25.9 percent of all food spending was on food away from home; by 2012, that share rose to its highest level of 43.1 percent. A number of factors contributed to the trend of increased dining out since the 1970s, including a larger share of women employed outside the home, more two-earner households, higher incomes, more affordable and convenient fast food outlets, increased advertising and promotion by large foodservice chains, and the smaller size of U.S. households.

Between 1977-78 and 2005-08, U.S. consumption of food prepared away from home increased from 18 to 32 percent of total calories. Meals and snacks based on food prepared away from home contained more calories per eating occasion than those based on at-home food. Away-from-home food was also higher in nutrients that Americans over consume (such as fat and saturated fat) and lower in nutrients that Americans under consume (calcium, fiber, and iron). Inroads are being made to improve the quality of American's diets, but the rising popularity of eating out presents a challenge for Americans.

Fast-Food Alternatives

Eat These Healthy Choices

Non-Starchy Vegetables and Fruits

1. Salad with low-fat dressings.

2. Grilled, steamed or stir-fried veggies.

3. Fresh fruits.

4. Edamame, cucumber salad.

Limit These Less Healthy Choices

1. Cream veggies, cheese vegetables.

2. Mayonnaise-based salads.

3. Fried or tempura veggies.

4. Fruits canned in sugar or syrup.

5. Salads with fried or crisp noodles.

Eat These Healthy Choices

Whole Grains and/or Starchy Vegetables

1. Baked potato.

2. Steamed brown rice.

3. Herb-seasoned squash, peas, corn, yams.

4. Beans without added fat: green, kidney, black, garbanzo.

5. Small whole grain bread (pumpernickel, rye).

6. Small whole grain dinner roll, English muffin, breadstick or French baguette.

7. Whole grain crackers.

8. Pasta primavera.

Limit These Less Healthy Choices

1. French fries or onion rings.

2. Fried rice.

3. Butter, fried, creamed veggies.

4. Refried beans and/or beans with added fat.

5. Croissants.

6. Biscuits, cornbread, muffins or garlic bread.

7. Tortilla chips or buttered popcorn.

8. Alfredo or cream sauce pasta.

Eat These Healthy Choices

Lean Meat/Protein

1. Grilled, roasted, smoked chicken (white meat/no skin).

2. Grilled, boiled, broiled, baked, smoked fish.

3. Fish and chicken tacos.

4. Grilled, broiled sirloin, filet steak.

5. Turkey, roast beef, lean ham, veggie burger, turkey burger, turkey dogs.

6. Pork tenderloin, grilled lean pork.

7. Steamed or baked tofu.

Limit These Less Healthy Choices

1. Fried, breaded, popcorn chicken and wings.

2. Fried or breaded fish.

3. Beef tacos.

4. Rib eye, prime rib.

5. Large or double hamburgers or cheeseburgers, bologna, hot dogs, pastrami, corned beef Fried pork.

6. Deep-fried tofu.

Combination and Miscellaneous Foods

Not everything fits neatly in the sections of the Healthy Plate, for example a lean roast beef sandwich can fit in the category of lean protein (roast beef) with the whole grain bread fitting in the healthy grain section. Here are some combo foods and some miscellaneous items that do not fit perfectly in a section of the Healthy Plate.

Table 24.1. Combination and Miscellaneous Foods:

Eat These Healthy Choices	Limit These Less Healthy Choices
1. Stir fry with vegetables and lean meat 2. Pasta primavera or vegetable pasta salad 3. Thin-crust veggie pizza with less cheese 4. Meatless, low-fat cheese lasagna Stuffed bell peppers with lean beef 5. Egg on English muffin 6. Whole grain 6-inch sub–more veggies, less sauces 7. Antipasto with vegetables	1. Pot pies 2. Macaroni and cheese 3. Meat-lovers pizza, thick-crust or butter-crust pizza with extra cheese 4. Meat and cheese lasagna 5. Shepherd's pie 6. Burrito with steak 7. Foot-long sub with cheese and sauces 8. Antipasto with meat
Dairy: Free (skim) or low-fat (1%) varieties of: 1. Milk fat 2. Cottage cheese 3. Cheese 4. Sherbet, sorbet 5. Yogurt parfait	1. Whole milk (4% fat) 2. Cottage cheese (4% fat) 3. Cheeses 4. Ice cream 5. Milkshake
Appetizers: 1. Clear or tomato-based soups 2. Salad with low-fat dressing 3. Shrimp with cocktail sauce 4. Raw vegetable sticks 5. Steamed vegetable or chicken dumplings 6. Egg drop, miso, wonton or hot and sour soups	1. Chowder or cream soups 2. Mozzarella sticks 3. Nachos, onion rings, potato skins 4. Fried/tempura vegetables 5. Fried chicken wings 6. Fried egg roll or wonton
Desserts: 1. Soft-serve ice cream 2. Soft-serve frozen yogurt 3. Fruit 4. Low-fat yogurt 5. Sugar-free gelatin 6. Sugar-free pudding	1. Sundaes 2. Cheesecake 3. Banana splits 4. Fried ice cream 5. Cakes, pies, and brownies 6. Cookies

Table 24.1. Continued

Eat These Healthy Choices	Limit These Less Healthy Choices
Beverages: 1. Water, seltzer 2. Low-fat milk 3. Coffee 4. Unsweetened tea 5. Sugar-free drinks 6. 100% juice	1. Beer 2. Sugar-sweetened soda 3. Sport drinks 4. Sweetened tea 5. Alcoholic beverages 6. Juice drinks
Condiments: 1. Light dressing 2. Butter spray, olive oil 3. Pickles 4. Mustard 5. Ketchup 6. Vinegar 7. Hot sauce 8. Low-fat sour cream or fresh salsa 9. Fresh fruit jelly 10. Sauces such as rice-wine vinegar, ponzu, wasabi, ginger, and low sodium soy sauce	1. Mayonnaise 2. Butter 3. Bacon bits or Chinese noodles 4. Tartar sauce or mayo 5. Thousand Island dressing 6. High-calorie dips 7. Gravy 8. Sour cream 9. Regular jelly or spreads 10. Coconut milk, sweet and sour sauce, regular soy sauce

Tips for Making Healthier Fast-Food Choices

- Make careful menu selections—pay attention to menu descriptions

- Avoid dishes labeled deep-fried, pan-fried, basted, batter-dipped, breaded, creamy, crispy, scalloped, Alfredo, au gratin or in cream sauce.

- Order items with more vegetables and choose lean proteins that are baked, broiled or grilled rather than fried.

- Drink water with your meal

- Many beverages are a huge source of hidden calories. Try adding a little lemon to your water or ordering unsweetened iced tea.

- "Undress" your food

- Leave off the cheese and hold the mayo!

- Avoid creamy dressings, spreads, cheeses, and sour cream.

- If you add condiments, like ketchup, use small amounts.

- Do NOT Super-Size!

- Say "No" to "Would you like fries (or pie or cookies) with that?"

Eating Healthy at Restaurants

Eating out can be fun and convenient. But restaurant meals can be super-big and come with lots of extra calories, sugar, sodium, and fat.

Check out one example: Let's say you eat a double burger, fries, and a shake.

- You will have eaten almost 2,000 calories, which is around the total number of calories you probably should eat in a whole day.

- You will have eaten around a day's worth of saturated fat, which is a type of fat that is bad for your heart.

- You'll be eating more sodium than is recommended for the whole day.

One great step is to try to limit how often you eat fast food. And when you eat out, learn about your choices. That should be easier now that some restaurants have started listing nutrition information on menus. More restaurants will start offering the info, too, because the government has passed a law that will require many of them to do this.

To get started, you can look at a couple of healthier options from your favorite food places. These choices have fewer calories and less saturated fat (which is an unhealthy kind of fat) than other items.

Keep in mind that although salads are often a healthier choice at restaurants, adding lots of regular salad dressing can make the calorie level much higher. If you're trying to keep your weight healthy, choose a "light" dressing and ask for it on the side.

Chapter 25

Sports Nutrition

Chapter Contents

Section 25.1

Nutrition for Athletes

This section includes excerpts from "A Guide to Eating for Sports," ©
1995–2016. The Nemours Foundation/KidsHealth®. Reprinted with
permission

Eat Extra for Excellence

There's a lot more to eating for sports than chowing down on carbs
or chugging sports drinks. The good news is that eating to reach your
peak performance level likely doesn't require a special diet or supplements. It's all about working the right foods into your fitness plan in
the right amounts.

Teen athletes have unique nutrition needs. Because athletes work
out more than their less-active peers, they generally need extra calories to fuel both their sports performance and their growth. Depending
on how active they are, teen athletes may need anywhere from 2,000
to 5,000 total calories per day to meet their energy needs.

So what happens if teen athletes don't eat enough? Their bodies
are less likely to achieve peak performance and may even break down
rather than build up muscles. Athletes who don't take in enough calories every day won't be as fast and as strong as they could be and may
not be able to maintain their weight. And extreme calorie restriction
can lead to growth problems and other serious health risks for both
girls and guys, including increased risk for fractures and other injuries.

Athletes and Dieting

Since teen athletes need extra fuel, it's usually a bad idea to diet.
Athletes in sports where weight is emphasized—such as wrestling,
swimming, dance or gymnastics—might feel pressure to lose weight,
but they need to balance that choice with the possible negative side
effects mentioned above.

If a coach, gym teacher or teammate says that you need to go on
a diet, talk to your doctor first or visit a dietitian who specializes in
teen athletes. If a health professional you trust agrees that it's safe to
diet, then he or she can work with you to develop a plan that allows

you get the proper amount of nutrients, and perform your best while also losing weight.

Eat a Variety of Foods

You may have heard about "carb loading" before a game. But when it comes to powering your game for the long haul, it's a bad idea to focus on only one type of food.

Carbohydrates are an important source of fuel, but they're *only one* of many foods an athlete needs. It also takes vitamins, minerals, protein, and fats to stay in peak playing shape.

Muscular Minerals and Vital Vitamins

Calcium helps build the strong bones that athletes depend on, and iron carries oxygen to muscles. Most teens don't get enough of these minerals, and that's especially true of teen athletes because their needs may be even higher than those of other teens.

To get the iron you need, eat lean (not much fat) meat, fish, and poultry; green, leafy vegetables; and iron-fortified cereals. Calcium—a must for protecting against stress fractures—is found in dairy foods, such as low-fat milk, yogurt, and cheese.

In addition to calcium and iron, you need a whole bunch of other vitamins and minerals that do everything from help you access energy to keep you from getting sick. Eating a balanced diet, including lots of different fruits and veggies, should provide the vitamins and minerals needed for good health and sports performance.

Protein Power

Athletes may need more protein than less-active teens, but most teen athletes get plenty of protein through regular eating. It's a myth that athletes need a huge daily intake of protein to build large, strong muscles. Muscle growth comes from regular training and hard work. And taking in too much protein can actually harm the body, causing dehydration, calcium loss, and even kidney problems.

Good sources of protein are fish, lean meats and poultry, eggs, dairy, nuts, soy, and peanut butter.

Carb Charge

Carbohydrates provide athletes with an excellent source of fuel. Cutting back on carbs or following low-carb diets isn't a good idea for athletes because restricting carbohydrates can cause a person to feel tired and worn out, which ultimately affects performance.

Good sources of carbohydrates include fruits, vegetables, and grains. Choose whole grains (such as brown rice, oatmeal, whole-wheat bread) more often than their more processed counterparts like white rice and white bread. That's because whole grains provide both the energy athletes need to perform and the fiber and other nutrients they need to be healthy.

Sugary carbs such as candy bars or sodas are less healthy for athletes because they don't contain any of the other nutrients you need. In addition, eating candy bars or other sugary snacks just before practice or competition can give athletes a quick burst of energy and then leave them to "crash" or run out of energy before they've finished working out.

Fat Fuel

Everyone needs a certain amount of fat each day, and this is particularly true for athletes. That's because active muscles quickly burn through carbs and need fats for long-lasting energy. Like carbs, not all fats are created equal. Experts advise athletes to concentrate on eating healthier fats, such as the unsaturated fat found in most vegetable oils, some fish, and nuts and seeds. Try to not to eat too much trans fat–like partially hydrogenated oils–and saturated fat, that is found in high fat meat and high fat dairy products, like butter.

Choosing when to eat fats is also important for athletes. Fatty foods can slow digestion, so it's a good idea to avoid eating these foods for a few hours before and after exercising.

Shun Supplements

Protein and energy bars don't do a whole lot of good, but they won't really do you much harm either. Energy drinks have lots of caffeine, though, so no one should drink them before exercising.

Other types of supplements can really do some damage.

Anabolic steroids can seriously mess with a person's hormones, causing side effects like testicular shrinkage and baldness in guys and facial hair growth in girls. Steroids can cause mental health problems, including depression and serious mood swings.

Some supplements contain hormones that are related to testosterone (such as dehydroepiandrosterone or DHEA for short). These supplements can have similar side effects to anabolic steroids. Other sports supplements (like creatine, for example) have not been tested in people younger than 18. So the risks of taking them are not yet known.

Salt tablets are another supplement to watch out for. People take them to avoid dehydration, but salt tablets can actually lead to dehydration. In large amounts, salt can cause nausea, vomiting, cramps, and diarrhea and may damage the lining of the stomach. In general, you are better off drinking fluids in order to maintain hydration. Any salt you lose in sweat can usually be made up with sports drinks or food eaten after exercise.

Ditch Dehydration

Speaking of dehydration, **water** is just as important to unlocking your game power as food. When you sweat during exercise, it's easy to become overheated, headachy, and worn out—especially in hot or humid weather. Even mild dehydration can affect an athlete's physical and mental performance.

There's no one-size-fits-all formula for how much water to drink. How much fluid each person needs depends on the individual's age, size, level of physical activity, and environmental temperature.

Experts recommend that athletes drink before and after exercise as well as every 15 to 20 minutes during exercise. Don't wait until you feel thirsty, because thirst is a sign that your body has needed liquids for a while. But don't force yourself to drink more fluids than you may need either. It's hard to run when there's a lot of water sloshing around in your stomach!

If you like the taste of sports drinks better than regular water, then it's OK to drink them. But it's important to know that a sports drink is really no better for you than water unless you are exercising for more than 60 to 90 minutes or in really hot weather. The additional carbohydrates and electrolytes may improve performance in these conditions, but otherwise your body will do just as well with water.

Avoid drinking carbonated drinks or juice because they could give you a stomachache while you're competing.

Never drink energy drinks before exercising. Energy drinks contain a large amount of caffeine and other ingredients that have caffeine-like effects.

Caffeine

Caffeine is a diuretic. That means it causes a person to urinate (pee) more. It's not clear whether this causes dehydration or not, but to be safe, it's wise to stay away from too much caffeine. That's especially true if you'll be exercising in hot weather.

When it comes to caffeine and exercise, it's good to weigh any benefits against potential problems. Although some studies find that caffeine may help adults perform better in endurance sports, other studies show too much caffeine may hurt.

Caffeine increases heart rate and blood pressure. Too much caffeine can leave an athlete feeling anxious or jittery. Caffeine can also cause trouble sleeping. All of these can drag down a person's sports performance. Plus, taking certain medications—including supplements—can make caffeine's side effects seem even worse.

Never drink energy drinks before exercising. These products contain a large amount of caffeine and other ingredients that have caffeine-like effects.

Game-Day Eats

Your performance on game day will depend on the foods you've eaten over the past several days and weeks. But you can boost your performance even more by paying attention to the food you eat on game day. Strive for a game-day diet rich in carbohydrates, moderate in protein, and low in fat.

Here are some guidelines on what to eat and when:

- **Eat a meal 2 to 4 hours before the game or event:** Choose a protein and carbohydrate meal (like a turkey or chicken sandwich, cereal and milk, chicken noodle soup and yogurt or pasta with tomato sauce).

- **Eat a snack less than 2 hours before the game:** If you haven't had time to have a pre-game meal, be sure to have a light snack such as low-fiber fruits or vegetables (like plums, melons, cherries, carrots), crackers, a bagel or low-fat yogurt.

Consider not eating anything for the hour before you compete or have practice because digestion requires energy—energy that you want to use to win. Also, eating too soon before any kind of activity can leave food in the stomach, making you feel full, bloated, crampy, and sick.

Everyone is different, so get to know what works best for you. You may want to experiment with meal timing and how much to eat on practice days so that you're better prepared for game day.

Want to get an eating plan personalized for you? Check the U.S. government's website ChooseMyPlate.gov, which tells a person how much to eat from different food groups based on age, gender, and activity level.

Section 25.2

Performance-Enhancing Sports Supplements

This section includes excerpts from "Sports Supplements,"
© 1995–2016. The Nemours Foundation/KidsHealth®.
Reprinted with permission

Sports Supplements

If you're a competitive athlete or a fitness buff, improving your sports performance is probably on your mind. Lots of people wonder if taking sports supplements could offer fast, effective results without so much hard work. But do sports supplements really work? And are they safe?

What Are Sports Supplements?

Sports supplements (also called ergogenic aids) are products used to enhance athletic performance that may include vitamins, minerals, amino acids, herbs or botanicals (plants)—or any concentration, extract or combination of these. These products are generally available over the counter without a prescription.

Sports supplements are considered dietary supplements. Dietary supplements do not require U.S. Food and Drug Administration (FDA) approval before they come on the market. Supplement manufacturers do have to follow the FDA's current good manufacturing practices to ensure quality and safety of their product, though. And the FDA is responsible for taking action if a product is found to be unsafe after it has gone on the market.

Critics of the supplement industry point out cases where manufacturers haven't done a good job of following standards. They also mention instances where the FDA hasn't enforced regulations. Both of these can mean that supplements contain variable amounts of ingredients or even ingredients not listed on the label.

Some over-the-counter medicines and prescription medications, including anabolic steroids, are used to enhance performance but they are not considered supplements. Although medications are FDA approved, using medicines—even over-the-counter ones—in ways other than their intended purpose puts the user at risk of serious side effects. For example, teen athletes who use medications like human growth hormone (hGH) that haven't been prescribed for them can have problems with growth, and may develop diabetes and heart problems.

Lots of sports organizations have developed policies on sports supplements. The National Football League (NFL), the National Collegiate Athletic Association (NCAA), and the International Olympic Committee (IOC) have banned the use of steroids, ephedra, and androstenedione by their athletes, and competitors who use them face fines, ineligibility, and suspension from their sports.

The National Federation of State High School Associations (NFHS) strongly recommends that student athletes consult with their doctor before taking any supplement.

How Some Common Supplements Affect the Body?

Whether you hear about sports supplements from your teammates in the locker room or the sales clerk at your local vitamin store, chances are you're not getting the whole story about how supplements work, if they are really effective, and the risks you take by using them.

Androstenedione and DHEA

Androstenedione (also known as andro) and dehydroepiandrosterone (also known as DHEA) are prohormones or "natural steroids" that can be broken down into testosterone. Andro used to be available over the counter, but now requires a prescription.

When researchers studied these prohormones in adult athletes, DHEA and andro did not increase muscle size, improve strength or enhance performance.

Andro and DHEA can cause hormone imbalances in people who use them. Both can have the same effects as taking anabolic steroids and may lead to dangerous side effects like testicular cancer, infertility, stroke, and an increased risk of heart disease. As with anabolic steroids, teens who use andro while they are still growing may not reach

316

their full adult height. Natural steroid supplements can also cause breast development and shrinking of testicles in guys.

Creatine

Creatine is already manufactured by the body in the liver, kidneys, and pancreas. It also occurs naturally in foods such as meat and fish. Creatine supplements are available over the counter.

People who take creatine usually take it to improve strength, but the long-term and short-term effects of creatine use haven't been studied in teens and kids. Research in adults found that creatine is most effective for athletes doing intermittent high-intensity exercise with short recovery intervals, such as sprinting and power lifting. However, researchers found no effect on athletic performance in nearly a third of athletes studied. Creatine has not been found to increase endurance or improve aerobic performance.

The most common side effects of creatine supplements include weight gain, diarrhea, abdominal pain, and muscle cramps. People with kidney problems should not use creatine because it may affect kidney function. The American College of Sports Medicine recommends that people younger than 18 years old do not use creatine. If you are considering using creatine, talk with your doctor about the risks and benefits, as well as appropriate dosing.

Fat Burners

Fat burners (sometimes known as **thermogenics**) were often made with an herb called ephedra, also known as ephedrine or ma huang, which acts as a stimulant and increases metabolism. Some athletes use fat burners to lose weight or to increase energy—but ephedra-based products can be one of the most dangerous supplements. Evidence has shown that it can cause heart problems, stroke, and occasionally even death.

Because athletes and others have died using this supplement, ephedra has been taken off the market. Since the ban, "ephedra-free" products have emerged, but they often contain ingredients with ephedra-like properties, including bitter orange or country mallow. Similar to ephedra, these supplements can cause high blood pressure, heart attack, stroke, and seizures.

Many of these products also contain caffeine, along with other caffeine sources (such as yerba mate and guarana). This combination may lead to restlessness, anxiety, racing heart, irregular heartbeat, and increases the chance of having a life-threatening side effect.

Will Supplements Make Me a Better Athlete?

Sports supplements haven't been tested on teens and kids. But studies on adults show that the claims of many supplements are weak at best. Most won't make you any stronger, and none will make you any faster or more skillful.

Many factors go into your abilities as an athlete—including your diet, how much sleep you get, genetics and heredity, and your training program. But the fact is that using sports supplements may put you at risk for serious health conditions.

So instead of turning to supplements to improve your performance, concentrate on nutrition and training, including strength and conditioning programs.

Tips for Dealing with Athletic Pressure and Competition

Ads for sports supplements often use persuasive before and after pictures that make it look easy to get a muscular, toned body. But the goal of supplement advertisers is to make money by selling more supplements, and many claims may be misleading.

Teens and kids may seem like an easy sell on supplements because they may feel dissatisfied or uncomfortable with their still-developing bodies, and many supplement companies try to convince teens that supplements are an easy solution.

Don't waste your money on expensive and dangerous supplements. Instead, try these tips for getting better game:

- **Make downtime a priority**. Studies show that teens need more than 8 hours of sleep a night, and sleep is important for athletes. Organize time for sleep into your schedule by doing as much homework as possible on the weekend or consider cutting back on after-school job hours during your sports season.

- **Learn to relax.** Your school, work, and sports schedules may have you sprinting from one activity to the next, but taking a few minutes to relax can be helpful. Meditating or visualizing your success during the next game may improve your performance; sitting quietly and focusing on your breathing can give you a brief break and prepare you for your next activity.

- **Choose good eats**. Fried, fatty or sugary foods will interfere with your performance. Instead, focus on eating foods such as lean meats, whole grains, vegetables, fruits, and low-fat dairy products. Celebrating with the team at the local pizza place after a big game is fine once in a while. But for most meals and snacks, choose healthy foods to keep your weight in a healthy range and your performance at its best.

- **Get enough fuel**. Sometimes people skip breakfast or have an early lunch, then try to play a late afternoon game. Not getting enough food to fuel an activity can quickly wear you out—and even place you at risk for injury or muscle fatigue. Be sure to eat lunch on practice and game days. If you feel hungry before the game, pack easy-to-carry, healthy snacks in your bag, such as fruit, trail mix or string cheese. It's important to eat well after a workout.

- **Avoid harmful substances**. Smoking will diminish your lung capacity and your ability to breathe, alcohol can make you sluggish and tired, and can impair your hand-eye coordination and reduce your alertness. And you can kiss your team good-bye if you get caught using drugs or alcohol—many schools have a no-tolerance policy for harmful substances.

- **Train harder and smarter**. If you get out of breath easily during your basketball game and you want to increase your endurance, work on improving your cardiovascular conditioning. If you think more leg strength will help you excel on the soccer field, consider weight training to increase your muscle strength. Before changing your program, though, get advice from your doctor.

- **Consult a professional**. If you're concerned about your weight or whether your diet is helping your performance, talk to your doctor or a registered dietitian who can evaluate your nutrition and steer you in the right direction. Coaches can help too. And if you're still convinced that supplements will help you, talk to your doctor or a sports medicine specialist. The doc will be able to offer alternatives to supplements based on your body and sport.

Chapter 26

Alcohol Use

Chapter Contents

Section 26.1

Recommendations for the Consumption of Alcohol

This section includes text excerpted from "Alcohol," Office of Disease Prevention and Health Promotion (ODPHP), U.S. Department of Health and Human Services (HHS), 2015.

If alcohol is consumed, it should be in moderation—up to one drink per day for women and up to two drinks per day for men—and only by adults of legal drinking age. For those who choose to drink, moderate alcohol consumption can be incorporated into the calorie limits of most healthy eating patterns. The *Dietary Guidelines* does not recommend that individuals who do not drink alcohol start drinking for any reason; however, it does recommend that all foods and beverages consumed be accounted for within healthy eating patterns. Alcohol is not a component of the ChooseMyPlate.gov, U.S. Department of Agriculture (USDA) Food Patterns. Thus, if alcohol is consumed, the calories from alcohol should be accounted for so that the limits on calories for other uses and total calories are not exceeded.

For the purposes of evaluating amounts of alcohol that may be consumed, the *Dietary Guidelines* includes drink-equivalents. One alcoholic drink-equivalent is described as containing 14 g (0.6 fl oz) of pure alcohol. The following are reference beverages that are one alcoholic drink-equivalent: 12 fluid ounces of regular beer (5% alcohol), 5 fluid ounces of wine (12% alcohol) or 1.5 fluid ounces of 80 proof distilled spirits (40% alcohol).

Packaged (e.g., canned beer, bottled wine) and mixed beverages (e.g., margarita, rum and soda, mimosa, sangria) vary in alcohol content. For this reason it is important to determine how many alcoholic drink-equivalents are in the beverage and limit intake. Table 26.1 lists reference beverages that are one drink-equivalent and provides examples of alcoholic drink-equivalents in other alcoholic beverages.

Table 26.1. Alcoholic Drink-Equivalents[a] of Select Beverages

Drink Description	Drink-Equivalents[b]
Beer, beer coolers, and malt beverages	
12 fl oz at 4.2% alcohol[c]	0.8
12 fl oz at 5% alcohol (reference beverage)	1
16 fl oz at 5% alcohol	1.3
12 fl oz at 7% alcohol	1.4
12 fl oz at 9% alcohol	1.8
Wine	
5 fl oz at 12% alcohol (reference beverage)	1
9 fl oz at 12% alcohol	1.8
5 fl oz at 15% alcohol	1.3
5 fl oz at 17% alcohol	1.4
Distilled spirits	
1.5 fl oz 80 proof distilled spirits (40% alcohol) (reference beverage)	1
Mixed drink with more than 1.5 fl oz 80 proof distilled spirits (40% alcohol)	> 1[d]

[a] One alcoholic drink-equivalent is defined as containing 14 grams (0.6 fl oz) of pure alcohol. The following are reference beverages that are one alcoholic drink-equivalent: 12 fluid ounces of regular beer (5% alcohol), 5 fluid ounces of wine (12% alcohol) or 1.5 fluid ounces of 80 proof distilled spirits (40% alcohol). Drink-equivalents are not intended to serve as a standard drink definition for regulatory purposes.

[b] To calculate drink-equivalents, multiply the volume in ounces by the alcohol content in percent and divide by 0.6 ounces of alcohol per drink-equivalent. For example: 16 fl oz beer at 5% alcohol: (16 fl oz)(0.05)/0.6 fl oz = 1.3 drink-equivalents.

[c] Light beer represents a substantial proportion of alcoholic beverages consumed in the United States. Light beer is approximately 4.2% alcohol or 0.8 alcoholic drink-equivalents in 12 fluid ounces.

[d] Depending on factors, such as the type of spirits and the recipe, one mixed drink can contain a variable number of drink-equivalents.

When determining the number of drink-equivalents in an alcoholic beverage, the variability in alcohol content and portion size must be considered together. As an example, the amount of alcohol in a beer may be higher than 5 percent and, thus, 12 ounces would be greater than one drink-equivalent. In addition to the alcohol content, the portion size may be many times larger than the reference beverage. For example, portion sizes for beer may be higher than 12 ounces and, thus, even if the alcohol content is 5 percent, the beverage would be greater than one drink-equivalent. The same is true for wine and mixed drinks with distilled spirits.

Alcoholic Beverages and Calories

Alcoholic beverages may contain calories from both alcohol and other ingredients. If they are consumed, the contributions from calories from alcohol and other dietary components (e.g., added sugars, solid fats) from alcoholic beverages should be within the various limits of healthy eating patterns. One drink-equivalent contains 14 grams of pure alcohol, which contributes 98 calories to the beverage. The total calories in a beverage may be more than those from alcohol alone, depending on the type, brand, ingredients, and portion size. For example, 12 ounces of regular beer (5% alcohol) may have about 150 calories, 5 ounces of wine (12% alcohol) may have about 120 calories, and 7 ounces of a rum (40% alcohol) and cola may have about 155 calories, each with 98 calories coming from pure alcohol.

Excessive Drinking

In comparison to moderate alcohol consumption, high-risk drinking is the consumption of 4 or more drinks on any day or 8 or more drinks per week for women and 5 or more drinks on any day or 15 or more drinks per week for men. Binge drinking is the consumption within about 2 hours of 4 or more drinks for women and 5 or more drinks for men.

Excessive alcohol consumption—which includes binge drinking (4 or more drinks for women and 5 or more drinks for men within about 2 hours); heavy drinking (8 or more drinks a week for women and 15 or more drinks a week for men); and any drinking by pregnant women or those under 21 years of age—has no benefits. Excessive drinking is responsible for 88,000 deaths in the United States each year, including 1 in 10 deaths among working age adults (age 20-64 years). In 2006, the estimated economic cost to the United States of excessive drinking was $224 billion. Binge drinking accounts for over half of the deaths and three-fourths of the economic costs due to excessive drinking.

Excessive drinking increases the risk of many chronic diseases and violence and, over time, can impair short- and long-term cognitive function. Over 90 percent of U.S. adults who drink excessively report binge drinking, and about 90 percent of the alcohol consumed by youth under 21 years of age in the United States is in the form of binge drinks. Binge drinking is associated with a wide range of health and social problems, including sexually transmitted diseases, unintended pregnancy, accidental injuries, and violent crime.

Those Who Should Not Consume Alcohol

Many individuals should not consume alcohol, including individuals who are taking certain over-the-counter or prescription medications or who have certain medical conditions, those who are recovering from alcoholism or are unable to control the amount they drink, and anyone younger than age 21 years. Individuals should not drink if they are driving, planning to drive or are participating in other activities requiring skill, coordination, and alertness.

Women who are or who may be pregnant should not drink. Drinking during pregnancy, especially in the first few months of pregnancy, may result in negative behavioral or neurological consequences in the offspring. No safe level of alcohol consumption during pregnancy has been established. Women who are breastfeeding should consult with their healthcare provider regarding alcohol consumption.

Alcohol and Caffeine

Mixing alcohol and caffeine is not generally recognized as safe by the FDA. People who mix alcohol and caffeine may drink more alcohol and become more intoxicated than they realize, increasing the risk of alcohol-related adverse events. Caffeine does not change blood alcohol content levels, and thus, does not reduce the risk of harms associated with drinking alcohol.

Section 26.2

Revisiting Red Wine's Health Claims

This section contains text excerpted from the following
sources: Text under the heading "Resveratrol's Health Claims"
is excerpted from "Revisiting Resveratrol's Health Claims,"
National Institutes of Health (NIH), May 20, 2014; Text under
the heading "NIH Researchers Find Resveratrol Helps Protect
against Cardiovascular Disease in Animal Study" is excerpted
from "NIH Researchers Find Resveratrol Helps Protect against
Cardiovascular Disease in Animal Study," National Institute
on Aging (NIA), June 3, 2014.

Resveratrol's Health Claims

A study gives insight into how resveratrol—a compound found in
grapes, red wine, and nuts—may ward off several age-related diseases.
The findings could help in the development of drugs to curtail some of
the health problems that arise as we get older.

Certain metabolic diseases, including type 2 diabetes and heart
disease, tend to strike as we age. In animal studies, severely restricting calories can help prevent some of these diseases. Over a decade
ago, researchers found that resveratrol can mimic calorie restriction
in some ways and extend the lifespans of yeast, worms, flies, and fish.

Resveratrol affects the activity of enzymes called sirtuins. Sirtuins
control several biological pathways and are known to be involved in
the aging process. Resveratrol is only one of many natural and synthetic sirtuin-activating compounds (STACs) now known. Whether
these STACs directly interact with sirtuins or affect them indirectly,
however, has been a subject of debate.

A research team led by Dr. David Sinclair of Harvard Medical
School—including researchers from NIH's National Heart, Lung,
and Blood Institute (NHLBI)—set out to explore whether STACs can
directly activate the sirtuin SIRT1. The study, funded in part by NIH's
National Institute on Aging (NIA), appeared on March 8, 2013, in
Science.

SIRT1 works in the cell by removing an acetyl chemical group from
its protein substrates. Previous research found that STACs increased

SIRT1 activity toward substrates tagged with fluorescent compounds. However, they didn't affect SIRT1 activity on untagged substrates. The scientists hypothesized that the fluorescent chemical group, typically used to track cells, might mimic some property that SIRT1 requires for its activity.

The scientists tested SIRT1 substrates tagged with compounds similar to the fluorescent tags. They discovered that STAC activation of SIRT1 depends on the presence of certain amino acids at particular positions on SIRT1 substrates. When they removed or changed these amino acids, the effect of STACs on SIRT1 activity was abolished.

The researchers screened for SIRT1 mutant proteins that couldn't be activated by resveratrol. One mutant, with a lysine instead of a glutamate at one particular position, blunted the enzyme's activation by more than 100 chemically diverse STACs. The glutamate normally found at this position in SIRT1 is conserved in species ranging from flies to humans. The lysine substitution didn't significantly alter any aspect of the enzyme's activity other than its activation by STACs.

STACs ultimately increase the activity of mitochondria, the organelles that produce the cell's energy. Some believe that this may be how STACs affect age-related diseases. In mouse cells with the mutant SIRT1, the effects of STACs on mitochondria were blocked.

"Now that we know the exact location on SIRT1 where and how resveratrol works, we can engineer even better molecules that more precisely and effectively trigger the effects of resveratrol," Sinclair says.

The scientists found no evidence for the involvement of other biological pathways that were previously linked to the effects of STACs. These results suggest that resveratrol and other STACs act, at least in part, through direct interactions with SIRT1 and its substrates. Further research will be needed to understand which of these pathways are responsible for the effects of STACs in the body.

NIH Researchers Find Resveratrol Helps Protect against Cardiovascular Disease in Animal Study

Resveratrol may protect against certain cardiovascular problems, according to an NIA study in nonhuman primates. Specifically, researchers found resveratrol prevented arterial stiffening and inflammation in monkeys on a high fat, high sugar diet. It also reduced fatty build up and calcification of the arteries, a condition known as atherosclerosis. These issues are common among older adults.

Positive effects of resveratrol were most profound after a year of supplementation. The compound did not, however, prevent all negative effects associated with a high fat, high sugar diet. For instance, it did not affect blood pressure or "bad" cholesterol (low density lipoprotein, LDL) nor did it prevent increase in body weight.

Researchers evaluated resveratrol's effects on arterial stiffness using a standard clinical test called pulse wave velocity (PWV). It measures how quickly blood can flow through the arteries from the heart to the rest of the body. Stiffer arteries create quicker waves of motion. Increased PWV commonly leads to high blood pressure, and, in humans, predicts an increased risk of developing (and death from) heart disease.

Researchers emphasize that their results are not immediately translatable to humans. Multiple studies on resveratrol in animal models, however, have presented ample evidence to support the next phase of investigation, a human study.

Part Five

Nutrition-Related
Health Concerns

Chapter 27

Metabolic Syndrome

What Is Metabolic Syndrome?

Metabolic syndrome is the name for a group of risk factors that raises your risk for heart disease and other health problems, such as diabetes and stroke.

The term "metabolic" refers to the biochemical processes involved in the body's normal functioning. Risk factors are traits, conditions or habits that increase your chance of developing a disease.

In this chapter, "heart disease" refers to coronary heart disease (CHD). CHD is a condition in which a waxy substance called plaque builds up inside the coronary (heart) arteries.

Plaque hardens and narrows the arteries, reducing blood flow to your heart muscle. This can lead to chest pain, a heart attack, heart damage or even death.

Metabolic Risk Factors

The five conditions described below are metabolic risk factors. You can have any one of these risk factors by itself, but they tend to occur together. You must have at least three metabolic risk factors to be diagnosed with metabolic syndrome.

1. A large waistline. This also is called abdominal obesity or "having an apple shape." Excess fat in the stomach area is a

This chapter includes text excerpted from "What Is Metabolic Syndrome?" National Heart, Lung, and Blood Institute (NHLBI), November 6, 2015.

331

greater risk factor for heart disease than excess fat in other parts of the body, such as on the hips.

2. A high triglyceride level (or you're on medicine to treat high triglycerides). Triglycerides are a type of fat found in the blood.

3. A low High-density lipoprotein (HDL) cholesterol level (or you're on medicine to treat low HDL cholesterol). HDL sometimes is called "good" cholesterol. This is because it helps remove cholesterol from your arteries. A low HDL cholesterol level raises your risk for heart disease.

4. High blood pressure (or you're on medicine to treat high blood pressure). Blood pressure is the force of blood pushing against the walls of your arteries as your heart pumps blood. If this pressure rises and stays high over time, it can damage your heart and lead to plaque buildup.

5. High fasting blood sugar (or you're on medicine to treat high blood sugar). Mildly high blood sugar may be an early sign of diabetes.

Overview

Your risk for heart disease, diabetes, and stroke increases with the number of metabolic risk factors you have. The risk of having metabolic syndrome is closely linked to overweight and obesity and a lack of physical activity.

Insulin resistance also may increase your risk for metabolic syndrome. Insulin resistance is a condition in which the body can't use its insulin properly. Insulin is a hormone that helps move blood sugar into cells where it's used for energy. Insulin resistance can lead to high blood sugar levels, and it's closely linked to overweight and obesity. Genetics (ethnicity and family history) and older age are other factors that may play a role in causing metabolic syndrome.

Outlook

Metabolic syndrome is becoming more common due to a rise in obesity rates among adults. In the future, metabolic syndrome may overtake smoking as the leading risk factor for heart disease.

It is possible to prevent or delay metabolic syndrome, mainly with lifestyle changes. A healthy lifestyle is a lifelong commitment. Successfully controlling metabolic syndrome requires long-term effort and teamwork with your healthcare providers.

Chapter 28

Sugar and Added Sweeteners

Chapter Contents

Section 28.1

Nutritive and Nonnutritive Sweeteners

This section contains text excerpted from the following sources: Text
in this section begins with excerpts from "Nutritive and Nonnutritive
Sweetener Resources," National Agricultural Library (NAL), U.S.
Department of Agriculture (USDA), May 20, 2016; Text under
the heading "Added Sugars" is excerpted from "Added Sugars,"
ChooseMyPlate.gov, U.S. Department of Agriculture (USDA),
January 7, 2016; Text under the heading "Build a Healthy Plate
with Fewer Added Sugars" is excerpted from "Build a Healthy Plate
with Fewer Added Sugars," Food and Nutrition Service (FNS), U.S.
Department of Agriculture (USDA), June 2013.

Nutritive and nonnutritive sweeteners enhance the flavor and/or
texture of food. Nutritive sweeteners provide the body with calories,
while nonnutritive sweeteners are very low in calories or contain no
calories at all. They can both be added to food and beverages.

Nutritive Sweeteners

Nutritive sweeteners, also known as caloric sweeteners or sugars,
provide energy in the form of carbohydrates.

Some sugars are found naturally in foods. For example, fructose is
found in fresh fruits. By eating the whole fruit, you not only consume
fructose, but you feed your body fiber, vitamins, minerals, and phytonutrients that you do not get from sugar alone.

Many of the sugars in our diet come from "added sugars"-sugars
added to food prior to consumption or during preparation or processing.
Added sugars are used to enhance the flavor and texture of foods and
to increase shelf-life. Examples of added sugars include sucrose and
high-fructose corn syrup (HFCS).

Nonnutritive Sweeteners

Nonnutritive sweeteners are zero-or low-calorie alternatives to
nutritive sweeteners, such as table sugar. These sweeteners can be
added to both hot and cold beverages and some can be used for baking.

Nonnutritive sweeteners are much sweeter than sugar so only small amounts are needed. They provide fewer calories per gram than sugar because they are not completely absorbed by your digestive system. The U.S. Food and Drug Administration (FDA) has approved the use of the following nonnutritive sweeteners: acesulfame-K, aspartame, neotame, saccharin, sucralose, and stevia.

Added Sugars

To build a healthy eating style and stay within your calorie needs, choose foods and beverages with less added sugars. Added sugars are sugars and syrups that are added to foods or beverages when they are processed or prepared. This does not include natural sugars found in milk and fruits.

Most of us eat and drink too many added sugars from the following foods:

- beverages, such as regular soft drinks, energy or sports drinks, fruit drinks, sweetened coffee, and tea
- candy
- cakes
- cookies and brownies
- pies and cobblers
- sweet rolls, pastries, and donuts
- ice cream and dairy desserts
- sugars, jams, syrups, and sweet toppings

Reading the ingredient label on packaged foods can help to identify added sugars.

Table 28.1. Names for Added Sugar

anhydrous dextrose	brown sugar	confectioner's powdered sugar
corn syrup	corn syrup solids	dextrose
fructose	high-fructose corn syrup (HFCS)	honey
invert sugar	lactose	malt syrup
maltose	maple syrup	molasses

Table 28.1. Continued

nectars (e.g., peach or pear nectar)	pancake syrup	raw sugar
sucrose	sugar	white granulated sugar

You may also see other names such as cane juice, evaporated corn sweetener, crystal dextrose, glucose, liquid fructose, sugar cane juice, and fruit nectar

Build a Healthy Plate with Fewer Added Sugars

Sugars are found naturally in fruits, milk, yogurt, and cheese. However, the majority of sugars in typical American diets are "added sugars." You can help children stay healthier as they grow by providing them with foods and beverages with fewer added sugars. It is important to remember that:

- The extra calories in added sugars can make children feel full before they've had a chance to get the nutrients they need from other foods.

- The extra calories from added sugars also make it harder for children to grow at a healthy weight, and may contribute to weight gain.

- Added sugars are often called "empty calories" because they add calories to the diet without offering any nutrients.

- Sugar also increases the risk for dental cavities.

How to Serve Children Fewer Foods with Added Sugars?

Children are born preferring sweet flavors. When children regularly taste sugar and sweet flavors, they learn to prefer these sweet flavors more and more. Adding little or no sugar and choosing foods and beverages lower in "added sugars" can help children learn to like foods that are not as sweet. Here are some tips:

- Serve fresh fruit more often instead of fruit-based desserts, such as fruit pies, cobblers, and crisps.

- Offer raisins instead of chewy fruit snacks, candy or sweets.

- Purchase whole-grain breads and cereals with little or no added sugars. Low-sugar cereals should have no more than 6 grams of sugar per serving, according to the Nutrition Facts label. Top cereal or oatmeal with fruit to sweeten the taste.

- Offer fresh foods and less-processed foods.

- Choose not to offer sweets as rewards. By offering food as a reward for good behavior, children learn to think that some foods are "better" than other foods. Reward the children in your care with kind words and comforting hugs or give them nonfood items, like stickers, to make them feel special.

How Can I Encourage Kids to Eat a Balanced Variety of Foods without Added Sugars?

Some kids may need time to adjust to a less sweet flavor. Introduce less-sweetened versions of the same foods that were previously sweetened. Here are some ways to help kids eat fewer added sugars:

- Make food fun! Serve a festive drink with no more than ½-cup serving of fruit juice, once per day, and add an orange, lemon or lime wedge as a garnish. During the rest of the day, offer most fruit whole or cut up, to get more fiber.

- Cook together. Children learn about foods when they help prepare them. Instead of sweetened yogurt, have kids make their own "fruit and yogurt parfait" by topping nonfat plain yogurt with whole-grain cereal and fresh or frozen berries, banana slices, fruit canned in 100% juice or their favorite fruit.

Section 28.2

High Fructose Corn Syrup: Questions and Answers

This section includes text excerpted from "High Fructose Corn Syrup: Questions and Answers," U.S. Food and Drug Administration (FDA), November 5, 2014.

Where Does High Fructose Corn Syrup (HFCS) Come From?

High Fructose Corn Syrup (HFCS) is derived from corn starch. Starch itself is a chain of glucose (a simple sugar) molecules joined together.

When corn starch is broken down into individual glucose molecules, the end product is corn syrup, which is essentially 100% glucose.

To make HFCS, enzymes are added to corn syrup in order to convert some of the glucose to another simple sugar called fructose, also called "fruit sugar" because it occurs naturally in fruits and berries.

HFCS is 'high' in fructose compared to the pure glucose that is in corn syrup. Different formulations of HFCS contain different amounts of fructose.

How Much Fructose Is in HFCS?

The most common forms of HFCS contain either 42 percent or 55 percent fructose, as described in the Code of Federal Regulations (21 CFR 184.1866), and these are referred to in the industry as HFCS 42 and HFCS 55. The rest of the HFCS is glucose and water. HFCS 42 is mainly used in processed foods, cereals, baked goods, and some beverages. HFCS 55 is used primarily in soft drinks.

Sucrose (sugar), the most well-known sweetener, is made by crystallizing sugar cane or beet juice. Sucrose is also made up of the same two simple sugars, glucose and fructose, joined together to form a single molecule containing one glucose molecule and one fructose molecule, an exact one-to-one ratio.

The proportion of fructose to glucose in both HFCS 42 and HFCS 55 is similar to that of sucrose. The primary differences between sucrose and the common forms of HFCS are:

- HFCS contains water.

- In sucrose, a chemical bond joins the glucose and fructose. Once one eats, stomach acid and gut enzymes rapidly break down this chemical bond.

- In HFCS, no chemical bond joins the glucose and fructose.

Other nutritive sweeteners can vary in their fructose content (by "nutritive," we mean that the sweetener contains calories). Honey is a common nutritive sweetener with an approximately one-to-one ratio of fructose to glucose. Fruit and nectar-based sweeteners may have more fructose than glucose, especially those that come from apples and pears.

Is HFCS Less Safe than Other Sweeteners?

U.S. Food and Drug Administration (FDA) receives many inquiries asking about the safety of HFCS, often referring to studies about how humans metabolize fructose or fructose-containing sweeteners. These studies are based on the observation that there are some differences between how we metabolize fructose and other simple sugars.

We are not aware of any evidence, including the studies mentioned above, that there is a difference in safety between foods containing HFCS 42 or HFCS 55 and foods containing similar amounts of other nutritive sweeteners with approximately equal glucose and fructose content, such as sucrose, honey or other traditional sweeteners. The *Dietary Guidelines for Americans* recommend that everyone limit consumption of all added sugars, including HFCS and sucrose. FDA participated in the development of the *Dietary Guidelines* and fully supports this recommendation.

Section 28.3

High Intensity Sweeteners Used in Food

This section includes text excerpted from "Additional
Information about High-Intensity Sweeteners Permitted
for Use in Food in the United States," U.S. Food and
Drug Administration (FDA), May 26, 2015.

High-Intensity Sweeteners Permitted for Use in Food in the United States

High-intensity sweeteners are commonly used as sugar substitutes or sugar alternatives because they are many times sweeter than sugar but contribute only a few to no calories when added to foods. High-intensity sweeteners, like all other ingredients added to food in the United States, must be safe for consumption.

- Saccharin

- Aspartame

- Acesulfame potassium (Ace-K)

- Sucralose

- Neotame

- Advantame

- Steviol glycosides

- Luo Han Guo fruit extracts

Saccharin

Saccharin is approved for use in food as a non-nutritive sweetener. Saccharin brand names include Sweet and Low®, Sweet Twin®, Sweet'N Low®, and Necta Sweet®. It is 200 to 700 times sweeter than table sugar (sucrose), and it does not contain any calories.

First discovered and used in 1879, saccharin is currently approved for use, under certain conditions, in beverages, fruit juice drinks, and bases or mixes when prepared for consumption in accordance with directions, as a sugar substitute for cooking or table use, and in processed foods. Saccharin is also approved for use for certain technological purposes.

In the early 1970s, saccharin was linked with the development of bladder cancer in laboratory rats, which led Congress to mandate additional studies of saccharin and the presence of a warning label on saccharin-containing products until such warning could be shown to be unnecessary. Since then, more than 30 human studies demonstrated that the results found in rats were not relevant to humans, and that saccharin is safe for human consumption. In 2000, the National Toxicology Program of the National Institutes of Health concluded that saccharin should be removed from the list of potential carcinogens. Products containing saccharin no longer have to carry the warning label.

Aspartame

Aspartame is approved for use in food as a nutritive sweetener. Aspartame brand names include Nutrasweet®, Equal®, and Sugar Twin®. It does contain calories, but because it is about 200 times sweeter than table sugar, consumers are likely to use much less of it.

U.S. Food and Drug Administration (FDA) approved aspartame in 1981 for uses, under certain conditions, as a tabletop sweetener, in chewing gum, cold breakfast cereals, and dry bases for certain foods (i.e., beverages, instant coffee and tea, gelatins, puddings, and fillings, and dairy products and toppings). In 1983, FDA approved the use of aspartame in carbonated beverages and carbonated beverage syrup bases, and in 1996, FDA approved it for use as a "general purpose sweetener." It is not heat stable and loses its sweetness when heated, so it typically isn't used in baked goods.

Aspartame is one of the most exhaustively studied substances in the human food supply, with more than 100 studies supporting its safety.

FDA scientists have reviewed scientific data regarding the safety of aspartame in food and concluded that it is safe for the general population under certain conditions. However, people with a rare hereditary disease known as phenylketonuria (PKU) have a difficult time metabolizing phenylalanine, a component of aspartame, and should control their intake of phenylalanine from all sources, including aspartame. Labels of aspartame-containing foods and beverages must include a statement that informs individuals with PKU that the product contains phenylalanine.

Acesulfame Potassium (Ace-K)

Acesulfame potassium is approved for use in food as a non-nutritive sweetener. It is included in the ingredient list on the food label as acesulfame K, acesulfame potassium or Ace-K. Acesulfame potassium is sold under the brand names Sunett® and Sweet One®. It is about 200 times sweeter than sugar and is often combined with other sweeteners.

FDA approved acesulfame potassium for use in specific food and beverage categories in 1988, and in 2003 approved it as a general purpose sweetener and flavor enhancer in food, except in meat and poultry, under certain conditions of use. It is heat stable, meaning that it stays sweet even when used at high temperatures during baking, making it suitable as a sugar substitute in baked goods.

Acesulfame potassium is typically used in frozen desserts, candies, beverages, and baked goods. More than 90 studies support its safety.

Sucralose

Sucralose is approved for use in food as a non-nutritive sweetener. Sucralose is sold under the brand name Splenda®. Sucralose is about 600 times sweeter than sugar.

FDA approved sucralose for use in 15 food categories in 1998 and for use as a general purpose sweetener for foods in 1999, under certain conditions of use. Sucralose is a general purpose sweetener that can be found in a variety of foods including baked goods, beverages, chewing gum, gelatins, and frozen dairy desserts. It is heat stable, meaning that it stays sweet even when used at high temperatures during baking, making it suitable as a sugar substitute in baked goods.

Sucralose has been extensively studied and more than 110 safety studies were reviewed by FDA in approving the use of sucralose as a general purpose sweetener for food.

Neotame

Neotame is approved for use in food as a non-nutritive sweetener. Neotame is sold under the brand name Newtame®, and is approximately 7,000 to 13,000 times sweeter than table sugar.

FDA approved neotame for use as a general purpose sweetener and flavor enhancer in foods (except in meat and poultry), under certain conditions of use, in 2002. It is heat stable, meaning that it stays sweet even when used at high temperatures during baking, making it suitable as a sugar substitute in baked goods.

In determining the safety of neotame, FDA reviewed data from more than 113 animal and human studies designed to identify possible toxic effects, including effects on the immune system, reproductive system, and nervous system.

Advantame

Advantame is approved for use in food as a non-nutritive sweetener. It is approximately 20,000 times sweeter than table sugar (sucrose).

FDA approved advantame for use as a general purpose sweetener and flavor enhancer in foods (except in meat and poultry), under certain conditions of use, in 2014. It is heat stable, meaning that it stays sweet even when used at high temperatures during baking, making it suitable as a sugar substitute in baked goods.

In determining the safety of advantame, FDA reviewed data from 37 animal and human studies designed to identify possible toxic effects, including effects on the immune system, reproductive and developmental systems, and nervous system. FDA also reviewed pharmacokinetic and carcinogenicity studies, as well as several additional exploratory and screening studies.

Steviol Glycosides

Steviol glycosides are natural constituents of the leaves of Stevia rebaudiana (Bertoni) Bertoni, a plant native to parts of South America and commonly known as Stevia. They are non-nutritive sweeteners and are reported to be 200 to 400 times sweeter than table sugar.

FDA has received many GRAS Notices for the use of high-purity (95% minimum purity) steviol glycosides including Rebaudioside A (also known as Reb A), Stevioside, Rebaudioside D or steviol glycoside mixture preparations with Rebaudioside A and/or Stevioside as predominant components. FDA has not questioned the notifiers' GRAS determinations for these high-purity stevia derived sweeteners under the intended conditions of use identified in the GRAS notices submitted to FDA.

The use of stevia leaf and crude stevia extracts is not considered GRAS and their import into the United States is not permitted for use as sweeteners.

Luo Han Guo Fruit Extracts

Siraitia grosvenorii Swingle fruit extract (SGFE) contains varying levels of mogrosides, which are the non-nutritive constituents of the fruit primarily responsible for the characteristic sweetness of SGFE. SGFE, depending on the mogroside content, is reported to be 100 to 250 times sweeter than sugar. *Siraitia grosvenorii* Swingle, commonly known as Luo Han Guo or monk fruit, is a plant native to Southern China.

FDA has received GRAS Notices for SGFE. FDA has not questioned the notifiers' GRAS determination for SGFE under the intended conditions of use identified in the GRAS notices submitted to FDA.

What Is the Difference between Nutritive and Nonnutritive High-Intensity Sweeteners?

Nutritive sweeteners add caloric value to the foods that contain them, while non-nutritive sweeteners are very low in calories or contain no calories at all. Specifically, aspartame, the only approved nutritive high-intensity sweetener, contains more than two percent of the calories in an equivalent amount of sugar, as opposed to non-nutritive sweeteners that contain less than two percent of the calories in an equivalent amount of sugar.

Why Do the Intended Conditions of Use of High-Intensity Sweeteners Sometimes Not Include Use in Meat and Poultry Products?

The intended conditions of use of some high-intensity sweeteners approved for use as food additives do not include use in meat and poultry products because the companies that sought FDA's approval for these substances did not request these uses. In the case of the high-intensity sweeteners that are subjects of GRAS notices (i.e., certain high-purity steviol glycosides and SGFE), the notifiers did not include use in meat and poultry products as an intended condition of use in the GRAS notices that they submitted for FDA's evaluation.

If a high-intensity sweetener is proposed for use in a meat or poultry product through a food additive petition, FDA would be responsible for reviewing the safety of the high-intensity sweetener under the proposed conditions of use, and the Food Safety and Inspection Service (FSIS) of the U.S. Department of Agriculture (USDA) would be responsible for evaluating its suitability. If FDA is notified under the GRAS Notification Program that a high-intensity sweetener is GRAS for use in a meat or poultry product, FDA would evaluate whether the notice provides a sufficient basis for a GRAS determination and whether information in the notice or otherwise available to FDA raises issues that lead the agency to question whether the use of the high-intensity sweetener is GRAS. FDA would also forward the GRAS notice to FSIS to evaluate whether the intended use of the substance in meat or poultry products complies with the relevant statutes that are administered by FSIS

Section 28.4

Artificial Sweeteners and Health Research

This section contains text excerpted from the following sources:
Text beginning with the heading "Taking a New Look at Artificial Sweeteners" is excerpted from "Taking a New Look at Artificial Sweeteners," National Institutes of Health (NIH), October 7, 2014; Text under the heading "Artificial Sweeteners and Cancer Risk" is excerpted from "Diet," National Cancer Institute (NCI), April 29, 2015.

Taking a New Look at Artificial Sweeteners

Diet sodas and other treats sweetened with artificial sweeteners are often viewed as guilt-free pleasures. Because such foods are usually lower in calories than those containing natural sugars, many have considered them a good option for people who are trying to lose weight or keep their blood glucose levels in check. But some surprising new research suggests that artificial sweeteners might actually do the opposite, by changing the microbes living in our intestines.

To explore the impact of various kinds of sweeteners on the zillions of microbes living in the human intestine (referred to as the gut microbiome), an Israeli research team first turned to mice. One group of mice was given water that contained one of two natural sugars: glucose or sucrose; the other group received water that contained one of three artificial sweeteners: saccharin (the main ingredient in Sweet'N Low®), sucralose (Splenda®) or aspartame (Equal®, Nutrasweet®). Both groups ate a diet of normal mouse chow.

To their surprise, the researchers discovered that many animals in the artificial sweetener groups—especially those that drank saccharin-sweetened water—developed a condition called glucose intolerance, which is characterized by high blood glucose levels and is an early warning sign of increased risk for developing type 2 diabetes. In contrast, the animals that drank sugar water remained healthy.

The result was puzzling. These mice weren't consuming natural sugars, so what was raising their blood glucose levels? The researchers had a hunch that the answer might lie in the gut microbiome—since those microbes play a vital role in digestion. Their suspicions were borne out. When they used DNA sequencing to analyze the artificial sweetener group's gut microbiome, they found a distinctly different collection of microbes than in the animals who drank sugar water.

The next step was to distinguish whether these changes in the microbiome resulted from high blood glucose or caused it. When the researchers used antibiotics to wipe out the artificial sweetener group's gut microbes, their blood glucose levels returned to normal—evidence that the gut microbes were actively causing glucose intolerance. Additional proof came from experiments in which the researchers transplanted microbes from both groups of mice into the intestines of a mouse strain that had been raised in a sterile environment from birth. The germ-free mice that received microbes from the artificial sweetener group developed glucose intolerance; those getting microbes from the sugar group did not.

But what about humans? The research team examined clinical data from 400 people taking part in an ongoing nutrition study. That analysis showed that, compared to people who didn't use artificial sweeteners, long-term users of artificial sweeteners tended to have higher blood glucose levels and other parameters often associated with metabolic diseases like diabetes, obesity, and fatty liver.

Next, the researchers asked seven healthy human volunteers, who had never previously consumed foods or beverages containing artificial sweeteners, to consume the daily maximum dose of saccharin allowed by the U.S. Food and Drug Administration (FDA) for six consecutive days. Of the seven volunteers, four developed glucose intolerance, while three maintained normal blood glucose regulation. The researchers then took intestinal microbes from human volunteers and transplanted them into germ-free mice. Microbes from humans with glucose intolerance also triggered glucose intolerance in the mice, while microbes from humans with normal blood glucose had no effect.

Previous studies have associated changes in the gut microbiome with obesity and diabetes in humans. But the latest findings, which still must be confirmed in larger studies and by other groups, advance our knowledge one step further by suggesting that artificial sweeteners may be one of what's likely to be an array of factors with the power to shape such changes.

Artificial Sweeteners and Cancer Risk

Many studies have looked at the possibility that specific dietary components or nutrients are associated with increases or decreases in cancer risk. Studies of cancer cells in the laboratory and of animal models have sometimes provided evidence that isolated compounds may be carcinogenic (or have anticancer activity).

But with few exceptions, studies of human populations have not yet shown definitively that any dietary component causes or protects against cancer. Sometimes the results of epidemiologic studies that compare the diets of people with and without cancer have indicated that people with and without cancer differ in their intake of a particular dietary component.

However, these results show only that the dietary component is associated with a change in cancer risk, not that the dietary component is responsible for, or causes, the change in risk. For example, study participants with and without cancer could differ in other ways besides their diet, and it is possible that some other difference accounts for the difference in cancer.

Studies have been conducted on the safety of several artificial sweeteners, including saccharin, aspartame, acesulfame potassium, sucralose, neotame, and cyclamate. There is no clear evidence that the artificial sweeteners available commercially in the United States are associated with cancer risk in humans.

Chapter 29

Empty Calories

What Are Empty Calories?

"Empty Calories" are the calories from solid fats and added sugars in foods and beverages. They add to total calories, but provide no vitamins or minerals. Allowing too many can fill you up without supplying the nutrients you need. Empty calories can also add more calories than you need.

Some examples of **empty calories** are:

- The **sugars or sweeteners** in soft drinks, fruit punch, candies, cakes, cookies, pies, and ice cream.

- The **solid fats** in cookies, cakes, pizza, cheese, sausages, fatty meats, butter, and stick margarine.

- Some foods–such as milk, yogurt, and cereals–provide important nutrients, but they can also contain some **empty calories**. For example, sweetened yogurt and sweetened breakfast cereals contain added sugars. Whole milk and cheese contain solid fat.

This chapter contains text excerpted from the following sources: Text under the heading "What Are Empty Calories?" is excerpted excerpts from "Empty Calories," ChooseMyPlate.gov, U.S. Department of Agriculture (USDA), March 30, 2016; Text under the heading "Discretionary Calories in the Context of the Sedentary Lifestyle and Typical Food Consumption of Americans" is excerpted from "Nutrition and Your Health: Dietary Guidelines for Americans: Discretionary Calories," Office of Disease Prevention and Health Promotion (ODPHP), U.S. Department of Health and Human Services (HHS), August 26, 2004. Reviewed June 2016.

Look for food choices that are low-fat, fat-free, unsweetened or with no-added sugars.

There is room for foods with some empty calories from added sugars or solid fats now and then. But most daily food choices should be low in empty calories.

Discretionary Calories in the Context of the Sedentary Lifestyle and Typical Food Consumption of Americans

Discretionary calories are calories remaining when an individual meets his or her recommended nutrient intake while consuming fewer calories than his or her daily energy requirement. Discretionary calories can be available only when individuals consume nutrient-dense, lower-energy density foods and maintain an adequate level of physical activity.

At present, Americans are consuming calories in excess of calorie needs (as manifest by the high prevalence of overweight and obesity) but are not meeting recommended nutrient intakes. This pattern of calorie intakes exceeding energy expenditure results because Americans often consume nutrient-poor and energy-dense foods and because they are increasingly sedentary. Therefore, Americans have few, if any, discretionary calories.

To make discretionary calories available or to increase the amount of discretionary calories, individuals need to

- increase their physical activity AND/OR

- consume nutrient-rich foods that are relatively low in energy density in a manner consistent with the dietary patterns recommended in this report.

When available, discretionary calories can be used to consume additional foods from the basic food groups and/or foods in the recommended food groups that are higher in solid fat and/or that contain added sugar.

Chapter 30

Excess Sodium

Is It Salt or Sodium?[1]

Sodium chloride is the chemical name for dietary salt. The words "salt" and "sodium" are not exactly the same, but consumers often use them interchangeably. The use of both terms may be seen on food packaging; for example, the Nutrition Facts label uses "sodium," whereas the front of the package may say "salt free." Ninety percent of the sodium we consume is in the form of salt.

Where Does Most of the Sodium in Our Diet Come from?[1]

Most of the sodium we eat comes from processed foods and foods prepared in restaurants. When sodium is added to processed foods, it cannot be removed. More than 40% of sodium intake comes from the following ten types of foods:

1. Breads and rolls

2. Cold cuts and cured meats such as deli or packaged ham or turkey

---

This chapter contains text excerpted from documents published by two public domain sources. Text under heading marked 1 is excerpted from "Sodium: Q&A," Centers for Disease Control and Prevention (CDC), April 2016; Text under heading marked 2 is excerpted from "Sodium: The Facts," Centers for Disease Control and Prevention (CDC), April 2016.

3. Pizza

4. Fresh and processed poultry

5. Soups

6. Sandwiches such as cheeseburgers

7. Cheese

8. Pasta dishes (not including macaroni and cheese)

9. Meat-mixed dishes such as meat loaf with tomato sauce

10. Snacks such as chips, pretzels, and popcorn

Sodium Consumption and Sodium in Our Food Supply[2]

- We all need a small amount of sodium to keep our bodies working properly.

- The *2015–2020 Dietary Guidelines for Americans* recommend that Americans consume less than 2,300 milligrams (mg) of sodium each day as part of a healthy eating pattern.

- The average daily sodium intake for Americans age 2 years and older is more than 3,400 mg.

- Americans are consuming substantially more sodium. Since the 1970s, the amount of sodium in our food has increased, and we are eating more food each day than in the past.

- The majority of the sodium consumed is from processed and restaurant foods; only a small portion is used in cooking or added at the table.

- Decreasing personal sodium intake can be hard, even for motivated persons.

- Sodium content can vary significantly within food categories. For example, a regular slice of frozen cheese pizza can range from 450 mg to 1200 mg, and some brands of breakfast sausage links have twice the sodium content of other brands.

- Nutrition labeling and package messaging are easily misunderstood by consumers.

Reducing Sodium, Reducing Cardiovascular Disease Burden[2]

High sodium intake raises blood pressure, and high blood pressure is a major cause of heart disease and stroke. Even if a person does not have high blood pressure, reducing sodium intake is important because the lower one's blood pressure in general, the lower the risk for heart disease and stroke. For American adults, the recommendation is to consume less than 2,300 mg of sodium each day. Reducing average population sodium consumption by 400 mg has been projected to prevent up to 28,000 deaths from any cause and save $7 billion in health care expenditures annually.

Can't Individuals Reduce Their Sodium Intake on Their Own?[2]

Although some foods are high in sodium, excess sodium intake also is from frequent consumption of foods with only moderate amounts of sodium, such as breads and poultry. Additionally, different brands of the same foods may have different sodium levels. For example, sodium in chicken noodle soup can vary by as much as 840 mg per serving. Americans also eat outside the home frequently, and many restaurant foods do not have nutrition labels, so consumers often underestimate the amount of sodium, calories, and fat in restaurant meals. For all of these reasons, lowering personal sodium intake can be difficult. Gradually lowering the sodium content of the entire food supply will create greater choice for consumers who want or need to reduce sodium intake.

What Does "Salt Sensitive" Mean? Who Is "Salt Sensitive"?[1]

Although nearly everyone can benefit from sodium reduction, some people are more salt sensitive than others—that is, they experience greater changes in blood pressure in relation to changes in sodium consumption. These individuals often include those who are older, black, have high blood pressure, have diabetes or have chronic kidney disease. No screening test exists for salt sensitive people.

Table Salt Provides Iodine. Will Reducing Salt Intake Lead to Iodine Deficiency?[1]

The majority of the sodium Americans consume comes from processed and restaurant foods. In the United States, salt used in food processing is not iodized. Reducing sodium in these foods would have minimal impact on iodine status in the population.

Other Potential Benefits of Reduced Sodium Consumption That Need Further Research[2]

- Reduced risk of gastro-esophageal cancer
- Reduced left ventricular mass
- Preserved bone mass

Chapter 31

Commercial Beverages

Chapter Contents

Section 31.1

Making Healthy Beverage Choices

This section includes text excerpted from "Rethink Your Drink," Centers for Disease Control and Prevention (CDC), September 23, 2015.

Rethink Your Drink

When it comes to weight loss, there's no lack of diets promising fast results. There are low-carb diets, high-carb diets, low-fat diets, grapefruit diets, cabbage soup diets, and blood type diets, to name a few. But no matter what diet you may try, to lose weight, you must take in fewer calories than your body uses. Most people try to reduce their caloric intake by focusing on food, but another way to cut calories may be to think about what you drink.

What Do You Drink? It Makes More Difference than You Think!

Calories in drinks are not hidden (they're listed right on the Nutrition Facts label), but many people don't realize just how many calories beverages can contribute to their daily intake. As you can see in the example below, calories from drinks can really add up. But there is good news: you have plenty of options for reducing the number of calories in what you drink.

Table 31.1. Options for Reducing the Number of Calories in Your Drink

Occasion	Instead of...	Calories	Try...	Calories
Morning coffee shop run	Medium café latte (16 ounces) made with whole milk	265	Small café latte (12 ounces) made with fat-free milk	125
Lunchtime combo meal	20-oz. bottle of nondiet cola with your lunch	227	Bottle of water or diet soda	0

Table 31.1. Continued

Occasion	Instead of...	Calories	Try...	Calories
Afternoon break	Sweetened lemon iced tea from the vending machine (16 ounces)	180	Sparkling water with natural lemon flavor (not sweetened)	0
Dinnertime	A glass of nondiet ginger ale with your meal (12 ounces)	124	Water with a slice of lemon or lime or seltzer water with a splash of 100% fruit juice	0 calories for the water with fruit slice or about 30 calories for seltzer water with 2 ounces of 100% orange juice.
Total beverage calories:		796		125-155
(USDA National Nutrient Database for Standard Reference)				

Substituting no-or low-calorie drinks for sugar-sweetened beverages cuts about 650 calories in the example above.

Of course, not everyone drinks the amount of sugar-sweetened beverages shown above.

Check the list below to estimate how many calories you typically take in from beverages.

Table 31.2. Estimated Calories Typically Taken from Beverages

Type of Beverage	Calories in 12 ounces	Calories in 20 ounces
Fruit punch	192	320
100% apple juice	192	300
100% orange juice	168	280
Lemonade	168	280
Regular lemon/lime soda	148	247
Regular cola	136	227
Sweetened lemon iced tea (bottled, not homemade)	135	225
Tonic water	124	207

Table 31.2. Estimated Calories Typically Taken from Beverages

Type of Beverage	Calories in 12 ounces	Calories in 20 ounces
Regular ginger ale	124	207
Sports drink	99	165
Fitness water	18	36
Unsweetened iced tea	2	3
Diet soda (with aspartame)	0*	0*
Carbonated water (unsweetened)	0	0
Water	0	0

##*Some diet soft drinks can contain a small number of calories that are not listed on the nutrition facts label. (USDA National Nutrient Database for Standard Reference)

Milk contains vitamins and other nutrients that contribute to good health, but it also contains calories. Choosing low-fat or fat-free milk is a good way to reduce your calorie intake and still get the nutrients that milk contains.

Table 31.3. Choosing Low-Fat or Fat-Free Milk

Type of Milk	Calories per cup (8 ounces)
Chocolate milk (whole)	208
Chocolate milk (2% reduced-fat)	190
Chocolate milk (1% low-fat)	158
Whole Milk (unflavored)	150
2% reduced-fat milk (unflavored)	120
1% low-fat milk (unflavored)	105
Fat-free milk (unflavored)	90

*Some diet soft drinks can contain a small number of calories that are not listed on the nutrition facts label. (USDA National Nutrient Database for Standard Reference)

Learn to Read Nutrition Facts Labels Carefully

Be aware that the Nutrition Facts label on beverage containers may give the calories for only part of the contents. The example below shows the label on a 20-oz. bottle. As you can see, it lists the number of calories in an 8-oz. serving (100) even though the bottle contains 20 oz. or 2.5 servings. To figure out how many calories are in the whole bottle, you need to multiply the number of calories in one serving by the number of servings in the bottle (100 x 2.5). You can see that the contents of the entire bottle actually contain 250 calories even though what the label calls a "serving" only contains 100. This shows that you need to look closely at the serving size when comparing the calorie content of different beverages.

Sugar by Any Other Name: How to Tell Whether Your Drink Is Sweetened?

Sweeteners that add calories to a beverage go by many different names and are not always obvious to anyone looking at the ingredients list. Some common caloric sweeteners are listed below. If these appear in the ingredients list of your favorite beverage, you are drinking a sugar-sweetened beverage.

- High-fructose corn syrup
- Fructose
- Fruit juice concentrates
- Honey
- Sugar
- Syrup
- Corn syrup
- Sucrose
- Dextrose

High-Calorie Culprits in Unexpected Places

Coffee drinks and blended fruit smoothies sound innocent enough, but the calories in some of your favorite coffee-shop or smoothie-stand items may surprise you. Check the Website or in-store nutrition information of your favorite coffee or smoothie shop to find out how many calories are in different menu items. And when a smoothie or coffee craving kicks in, here are some tips to help minimize the caloric damage:

At the Coffee Shop:

- Request that your drink be made with fat-free or low-fat milk instead of whole milk
- Order the smallest size available.
- Forgo the extra flavoring—the flavor syrups used in coffee shops, like vanilla or hazelnut, are sugar-sweetened and will add calories to your drink.

- Skip the whip. The whipped cream on top of coffee drinks adds calories and fat.

- Get back to basics. Order a plain cup of coffee with fat-free milk and artificial sweetener or drink it black.

At the Smoothie Stand:

- Order a child's size if available.

- Ask to see the nutrition information for each type of smoothie and pick the smoothie with the fewest calories.

- Hold the sugar. Many smoothies contain added sugar in addition to the sugar naturally in fruit, juice or yogurt. Ask that your smoothie be prepared without added sugar: the fruit is naturally sweet.

Better Beverage Choices Made Easy

Now that you know how much difference a drink can make, here are some ways to make smart beverage choices:

- Choose water, diet or low-calorie beverages instead of sugar-sweetened beverages.

- For a quick, easy, and inexpensive thirst-quencher, carry a water bottle and refill it throughout the day.

- Don't "stock the fridge" with sugar-sweetened beverages. Instead, keep a jug or bottles of cold water in the fridge.

- Serve water with meals.

- Make water more exciting by adding slices of lemon, lime, cucumber or watermelon or drink sparkling water.

- Add a splash of 100% juice to plain sparkling water for a refreshing, low-calorie drink.

- When you do opt for a sugar-sweetened beverage, go for the small size. Some companies are now selling 8-oz. cans and bottles of soda, which contain about 100 calories.

- Be a role model for your friends and family by choosing healthy, low-calorie beverages.

Section 31.2

Energy Drinks, Caffeine, and Health

This section includes text excerpted from "Energy Drinks,"
National Center for Complementary and Integrative
Health (NCCIH), May 23, 2016.

Energy drinks are widely promoted as products that increase alertness and enhance physical and mental performance. Marketing targeted at young people has been quite effective. Next to multivitamins, energy drinks are the most popular dietary supplement consumed by American teens and young adults. Males between the ages of 18 and 34 years consume the most energy drinks, and almost one-third of teens between 12 and 17 years drink them regularly.

Caffeine is the major ingredient in most energy drinks—a 24-oz energy drink may contain as much as 500 mg of caffeine (similar to that in four or five cups of coffee). Energy drinks also may contain guarana (another source of caffeine sometimes called Brazilian cocoa), sugars, taurine, ginseng, B vitamins, glucuronolactone, yohimbe, carnitine, and bitter orange.

Consuming energy drinks also increases important safety concerns. Between 2007 and 2011, the overall number of energy-drink related visits to emergency departments doubled, with the most significant increase (279 percent) in people aged 40 and older. A growing trend among young adults and teens is mixing energy drinks with alcohol. About 25 percent of college students consume alcohol with energy drinks, and they binge drink significantly more often than students who don't mix them. In 2011, 42 percent of all energy-drink related emergency department visits involved combining these beverages with alcohol or drugs (including illicit drugs, like marijuana, as well as central nervous system stimulants, like Ritalin or Adderall).

Bottom Line

- Although there's very limited data that caffeine-containing energy drinks may temporarily improve alertness and physical endurance, evidence that they enhance strength or power is lacking.

- There's not enough evidence to determine the effects of additives other than caffeine in energy drinks.

- The amounts of caffeine in energy drinks vary widely, and the actual caffeine content may not be identified easily.

Safety

- Large amounts of caffeine may cause serious heart and blood vessel problems such as heart rhythm disturbances and increases in heart rate and blood pressure. Caffeine also may harm children's still-developing cardiovascular and nervous systems.

- Caffeine use may be associated with palpitations, anxiety, sleep problems, digestive problems, elevated blood pressure, and dehydration.

- Guarana, commonly added to energy drinks, contains caffeine. Therefore, the addition of guarana increases the drink's total caffeine content.

- Young adults who combine caffeinated drinks with alcohol may not be able to tell how intoxicated they are.

- Excessive energy drink consumption may disrupt teens' sleep patterns and may fuel risk-taking behavior.

- Many energy drinks contain as much as 25–50 g of simple sugars; this may be problematic for people who are diabetic or prediabetic.

Chapter 32

Food Additives and Irradiation

Chapter Contents

Section 32.1

Food Ingredients, Additives, and Colors

This section includes text excerpted from "Overview of Food
Ingredients, Additives, and Colors," U.S. Food and Drug
Administration (FDA), December 2, 2014.

For centuries, ingredients have served useful functions in a variety
of foods. Our ancestors used salt to preserve meats and fish, added
herbs and spices to improve the flavor of foods, preserved fruit with
sugar, and pickled cucumbers in a vinegar solution. Today, consumers demand and enjoy a food supply that is flavorful, nutritious, safe,
convenient, colorful, and affordable. Food additives and advances in
technology help make that possible.

There are thousands of ingredients used to make foods. The U.S.
Food and Drug Administration (FDA) maintains a list of over 3000
ingredients in its database "Everything Added to Food in the United
States," many of which we use at home every day (e.g., sugar, baking
soda, salt, vanilla, yeast, spices, and colors).

Still, some consumers have concerns about additives because they
may see the long, unfamiliar names and think of them as complex
chemical compounds. In fact, every food we eat-whether a just-picked
strawberry or a homemade cookie-is made up of chemical compounds
that determine flavor, color, texture, and nutrient value. All food
additives are carefully regulated by federal authorities and various
international organizations to ensure that foods are safe to eat and
are accurately labeled.

The purpose of this section is to provide helpful background information about food and color additives: what they are, why they are
used in foods, and how they are regulated for safe use.

Why Are Food and Color Ingredients Added to Food?

Additives perform a variety of useful functions in foods that consumers often take for granted. Some additives could be eliminated if
we were willing to grow our own food, harvest and grind it, spend many
hours cooking and canning or accept increased risks of food spoilage.

But most consumers today rely on the many technological, aesthetic, and convenient benefits that additives provide.

Following are three main reasons why ingredients are added to foods:

1. To Maintain or Improve Safety and Freshness: Preservatives slow product spoilage caused by mold, air, bacteria, fungi or yeast. In addition to maintaining the quality of the food, they help control contamination that can cause foodborne illness, including life-threatening botulism. One group of preservatives—antioxidants—prevents fats and oils and the foods containing them from becoming rancid or developing an off-flavor. They also prevent cut fresh fruits such as apples from turning brown when exposed to air.

2. To Improve or Maintain Nutritional Value: Vitamins and minerals (and fiber) are added to many foods to make up for those lacking in a person's diet or lost in processing or to enhance the nutritional quality of a food. Such fortification and enrichment has helped reduce malnutrition in the U.S. and worldwide. All products containing added nutrients must be appropriately labeled.

3. Improve Taste, Texture, and Appearance: Spices, natural and artificial flavors, and sweeteners are added to enhance the taste of food. Food colors maintain or improve appearance. Emulsifiers, stabilizers, and thickeners give foods the texture and consistency consumers expect. Leavening agents allow baked goods to rise during baking. Some additives help control the acidity and alkalinity of foods, while other ingredients help maintain the taste and appeal of foods with reduced fat content.

What Is a Food Additive?

In its broadest sense, a food additive is any substance added to food. Legally, the term refers to "any substance the intended use of which results or may reasonably be expected to result—directly or indirectly—in its becoming a component or otherwise affecting the characteristics of any food." This definition includes any substance used in the production, processing, treatment, packaging, transportation or storage of food. The purpose of the legal definition, however, is to impose a premarket approval requirement. Therefore, this definition excludes ingredients whose use is generally recognized as safe (where government approval is not needed), those ingredients approved for use by FDA or the U.S. Department of Agriculture (USDA) prior to the food additives provisions of law, and color additives and pesticides where other legal premarket approval requirements apply.

Direct food additives are those that are added to a food for a specific purpose in that food. For example, xanthan gum—used in salad dressings, chocolate milk, bakery fillings, puddings, and other foods to add texture—is a direct additive. Most direct additives are identified on the ingredient label of foods.

Indirect food additives are those that become part of the food in trace amounts due to its packaging, storage or other handling. For instance, minute amounts of packaging substances may find their way into foods during storage. Food packaging manufacturers must prove to the U.S. Food and Drug Administration (FDA) that all materials coming in contact with food are safe before they are permitted for use in such a manner.

What Is a Color Additive?

A color additive is any dye, pigment or substance which when added or applied to a food, drug or cosmetic or to the human body, is capable (alone or through reactions with other substances) of imparting color. FDA is responsible for regulating all color additives to ensure that foods containing color additives are safe to eat, contain only approved ingredients and are accurately labeled.

Color additives are used in foods for many reasons:

1. to offset color loss due to exposure to light, air, temperature extremes, moisture, and storage conditions

2. to correct natural variations in color

3. to enhance colors that occur naturally

4. to provide color to colorless and "fun" foods

Without color additives, colas wouldn't be brown, margarine wouldn't be yellow and mint ice cream wouldn't be green. Color additives are now recognized as an important part of practically all processed foods we eat.

FDA's permitted colors are classified as subject to certification or **exempt from certification**, both of which are subject to rigorous safety standards prior to their approval and listing for use in foods.

- **Certified colors** are synthetically produced (or human made) and used widely because they impart an intense, uniform color, are less expensive, and blend more easily to create a variety of hues. There are nine certified color additives approved for use in the United States. Certified food colors generally do not add undesirable flavors to foods.

- Colors that are **exempt from certification** include pigments derived from natural sources such as vegetables, minerals or animals. Nature derived color additives are typically more expensive than certified colors and may add unintended flavors to foods. Examples of exempt colors include annatto extract (yellow), dehydrated beets (bluish-red to brown), caramel (yellow to tan), beta-carotene, (yellow to orange) and grape skin extract (red, green).

How Are Additives Approved for Use in Foods?

Food and color additives are more strictly studied, regulated, and monitored than at any other time in history. FDA has the primary legal responsibility for determining their safe use. To market a new food or color additive (or before using an additive already approved for one use in another manner not yet approved), a manufacturer or other sponsor must first petition FDA for its approval. These petitions must provide evidence that the substance is safe for the ways in which it will be used. As a result of recent legislation, since 1999, indirect additives have been approved via a premarket notification process requiring the same data as was previously required by petition.

When evaluating the safety of a substance and whether it should be approved, FDA considers:

1. the composition and properties of the substance;

2. the amount that would typically be consumed;

3. immediate and long-term health effects; and

4. various safety factors.

The evaluation determines an appropriate level of use that includes a built-in safety margin-a factor that allows for uncertainty about the levels of consumption that are expected to be harmless. In other words, the levels of use that gain approval are much lower than what would be expected to have any adverse effect.

Because of inherent limitations of science, FDA can never be *absolutely* certain of the absence of any risk from the use of any substance. Therefore, FDA must determine-based on the best science available-if there is a *reasonable certainty of no harm* to consumers when an additive is used as proposed.

If an additive is approved, FDA issues regulations that may include the types of foods in which it can be used, the maximum amounts to be used, and how it should be identified on food labels. In 1999, procedures changed so that FDA now consults with USDA during the review process for ingredients that are proposed for use in meat and poultry products. Federal officials then monitor the extent of American's' consumption of the new additive and results of any new research on its safety to ensure its use continues to be within safe limits.

If new evidence suggests that a product already in use may be unsafe or if consumption levels have changed enough to require another look, federal authorities may prohibit its use or conduct further studies to determine if the use can still be considered safe.

Regulations known as Good Manufacturing Practices (GMP) limit the amount of food ingredients used in foods to the amount necessary to achieve the desired effect.

Table 32.1. Types of Food Ingredients

Types of Ingredients	What They Do	Examples of Uses	Names Found on Product Labels
Preservatives	Prevent food spoilage from bacteria, molds, fungi or yeast (antimicrobials); slow or prevent changes in color, flavor or texture and delay rancidity (antioxidants); maintain freshness	Fruit sauces and jellies, beverages, baked goods, cured meats, oils and margarines, cereals, dressings, snack foods, fruits and vegetables	Ascorbic acid, citric acid, sodium benzoate, calcium propionate, sodium erythorbate, sodium nitrite, calcium sorbate, potassium sorbate, BHA, BHT, EDTA, tocopherols (Vitamin E)
Sweeteners	Add sweetness with or without the extra calories	Beverages, baked goods, confections, table-top sugar, substitutes, many processed foods	Sucrose (sugar), glucose, fructose, sorbitol, mannitol, corn syrup, high fructose corn syrup, saccharin, aspartame, sucralose, acesulfame potassium (acesulfame-K), neotame

Table 32.1. Continued

Types of Ingredients	What They Do	Examples of Uses	Names Found on Product Labels
Color Additives	Offset color loss due to exposure to light, air, temperature extremes, moisture and storage conditions; correct natural variations in color; enhance colors that occur naturally; provide color to colorless and "fun" foods	Many processed foods, (candies, snack foods margarine, cheese, soft drinks, jams/jellies, gelatins, pudding and pie fillings)	FD&C Blue Nos. 1 and 2, FD&C Green No. 3, FD&C Red Nos. 3 and 40, FD&C Yellow Nos. 5 and 6, Orange B, Citrus Red No. 2, annatto extract, beta-carotene, grape skin extract, cochineal extract or carmine, paprika oleoresin, caramel color, fruit and vegetable juices, saffron (Note: Exempt color additives are not required to be declared by name on labels but may be declared simply as colorings or color added)
Flavors and Spices	Add specific flavors (natural and synthetic)	Pudding and pie fillings, gelatin dessert mixes, cake mixes, salad dressings, candies, soft drinks, ice cream, BBQ sauce	Natural flavoring, artificial flavor, and spices
Flavor Enhancers	Enhance flavors already present in foods (without providing their own separate flavor)	Many processed foods	Monosodium glutamate (MSG), hydrolyzed soy protein, autolyzed yeast extract, disodium guanylate or inosinate

Table 32.1. Continued

Types of Ingredients	What They Do	Examples of Uses	Names Found on Product Labels
Fat Replacers (and components of formulations used to replace fats)	Provide expected texture and a creamy "mouth-feel" in reduced-fat foods	Baked goods, dressings, frozen desserts, confections, cake and dessert mixes, dairy products	Olestra, cellulose gel, carrageenan, polydextrose, modified food starch, microparticulated egg white protein, guar gum, xanthan gum, whey protein concentrate
Nutrients	Replace vitamins and minerals lost in processing (enrichment), add nutrients that may be lacking in the diet (fortification)	Flour, breads, cereals, rice, macaroni, margarine, salt, milk, fruit beverages, energy bars, instant breakfast drinks	Thiamine hydrochloride, riboflavin (Vitamin B2), niacin, niacinamide, folate or folic acid, beta carotene, potassium iodide, iron or ferrous sulfate, alpha tocopherols, ascorbic acid, Vitamin D, amino acids (L-tryptophan, L-lysine, L-leucine, L-methionine)
Emulsifiers	Allow smooth mixing of ingredients, prevent separation Keep emulsified products stable, reduce stickiness, control crystallization, keep ingredients dispersed, and to help products dissolve more easily	Salad dressings, peanut butter, chocolate, margarine, frozen desserts	Soy lecithin, mono- and diglycerides, egg yolks, polysorbates, sorbitan monostearate

Table 32.1. Continued

Types of Ingredients	What They Do	Examples of Uses	Names Found on Product Labels
Stabilizers and Thickeners, Binders, Texturizers	Produce uniform texture, improve "mouth-feel"	Frozen desserts, dairy products, cakes, pudding and gelatin mixes, dressings, jams and jellies, sauces	Gelatin, pectin, guar gum, carrageenan, xanthan gum, whey
pH Control Agents and acidulants	Control acidity and alkalinity, prevent spoilage	Beverages, frozen desserts, chocolate, low acid canned foods, baking powder	Lactic acid, citric acid, ammonium hydroxide, sodium carbonate
Leavening Agents	Promote rising of baked goods	Breads and other baked goods	Baking soda, monocalcium phosphate, calcium carbonate
Anti-caking agents	Keep powdered foods free-flowing, prevent moisture absorption	Salt, baking powder, confectioner's sugar	Calcium silicate, iron ammonium citrate, silicon dioxide
Humectants	Retain moisture	Shredded coconut, marshmallows, soft candies, confections	Glycerin, sorbitol
Yeast Nutrients	Promote growth of yeast	Breads and other baked goods	Calcium sulfate, ammonium phosphate
Dough Strengtheners and Conditioners	Produce more stable dough	Breads and other baked goods	Ammonium sulfate, azodicarbonamide, L-cysteine
Firming Agents	Maintain crispness and firmness	Processed fruits and vegetables	Calcium chloride, calcium lactate
Enzyme Preparations	Modify proteins, polysaccharides and fats	Cheese, dairy products, meat	Enzymes, lactase, papain, rennet, chymosin
Gases	Serve as propellant, aerate or create carbonation	Oil cooking spray, whipped cream, carbonated beverages	Carbon dioxide, nitrous oxide

Section 32.2

Food Irradiation

This section includes text excerpted from "Food Irradiation:
What You Need to Know," U.S. Food and Drug Administration
(FDA), September 3, 2015.

Food irradiation (the application of ionizing radiation to food) is a technology that improves the safety and extends the shelf life of foods by reducing or eliminating microorganisms and insects. Like pasteurizing milk and canning fruits and vegetables, irradiation can make food safer for the consumer.

The U.S. Food and Drug Administration (FDA) is responsible for regulating the sources of radiation that are used to irradiate food. FDA approves a source of radiation for use on foods only after it has determined that irradiating the food is safe.

Why Irradiate Food?

Irradiation can serve many purposes.

- **Prevention of Foodborne Illness**–irradiation can be used to effectively eliminate organisms that cause foodborne illness, such as Salmonella and Escherichia coli (E. coli).

- **Preservation**–irradiation can be used to destroy or inactivate organisms that cause spoilage and decomposition and extend the shelf life of foods.

- **Control of Insects**–irradiation can be used to destroy insects in or on tropical fruits imported into the United States. Irradiation also decreases the need for other pest-control practices that may harm the fruit.

- **Delay of Sprouting and Ripening**–irradiation can be used to inhibit sprouting (e.g., potatoes) and delay ripening of fruit to increase longevity.

- **Sterilization**–irradiation can be used to sterilize foods, which can then be stored for years without refrigeration. Sterilized foods are useful in hospitals for patients with severely impaired immune systems, such as patients with AIDS or undergoing chemotherapy. Foods that are sterilized by irradiation are exposed to substantially higher levels of treatment than those approved for general use.

Debunking Irradiation Myths

Irradiation does not make foods radioactive, compromise nutritional quality or noticeably change the taste, texture or appearance of food. In fact, any changes made by irradiation are so minimal that it is not easy to tell if a food has been irradiated.

How Is Food Irradiated?

There are three sources of radiation approved for use on foods.

1. **Gamma rays** are emitted from radioactive forms of the element cobalt (Cobalt 60) or of the element cesium (Cesium 137). Gamma radiation is used routinely to sterilize medical, dental and household products and is also used for the radiation treatment of cancer.

2. **X-rays** are produced by reflecting a high-energy stream of electrons off a target substance (usually one of the heavy metals) into food. X-rays are also widely used in medicine and industry to produce images of internal structures.

3. **Electron beam** (or e-beam) is similar to X-rays and is a stream of high-energy electrons propelled from an electron accelerator into food.

Is Irradiated Food Safe to Eat?

FDA has evaluated the safety of irradiated food for more than thirty years and has found the process to be safe. The World Health Organization (WHO), the Centers for Disease Control and Prevention (CDC), and the U.S. Department of Agriculture (USDA) have also endorsed the safety of irradiated food.

What Foods Have Been Approved for Irradiation?

FDA has approved a variety of foods for irradiation in the United States including:

- Beef and Pork

- Crustaceans (e.g., lobster, shrimp, and crab)

- Fresh Fruits and Vegetables

- Lettuce and Spinach

- Molluscan Shellfish (e.g., oysters, clams, mussels, and scallops)

- Poultry

- Seeds for Sprouting (e.g., for alfalfa sprouts)

- Shell Eggs

- Spices and Seasonings

How Will I Know If My Food Has Been Irradiated?

FDA requires that irradiated foods bear the international symbol for irradiation. Look for the Radura symbol along with the statement "Treated with radiation" or "Treated by irradiation" on the food label. Bulk foods, such as fruits and vegetables, are required to be individually labeled or to have a label next to the sale container. FDA does not require that individual ingredients in multi-ingredient foods (e.g., spices) be labeled.

It is important to remember that irradiation is not a replacement for proper food-handling practices by producers, processors, and consumers. Irradiated foods need to be stored, handled and cooked in the same way as non-irradiated foods, because they could still become contaminated with disease-causing organisms after irradiation if the rules of basic food safety are not followed.

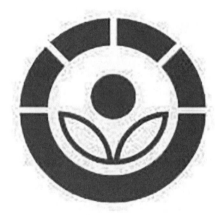

Figure 32.1. *Food Irradiation Logo*

Chapter 33

Food Safety

Chapter Contents

Section 33.1

How Food Gets Contaminated in the Production Chain?

This section includes text excerpted from "The Food Production Chain-How Food Gets Contaminated," Centers for Disease Control and Prevention (CDC), March 24, 2015.

It takes several steps to get food from the farm or fishery to the dining table. We call these steps the food production chain. Contamination can occur at any point along the chain—during production, processing, distribution or preparation.

Production

Production means growing the plants we harvest or raising the animals we use for food. Most food comes from domesticated animals and plants, and their production occurs on farms or ranches. Some foods are caught or harvested from the wild, such as some fish, mushrooms, and game.

Examples of Contamination in Production

- If a hen's reproductive organs are infected, the yolk of an egg can be contaminated in the hen before it is even laid.

- If the fields are sprayed with contaminated water for irrigation, fruits and vegetables can be contaminated before harvest.

- Fish in some tropical reefs may acquire a toxin from the smaller sea creatures they eat.

Processing

Processing means changing plants or animals into what we recognize and buy as food. Processing involves different steps for different kinds of foods. For produce, processing can be as simple as cleaning and sorting or it can involve trimming, slicing or shredding and bagging.

Milk is usually processed by pasteurizing it; sometimes it is made into cheese. Nuts may be roasted, chopped or ground (such as with peanut butter). For animals, the first step of processing is slaughter. Meat and poultry may then be cut into pieces or ground. They may also be smoked, cooked or frozen and may be combined with other ingredients to make a sausage or entrée, such as a potpie.

Examples of Contamination in Processing

- If contaminated water or ice is used to wash, pack or chill fruits or vegetables, the contamination can spread to those items.

- Peanut butter can become contaminated if roasted peanuts are stored in unclean conditions or come into contact with contaminated raw peanuts.

- During the slaughter process, pathogens on an animal's hide that came from the intestines can get into the final meat product.

Distribution

Distribution means getting food from the farm or processing plant to the consumer or a food service facility like a restaurant, cafeteria or hospital kitchen. This step might involve transporting foods just once, such as trucking produce from a farm to the local farmers' market. Or it might involve many stages. For instance, frozen hamburger patties might be trucked from a meat processing plant to a large supplier, stored for a few days in the supplier's warehouse, trucked again to a local distribution facility for a restaurant chain, and finally delivered to an individual restaurant.

Examples of Contamination in Distribution

- If refrigerated food is left on a loading dock for long time in warm weather, it could reach temperatures that allow bacteria to grow.

- Fresh produce can be contaminated if it is loaded into a truck that was not cleaned after transporting animals or animal products.

- The contents of a glass jar that breaks in transport can contaminate nearby foods.

Preparation

Preparation means getting the food ready to eat. This step may occur in the kitchen of a restaurant, home or institution. It may involve following a complex recipe with many ingredients, simply heating and serving a food on a plate or just opening a package and eating the food.

Examples of Contamination in Preparation

- If a food worker stays on the job while he or she is sick and does not wash his or her hands carefully after using the toilet, he or she can spread pathogens by touching food.

- If a cook uses a cutting board or knife to cut raw chicken and then uses the same knife or cutting board without washing it to slice tomatoes for a salad, the tomatoes can be contaminated by pathogens from the chicken.

- Contamination can occur in a refrigerator if meat juices get on other items that will be eaten raw.

Mishandling at Multiple Points

Sometimes, by the time a food causes illness, it has been mishandled in several ways along the food production chain. Once contamination occurs, further mishandling of food, such as undercooking the food or leaving it out on the counter at unsafe temperatures, can make an outbreak more likely. Many pathogens grow quickly in food held at room temperature; a tiny number can grow to a large number in just a few hours. Reheating or boiling food after it has been left at room temperature for a long time does not always make it safe because some pathogens produce toxins that are not destroyed by heating.

Section 33.2

Safe Food Preparation and Handling

This section includes text excerpted from "Safe Food Handling:
What You Need to Know," U.S. Food and Drug Administration
(FDA), February 9, 2015.

The food supply in the United States is among the safest in the world.
However, when certain disease-causing bacteria or pathogens contaminate food, they can cause foodborne illness, often called "food poisoning."

The Federal government estimates that there are about 48 million
cases of foodborne illness annually–the equivalent of sickening 1 in
6 Americans each year. And each year these illnesses result in an
estimated 128,000 hospitalizations and 3,000 deaths.

Since foodborne illness can be serious—or even fatal—it is important for you to know and practice safe food handling behaviors to help
reduce your risk of accidentally getting sick from contaminated food.

Four Steps to Food Safety

1. CLEAN: Wash hands and surfaces often

Bacteria can be spread throughout the kitchen and get onto hands,
cutting boards, utensils, counter tops and food.

To ensure that your hands and surfaces are clean, be sure to:

- Wash your hands with warm water and soap for at least 20
  seconds before and after handling food and after using the bathroom, changing diapers and handling pets.

- Wash your cutting boards, dishes, utensils and counter tops with
  hot soapy water after preparing each food item and before you go
  on to the next food.

- Consider using paper towels to clean up kitchen surfaces. If you
  use cloth towels wash them often in the hot cycle of your washing machine.

- Rinse fresh fruits and vegetables under running tap water,
  including those with skins and rinds that are not eaten.

379

- Rub firm-skin fruits and vegetables under running tap water or scrub with a clean vegetable brush while rinsing with running tap water.

- With canned goods, remember to clean lids before opening.

2. SEPARATE: Separate raw meats from other foods

Cross-contamination can occur when bacteria are spread from one food product to another. This is especially common when handling raw meat, poultry, seafood and eggs. The key is to keep these foods—and their juices—away from ready-to-eat foods.

To prevent cross-contamination, remember to:

- Separate raw meat, poultry, seafood and eggs from other foods in your grocery shopping cart, grocery bags and in your refrigerator.

- Use one cutting board for fresh produce and a separate one for raw meat, poultry and seafood.

- Never place cooked food on a plate that previously held raw meat, poultry, seafood or eggs.

- Don't reuse marinades used on raw foods unless you bring them to a boil first.

3. COOK: Cook to the right temperatures

Food is safely cooked when it reaches a high enough internal temperature to kill the harmful bacteria that cause illness. Refer to the Safe Cooking Temperatures Chart for the proper internal temperatures.

To ensure that your foods are cooked safely, always:

- Use a food thermometer to measure the internal temperature of cooked foods. Check the internal temperature in several places to make sure that the meat, poultry, seafood, eggs or dishes containing eggs are cooked to safe minimum internal temperatures as shown in the Safe Cooking Temperatures Chart.

- Cook ground meat or ground poultry until it reaches a safe internal temperature. Color is not a reliable indicator of doneness.

- Cook eggs until the yolk and white are firm. Only use recipes in which eggs are cooked or heated thoroughly.

- When cooking in a microwave oven, cover food, stir, and rotate for even cooking. If there is no turntable, rotate the dish by hand once or twice during cooking. Always allow standing time, which completes the cooking, before checking the internal temperature with a food thermometer. Food is done when it reaches the safe minimum internal temperature.

- Bring sauces, soups, and gravy to a boil when reheating.

4. CHILL: Refrigerate foods promptly

Refrigerate foods quickly because cold temperatures slow the growth of harmful bacteria. Do not over-stuff the refrigerator. Cold air must circulate to help keep food safe. Keeping a constant refrigerator temperature of 40°F or below is one of the most effective ways to reduce the risk of foodborne illness. Use an appliance thermometer to be sure the temperature is consistently 40°F or below and the freezer temperature is 0°F or below.

To chill foods properly:

- Refrigerate or freeze meat, poultry, eggs, seafood and other perishables within 2 hours of cooking or purchasing. Refrigerate within 1 hour if the temperature outside is above 90°F.

- Never thaw food at room temperature, such as on the counter top. Food must be kept at a safe temperature during thawing. There are three safe ways to defrost food: in the refrigerator, in cold water, and in the microwave. Food thawed in cold water or in the microwave should be cooked immediately.

- Always marinate food in the refrigerator.

- Divide large amounts of leftovers into shallow containers for quicker cooling in the refrigerator.

- Use or discard refrigerated food on a regular basis.

Is It Done Yet?

Table 33.1. Safe Cooking Temperatures

Safe cooking temperatures as measured with a food thermometer	
Food Type	**Internal temperature**
Ground Meat and Meat Mixtures	
Beef, Pork, Veal, Lamb	160oF
Turkey, Chicken	165oF
Fresh Beef, Pork, Veal, and Lamb	145oF with a 3 minute rest time
Poultry	

Table 33.1. Continued

Safe cooking temperatures as measured with a food thermometer	
Food Type	**Internal temperature**
Chicken and Turkey, Whole	165oF
Poultry Parts	165oF
Duck and Goose	165oF
Stuffing (cooked alone/in bird)	165oF
Ham	
Fresh (raw)	145oF with a 3 minute rest time
Pre-cooked (to reheat)	140oF
Eggs and Egg Dishes	
Eggs	Cook until yolk and white are firm
Egg Dishes	160oF
Seafood	
Fin Fish	145oF or flesh is opaque and separates easily with fork
Shrimp, Lobster and Crabs	Flesh pearly and opaque
Clams, Oysters and Mussels	Shells open during cooking
Scallops	Milky white or opaque and firm
Leftovers and Casseroles	165oF

Section 33.3

Food Safety: Mistakes and Myths

This section contains text excerpted from the following sources: Text beginning with the heading "Dangerous Food Safety Mistakes" is excerpted from "Dangerous Food Safety Mistakes," FoodSafety.gov, U.S. Department of Health and Human Services (HHS), July 1, 2011. Reviewed June 2016; Text beginning with the heading "Food Safety Myths Exposed" is excerpted from "Food Safety Myths Exposed," FoodSafety.gov, U.S. Department of Health and Human Services (HHS), July 1, 2011. Reviewed June 2016.

Dangerous Food Safety Mistakes

Sometimes a simple mistake can have grave consequences. What may seem like a small food safety mistake can cause serious illness with long-term consequences.

When it comes to some germs, such as Salmonella, all it takes is 15 to 20 cells in undercooked food to cause food poisoning. And just a tiny taste of food with botulinum toxin can cause paralysis and even death.

Here are some common food safety mistakes that have been proven to cause serious illness.

Tasting Food to See If It's Still Good

Why: You can't taste (or smell or see) the bacteria that cause food poisoning. Tasting only a tiny amount can cause serious illness.

Solution: Throw food out before harmful bacteria grows.

Putting Cooked Meat Back on a Plate That Held Raw Meat

Why: Germs from the raw meat can spread to the cooked meat.

Solution: Always use separate plates for raw meat and cooked meat. The same rule applies to poultry and seafood.

Thawing Food on the Counter

Why: Harmful germs can multiply extremely rapidly at room temperature.

Solution: Thaw food safely:

• In the refrigerator

• In cold water

• In the microwave

Letting Food Cool before Putting It in the Fridge

Why: Illness-causing bacteria can grow in perishable foods within two hours unless you refrigerate them

Solution: Refrigerate perishable foods within 2 hours (or within 1 hour if the temperature is over 90°F.

Eating Raw Cookie Dough (or Other Foods with Uncooked Eggs)

Why: Uncooked eggs may contain Salmonella or other harmful bacteria.

Solution: Always cook eggs thoroughly. Avoid foods that contain raw or undercooked eggs.

Marinating Meat or Seafood on the Counter

Why: Harmful germs in meat or seafood can multiply extremely rapidly at room temperature.

Solution: Always marinate meat or seafood in the refrigerator.

Using Raw Meat Marinade on Cooked Food

Why: Germs from the raw meat (or seafood) can spread to the cooked food.

Solution: You can reuse marinade only if you bring it to a boil just before using.

Undercooking Meat, Poultry, Seafood or Eggs

Why: Cooked food is safe only after it's been cooked to a high enough temperature to kill harmful bacteria

Solution: Use the Safe Minimum Cooking Temperatures chart and a food thermometer.

Not Washing Your Hands

Why: Germs on your hands can contaminate the food that you or others eat.

Solution: Wash hands the right way—for 20 seconds with soap and running water.

Food Safety Myths Exposed

We all do our best to serve our families food that's safe and healthy, but some common myths about food safety might surprise you.

Common Myths about Food Safety at Home

Myth #1: Food poisoning isn't that big of a deal. I just have to tough it out for a day or two and then it's over.

Fact: Many people don't know it, but some foodborne illnesses can actually lead to long-term health conditions, and 3,000 Americans a year die from foodborne illness. Get the facts on long-term effects of food poisoning.

Myth #2: When cleaning my kitchen, the more bleach I use, the better. More bleach kills more bacteria, so it's safer for my family.

Fact: There is actually no advantage to using more bleach than needed. To clean kitchen surfaces effectively, use just one teaspoon of liquid, unscented bleach to one quart of water.

Myth #3: I don't need to wash fruits or vegetables if I'm going to peel them.

Fact: Because it's easy to transfer bacteria from the peel or rind you're cutting to the inside of your fruits and veggies, it's important to wash all produce, even if you plan to peel it.

Myth #4: To get rid of any bacteria on my meat, poultry or seafood, I should rinse off the juices with water first.

Fact: Actually, rinsing meat, poultry or seafood with water can increase your chance of food poisoning by splashing juices (and any bacteria they might contain) onto your sink and counters. The best way to cook meat, poultry or seafood safely is to make sure you cook it to the right temperature.

Myth #5: The only reason to let food sit after it's been microwaved is to make sure you don't burn yourself on food that's too hot.

Fact: In fact, letting microwaved food sit for a few minutes ("standing time") helps your food cook more completely by allowing colder areas of food time to absorb heat from hotter areas of food.

Myth #6: If I really want my produce to be safe, I should wash fruits and veggies with soap or detergent before I use them.

Fact: In fact, it's best not to use soaps or detergents on produce, since these products can linger on foods and are not safe for consumption. Using clean running water is actually the best way to remove bacteria and wash produce safely.

Section 33.4

Food Safety: At Risk Groups

This section includes text excerpted from "Food Safety: It's Especially Important for At-Risk Groups," U.S. Food and Drug Administration (FDA), April 6, 2013.

The food supply in the United States is among the safest in the world. However, when certain disease-causing bacteria or pathogens contaminate food, they can cause foodborne illness, often called "food poisoning." The Federal government estimates that there are about 48 million cases of foodborne illness annually—the equivalent of sickening 1 in 6 Americans each year. And each year, these illnesses result in an estimated 128,000 hospitalizations and 3,000 deaths. Although everyone is susceptible, some people are at greater risk for developing foodborne illness.

Who's At-Risk?

If you—or someone you care for—are in one of these high-risk groups, it's especially important to practice safe food handling. Vulnerable people are not only at increased risk of contracting a foodborne illness, but are also more likely to have a lengthy illness, undergo hospitalization or even die.

Pregnant Women

Changes during pregnancy alter the mother's immune system, making pregnant women more susceptible to foodborne illness. Harmful bacteria can also cross the placenta and infect an unborn baby whose immune system is underdeveloped and not able to fight infection. Foodborne illness during pregnancy is serious and can lead to miscarriage, premature delivery, stillbirth, sickness or the death of a newborn baby.

Young Children

Young children are more at risk for foodborne illness because their immune systems are still developing.

Older Adults

As people age, their immune system and other organs become sluggish in recognizing and ridding the body of harmful bacteria and other pathogens that cause infections, such as foodborne illness. Many older adults have also been diagnosed with one or more chronic conditions, such as diabetes, arthritis, cancer or cardiovascular disease, and are taking at least one medication. The chronic disease process and/or the side effects of some medications may also weaken the immune system. In addition, stomach acid decreases as people get older, and stomach acid plays an important role in reducing the number of bacteria in the intestinal tract–and the risk of illness.

People with Immune Systems Weakened by Disease or Medical Treatment

The immune system is the body's natural reaction or response to "foreign invasion." In healthy people, a properly functioning immune system readily fights off harmful bacteria and other pathogens that cause infection. However, the immune systems of **transplant patients** and people with certain illnesses, such as **HIV/AIDS, cancer, and diabetes**, are often weakened from the disease process and/or the side effects of some treatments, making them susceptible to many types of infections—like those that can be brought on by harmful bacteria that cause foodborne illness. In addition, diabetes may lead to a slowing of the rate at which food passes through the stomach and intestines, allowing harmful foodborne pathogens an opportunity to multiply.

Foods to Avoid

If you are at greater risk of foodborne illness, **you are advised not to eat:**

- Raw or undercooked meat or poultry.

- Raw fish, partially cooked seafood (such as shrimp and crab), and refrigerated smoked seafood.

- Raw shellfish (including oysters, clams, mussels, and scallops) and their juices.

- Unpasteurized (raw) milk and products made with raw milk, like yogurt and cheese.

- Soft cheeses made from unpasteurized milk, such as Feta, Brie, Camembert, blue-veined, and Mexican-style cheeses (such as such as Queso Fresco, Panela, Asadero, and Queso Blanco).

- Raw or undercooked eggs or foods containing raw or under-cooked eggs, including certain homemade salad dressings (such as Caesar salad dressing), homemade cookie dough and cake batters, and homemade eggnog.

NOTE: Most pre-made foods from grocery stores, such as Caesar dressing, pre-made cookie dough or packaged eggnog are made with pasteurized eggs.

- Unwashed fresh vegetables, including lettuce/salads.

- Unpasteurized fruit or vegetable juices (these juices will carry a warning label).

- Hot dogs, luncheon meats (cold cuts), fermented and dry sausage, and other deli-style meats, poultry products, and smoked fish—unless they are reheated until steaming hot.

- Salads (without added preservatives) prepared on site in a deli-type establishment, such as ham salad, chicken salad or seafood salad.

- Unpasteurized, refrigerated pâtés or meat spreads.

- Raw sprouts (alfalfa, bean or any other sprout).

Foodborne Illness: Know the Symptoms

Symptoms of foodborne illness usually appear 12 to 72 hours after eating contaminated food, but may occur between 30 minutes and 4 weeks later. Symptoms include:

- Nausea, vomiting, diarrhea (may be bloody), and abdominal pain

- Flu Like symptoms such as fever, headache, and bodyache

If you suspect that you could have a foodborne illness, **contact your physician or healthcare provider right away!**

Section 33.5

Mold on Foods

This section includes text excerpted from "Molds on Food: Are They Dangerous?" Food Safety and Inspection Service (FSIS), U.S. Department of Agriculture (USDA), August 22, 2013.

What Are Molds?

Molds are microscopic fungi that live on plant or animal matter. No one knows how many species of fungi exist, but estimates range from tens of thousands to perhaps 300,000 or more. Most are filamentous (threadlike) organisms and the production of spores is characteristic of fungi in general. These spores can be transported by air, water or insects.

Unlike bacteria that are one-celled, molds are made of many cells and can sometimes be seen with the naked eye. Under a microscope, they look like skinny mushrooms. In many molds, the body consists of:

- root threads that invade the food it lives on,

- a stalk rising above the food, and

- spores that form at the ends of the stalks.

The spores give mold the color you see. When airborne, the spores spread the mold from place to place like dandelion seeds blowing across a meadow.

Molds have branches and roots that are like very thin threads. The roots may be difficult to see when the mold is growing on food and may be very deep in the food. Foods that are moldy may also have invisible bacteria growing along with the mold.

Are Some Molds Dangerous?

Yes, some molds cause allergic reactions and respiratory problems. And a few molds, in the right conditions, produce "mycotoxins," poisonous substances that can make you sick.

Are Molds Only on the Surface of Food?

No, you only see part of the mold on the surface of food—gray fur on forgotten bologna, fuzzy green dots on bread, white dust on Cheddar, coin-size velvety circles on fruits, and furry growth on the surface of jellies. When a food shows heavy mold growth, "root" threads have invaded it deeply. In dangerous molds, poisonous substances are often contained in and around these threads. In some cases, toxins may have spread throughout the food.

Where Are Molds Found?

Molds are found in virtually every environment and can be detected, both indoors and outdoors, year round. Mold growth is encouraged by warm and humid conditions. Outdoors, they can be found in shady, damp areas or places where leaves or other vegetation are decomposing. Indoors, they can be found where humidity levels are high.

Molds form spores which, when dry, float through the air and find suitable conditions where they can start the growth cycle again.

What Are Some Common Foodborne Molds?

Molds most often found on meat and poultry are *Alternaria, Aspergillus, Botrytis, Cladosporium, Fusarium, Geotrichum, Monilia, Manoscus, Mortierella, Mucor, Neurospora, Oidium, Oosproa, Penicillium, Rhizopus,* and *Thamnidium.* These molds can also be found on many other foods.

What Are Mycotoxins?

Mycotoxins are poisonous substances produced by certain molds found primarily in grain and nut crops, but are also known to be on celery, grape juice, apples, and other produce. There are many of them and scientists are continually discovering new ones. The Food and Agriculture Organization (FAO) of the United Nations estimates that 25% of the world's food crops are affected by mycotoxins, of which the most notorious are aflatoxins.

What is Aflatoxin?

Aflatoxin is a cancer-causing poison produced by certain fungi in or on foods and feeds, especially in field corn and peanuts. They are probably the best known and most intensively researched mycotoxins in the world. Aflatoxins have been associated with various diseases, such as aflatoxicosis in livestock, domestic animals, and humans throughout the world. Many countries try to limit exposure to aflatoxin by regulating and monitoring its presence on commodities intended for use as food and feed. The prevention of aflatoxin is one of the most challenging toxicology issues of present time.

How Does the U.S. Government Control Aflatoxins?

Aflatoxins are considered unavoidable contaminants of food and feed, even where good manufacturing practices have been followed. The U.S. Food and Drug Administration and the U.S. Department of Agriculture (USDA) monitor peanuts and field corn for aflatoxin and can remove any food or feed with unacceptable levels of it.

Is Mushroom Poisoning Caused by Molds?

No, it is due to the toxin produced by the fungi, which are in the same family as molds. Mushroom poisoning is caused by the consumption of raw or cooked mushrooms, which are higher-species of fungi. There is no general rule of thumb for distinguishing edible mushrooms from poisonous toadstools. The toxins that cause mushroom poisoning are produced naturally by the fungi. Most mushrooms that cause human poisoning cannot be made safe by cooking, canning, freezing or any other processing. The only way to avoid poisoning is not to eat poisonous mushrooms.

Are Any Food Molds Beneficial?

Yes, molds are used to make certain kinds of cheeses and can be on the surface of cheese or be developed internally. Blue veined cheese such as Roquefort, blue, Gorgonzola, and Stilton are created by the introduction of *P. roqueforti* or *Penicillium roqueforti* spores. Cheeses such as Brie and Camembert have white surface molds. Other cheeses have both an internal and a surface mold. The molds used to manufacture these cheeses are safe to eat.

Why Can Mold Grow in the Refrigerator?

While most molds prefer warmer temperatures, they can grow at refrigerator temperatures, too. Molds also tolerate salt and sugar better than most other food invaders. Therefore, molds can grow in refrigerated jams and jelly and on cured, salty meats — ham, bacon, salami, and bologna.

How Can You Minimize Mold Growth?

Cleanliness is vital in controlling mold. Mold spores from affected food can build up in your refrigerator, dishcloths, and other cleaning utensils.

- Clean the inside of the refrigerator every few months with 1 tablespoon of baking soda dissolved in a quart of water. Rinse with clear water and dry. Scrub visible mold (usually black) on rubber casings using 3 teaspoons of bleach in a quart of water.

- Keep dishcloths, towels, sponges, and mops clean and fresh. A musty smell means they're spreading mold around. Discard items you can't clean or launder.

- Keep the humidity level in the house below 40%.

Don't Buy Moldy Foods

Examine food well before you buy it. Check food in glass jars, look at the stem areas on fresh produce, and avoid bruised produce. Notify the store manager about mold on foods!

Fresh meat and poultry are usually mold free, but cured and cooked meats may not be. Examine them carefully. Exceptions: Some salamis—San Francisco, Italian, and Eastern European types—have a characteristic thin, white mold coating which is safe to consume; however, they shouldn't show any other mold. Dry-cured country hams normally have surface mold that must be scrubbed off before cooking.

Must Homemade Shelf-Stable Preserves be Water-Bath Processed?

Yes, molds can thrive in high-acid foods like jams, jellies, pickles, fruit, and tomatoes. But these microscopic fungi are easily destroyed by heat processing high-acid foods at a temperature of 212 °F in a boiling water canner for the recommended length of time. For more information about processing home-canned foods, go to the National Center for Home Food Preservation at: www.uga.edu/nchfp/.

How Can You Protect Food from Mold?

- When serving food, keep it covered to prevent exposure to mold spores in the air. Use plastic wrap to cover foods you want to stay moist—fresh or cut fruits and vegetables, and green and mixed salads.

- Empty opened cans of perishable foods into clean storage containers and refrigerate them promptly.

- Don't leave any perishables out of the refrigerator more than 2 hours.

- Use leftovers within 3 to 4 days so mold doesn't have a chance to grow.

How Should You Handle Food with Mold on It?

Buying small amounts and using food quickly can help prevent mold growth. But when you see moldy food:

- Don't sniff the moldy item. This can cause respiratory trouble.

- If food is covered with mold, discard it. Put it into a small paper bag or wrap it in plastic and dispose in a covered trash can that children and animals can't get into.

- Clean the refrigerator or pantry at the spot where the food was stored.

- Check nearby items the moldy food might have touched. Mold spreads quickly in fruits and vegetables.

Table 33.2. Moldy Food: When to Use, When to Discard

FOOD	HANDLING	REASON
Luncheon meats, bacon or hot dogs	Discard	Foods with high moisture content can be contaminated below the surface. Moldy foods may also have bacteria growing along with the mold.
Hard salami and dry-cured country hams	Use. Scrub mold off surface.	It is normal for these shelf-stable products to have surface mold.
Cooked leftover meat and poultry	Discard	Foods with high moisture content can be contaminated below the surface. Moldy foods may also have bacteria growing along with the mold.

Table 33.2. Continued

FOOD	HANDLING	REASON
Cooked casseroles	Discard	Foods with high moisture content can be contaminated below the surface. Moldy foods may also have bacteria growing along with the mold.
Cooked grain and pasta	Discard	Foods with high moisture content can be contaminated below the surface. Moldy foods may also have bacteria growing along with the mold.
Hard cheese (not cheese where mold is part of the processing)	Use. Cut off at least 1 inch around and below the mold spot (keep the knife out of the mold itself so it will not cross-contaminate other parts of the cheese). After trimming off the mold, re-cover the cheese in fresh wrap.	Mold generally cannot penetrate deep into the product.
Cheese made with mold (such as Roquefort, blue, Gorgonzola, Stilton, Brie, Camembert)	Discard soft cheeses such as Brie and Camembert if they contain molds that are not a part of the manufacturing process. If surface mold is on hard cheeses such as Gorgonzola and Stilton, cut off mold at least 1 inch around and below the mold spot and handle like hard cheese (above).	Molds that are not a part of the manufacturing process can be dangerous.
Soft cheese (such as cottage, cream cheese, Neufchatel, chevre, Bel Paese, etc.) Crumbled, shredded, and sliced cheeses (all types)	Discard	Foods with high moisture content can be contaminated below the surface. Shredded, sliced or crumbled cheese can be contaminated by the cutting instrument. Moldy soft cheese can also have bacteria growing along with the mold.

Table 33.2. Continued

FOOD	HANDLING	REASON
Yogurt and sour cream	Discard	Foods with high moisture content can be contaminated below the surface. Moldy foods may also have bacteria growing along with the mold.
Jams and jellies	Discard	The mold could be producing a mycotoxin. Microbiologists recommend against scooping out the mold and using the remaining condiment.
Fruits and vegetables, FIRM (such as cabbage, bell peppers, carrots, etc.)	Use. Cut off at least 1 inch around and below the mold spot (keep the knife out of the mold itself so it will not cross-contaminate other parts of the produce).	Small mold spots can be cut off FIRM fruits and vegetables with low moisture content. It's difficult for mold to penetrate dense foods.
Fruits and vegetables, SOFT (such as cucumbers, peaches, tomatoes, etc.)	Discard	SOFT fruits and vegetables with high moisture content can be contaminated below the surface.
Bread and baked goods	Discard	Porous foods can be contaminated below the surface.
Peanut butter, legumes and nuts	Discard	Foods processed without preservatives are at high risk for mold.

Section 33.6

Foodborne Illnesses

This section includes text excerpted from "Foodborne Illnesses:
What You Need to Know," U.S. Food and Drug
Administration (FDA), January 7, 2016.

While the American food supply is among the safest in the world,
the Federal government estimates that there are about **48 million
cases of foodborne illness annually**—the equivalent of sickening
1 in 6 Americans each year. And each year these illnesses result in an
estimated 128,000 hospitalizations and 3,000 deaths.

The table below includes foodborne disease-causing organisms that
frequently cause illness in the United States. As the chart shows, the
threats are numerous and varied, with symptoms ranging from relatively mild discomfort to very serious,life-threatening illness. While
the very young, the elderly, and persons with weakened immune systems are at greatest risk of serious consequences from most foodborne
illnesses, some of the organisms shown below pose grave threats to
all persons.

Table 33.3. Foodborne Illnesses: What You Need to Know

Organism	Common Name of Illness	Onset Time After Ingesting	Signs and Symptoms	Duration	Food Sources
Bacillus cereus	*B. cereus food poisoning*	10-16 hrs	Abdominal cramps, watery diarrhea, nausea	24-48 hours	Meats, stews, gravies, vanilla sauce
Campylobacter jejuni	Campylobacteriosis	2-5 days	Diarrhea, cramps, fever, and vomiting; diarrhea may be bloody	2-10 days	Raw and undercooked poultry, unpasteurized milk, contaminated water
Clostridium botulinum	Botulism	12-72 hours	Vomiting, diarrhea, blurred vision, double vision, difficulty in swallowing, muscle weakness. Can result in respiratory failure and death	Variable	Improperly canned foods, especially home-canned vegetables, fermented fish, baked potatoes in aluminum foil
Clostridium perfringens	Perfringens food poisoning	8–16 hours	Intense abdominal cramps, watery diarrhea	Usually 24 hours	Meats, poultry, gravy, dried or precooked foods, time and/ or temperature-abused foods

Table 33.3. Continued

Organism	Common Name of Illness	Onset Time After Ingesting	Signs and Symptoms	Duration	Food Sources
Cryptosporidium	Intestinal cryptosporidiosis	2-10 days	Diarrhea (usually watery), stomach cramps, upset stomach, slight fever	May be remitting and relapsing over weeks to months	Uncooked food or food contaminated by an ill food handler after cooking, contaminated drinking water
Cyclospora cayetanensis	Cyclosporiasis	1-14 days, usually at least 1 week	Diarrhea (usually watery), loss of appetite, substantial loss of weight, stomach cramps, nausea, vomiting, fatigue	May be remitting and relapsing over weeks to months	Various types of fresh produce (imported berries, lettuce, basil)
E. coli (Escherichia coli) producing toxin	*E. coli infection (common cause of "travelers' diarrhea")*	1-3 days	Watery diarrhea, abdominal cramps, some vomiting	3-7 or more days	Water or food contaminated with human feces
E. coli O157:H7	Hemorrhagic colitis or E. coli O157:H7 infection	1-8 days	Severe (often bloody) diarrhea, abdominal pain and vomiting. Usually, little or no fever is present. More common in children 4 years or younger. Can lead to kidney failure.	5-10 days	Undercooked beef (especially hamburger), unpasteurized milk and juice, raw fruits and vegetables (e.g. sprouts), and contaminated water

Table 33.3. Continued

Organism	Common Name of Illness	Onset Time After Ingesting	Signs and Symptoms	Duration	Food Sources
Hepatitis A	Hepatitis	28 days average (15-50 days)	Diarrhea, dark urine, jaundice, and flu-like symptoms, i.e., fever, headache, nausea, and abdominal pain	Variable, 2 weeks-3 months	Raw produce, contaminated drinking water, uncooked foods and cooked foods that are not reheated after contact with an infected food handler; shellfish from contaminated waters
Listeria monocytogenes	Listeriosis	9-48 hrs for gastro-intestinal symptoms, 2-6 weeks for invasive disease	Fever, muscle aches, and nausea or diarrhea. Pregnant women may have mild flu-like illness, and infection can lead to premature delivery or stillbirth. The elderly or immunocompromised patients may develop bacteremia or meningitis.	Variable	Unpasteurized milk, soft cheeses made with unpasteurized milk, ready-to-eat deli meats

Table 33.3. Continued

Organism	Common Name of Illness	Onset Time After Ingesting	Signs and Symptoms	Duration	Food Sources
Noroviruses	Variously called viral gastroenteritis, winter diarrhea, acute non-bacterial gastroenteritis, food poisoning, and food infection	12-48 hrs	Nausea, vomiting, abdominal cramping, diarrhea, fever, headache. Diarrhea is more prevalent in adults, vomiting more common in children.	12-60 hrs	Raw produce, contaminated drinking water, uncooked foods and cooked foods that are not reheated after contact with an infected food handler; shellfish from contaminated waters
Salmonella	Salmonellosis	6-48 hours	Diarrhea, fever, abdominal cramps, vomiting	4-7 days	Eggs, poultry, meat, unpateurized milk or juice, cheese, contaminated raw fruits and vegetables

Table 33.3. Continued

Organism	Common Name of Illness	Onset Time After Ingesting	Signs and Symptoms	Duration	Food Sources
Shigella	Shigellosis or Bacillary dysentery	4-7 days	Abdominal cramps, fever, and diarrhea. Stools may contain blood and mucus.	24-48 hrs	Raw produce, contaminated drinking water, uncooked foods and cooked foods that are not reheated after contact with an infected food handler
Staphylococcus aureus	Staphylococcal food poisoning	1-6 hours	Sudden onset of severe nausea and vomiting. Abdominal cramps. Diarrhea and fever may be present.	24-48 hours	Unrefrigerated or improperly refrigerated meats, potato and egg salads, cream pastries
Vibrio parahaemolyticus	*V. parahaemolyticusinfection*	4-96 hours	Watery (occasionally bloody) diarrhea, abdominal cramps, nausea, vomiting, fever	2-5 days	Undercooked or raw seafood, such as shellfish

401

Table 33.3. Continued

Organism	Common Name of Illness	Onset Time After Ingesting	Signs and Symptoms	Duration	Food Sources
Vibrio vulnificus	*V. vulnificusinfection*	1-7 days	Vomiting, diarrhea, abdominal pain, bloodborne infection. Fever, bleeding within the skin, ulcers requiring surgical removal. Can be fatal to persons with liver disease or weakened immune systems.	2-8 days	Undercooked or raw seafood, such as shellfish (especially oysters)

Chapter 34

The Health Consequences of Nutrition Misinformation

Why is Food and Nutrition Misinformation on the Rise?

Health fraud takes many forms, and one of the most common examples is nutrition fraud. Nutrition fraud refers to inaccurate, misleading, or exaggerated information about the content, ingredients, or expected results of food and nutritional products, including food items, supplements, diet plans, and devices. In the United States, nutrition fraud is a serious problem. Nutrition fraud is occurring with increasing frequency due to the large number of new food products and herbal, botanical, sports, and dietary supplements entering the market. The rise of food fads has also contributed to the increase of nutrition misinformation. Food fads are themselves based on misinformation and exaggerated claims that certain foods have special health benefits, or that certain foods are harmful and should be eliminated from the diet.

Nutrition misinformation spreads in many ways. Overzealous marketers promote new products through books, television talk shows, articles and advertisements in magazines and newspapers, and direct mail to consumers. Word of mouth also helps to spread misinformation among families, friends, and communities. Nutrition misinformation is difficult to control through government regulation, therefore consumers must thoughtfully evaluate information they receive about the nutritional properties of food and dietary supplements.

Sources of Food and Nutrition Misinformation

Consumers get information about food products and dietary supplements from a variety of sources. The media plays a role by providing information via television, newspapers, and magazines. Information reaches consumers directly from the food industry in the form of advertisements, celebrity endorsements, food labels and packaging, and other communications. Information is also passed via more informal means, through word of mouth among friends, coworkers, neighbors, and other community members. The Internet is also a primary source of information for many consumers.

Many channels of information about food and nutrition are not well regulated and must be evaluated carefully by consumers. For example, information appearing on web sites is generally not governed by any regulatory agency. On the Internet, misleading or false information often appears side-by-side with valid, science-based information. Discussions in Internet chat rooms and forums are a popular source of nutrition information, and these sources may be sponsored or influenced by people or organizations with a vested interest in promoting a certain product. The Internet can facilitate the spread of inaccurate information with alarming speed.

Types of Food and Nutrition Misinformation

Nutrition misinformation takes many forms. Food fads are a major source of misinformation about individual foods or food ingredients. A certain food, for example kale, may suddenly become wildly popular and heralded as a "super food" offering many health benefits. Or a food ingredient such as gluten can suddenly be labelled as bad, unhealthy, and even harmful for people to consume. Fad diets are another source of nutrition misinformation. Fad diets promote rapid weight loss through either eliminating "bad" foods or consuming only "good" foods. Examples of fad diets include low-carbohydrate eating plans and specific-food diets like the grapefruit diet.

Health fraud can generally be recognized by the use of extravagant claims touting the product or diet as a "miracle cure" or "secret to effortless weight loss." Health fraud usually involves the promotion of a product for financial gain that is unproven or doesn't work. In a similar way, misdirected health claims are statements intended to encourage consumers to make incorrect judgements about the nutritional content or health benefits of a food or product. One example of a misdirected health claim is a food that is advertised as low fat and therefore healthy, when it in fact is high in calories.

Consequences of Nutrition Misinformation

Consumers spend billions of dollars each year on food and nutrition products, dietary supplements, and weight-loss products. An overwhelming amount of information is circulated about the nutritional value and effects of various foods, supplements, diet products, and so on. In this environment, it can be difficult for consumers to make educated decisions about the potential value and merit of their purchasing decisions. When misinformation leads people to purchase products that don't work, are unproven, or promise unrealistic results, there can be serious health and economic consequences for consumers.

Short-Term and Long-Term Costs of Food and Nutrition Misinformation

Nutrition misinformation can result in both short- and long-term costs for individuals and for society as a whole. These costs can include physical harm if foods contain undocumented ingredients, toxic ingredients, or unknown/undocumented interactions with other substances such as prescription medications. Personal health products can result in physical harm if the use of these products replaces proper medical treatment. This is also the case when remedies fail to work, even if no harm is done.

All of these circumstances can also result in economic costs to consumers. The current overall annual cost of health fraud is estimated in the billions of dollars. Other costs which cannot be measured in dollars include a loss of faith in traditional sources of health and nutrition information and scientific findings. It is difficult to promote public health and gain public trust in an environment of persistent misinformation.

Communicating Evidence-Based Nutrition Information

Successful communication of accurate nutrition and health information depends on two factors: how the information is communicated and how well the information is understood. Health and nutrition information must be communicated with a careful balance between providing enough context and background for consumers to make educated decisions, and overwhelming consumers with too much scientific detail. Information that is provided in clear, easy to understand language can reduce consumer confusion while reinforcing the credibility of the source, whether that is a scientific report, a health professional, or other expert.

Agencies and regulatory bodies of the U.S. Federal Government play a role in communicating nutrition information to consumers through the U.S. Food and Drug Administration's (FDA) food labeling programs. The FDA has implemented standard labeling intended to make it easier for consumers to understand and compare the nutrition information of different products. Government agencies also work with various organizations to communicate health and nutrition information to consumers via web sites, publications, and the media. The media has the capability to effectively reach the largest number of consumers through television, radio, newspapers, and magazines.

The Role of Consumers in Interpreting Information

Ultimately, consumers bear the burden of evaluating health and nutrition information and making reasoned choices. Consumers must thoughtfully assess claims made in advertisements to determine whether a product will meet their specific needs, keeping in mind the trustworthiness and credibility of the information source. A wise consumer will attempt to validate information by checking with their doctor or other health professional, or by contacting the FDA, Better Business Bureau, or other consumer interest groups. In cases of direct marketing, consumers are wise to avoid making spontaneous purchases. A reputable seller will provide time for consumers to think about their purchase and verify information. A legitimate product will stand up to consumer evaluation.

How to Assess the Credibility of Information?

If in doubt that any product will perform as advertised, consumers should attempt to gather and verify product information. Some points to evaluate include:

- What or who is the source of the information? Is that source trustworthy and credible? Does the person or organization have any credentials, professional license, or certification?

- Is the information current?

- How much information is provided? Does it answer all your questions?

- Are there credible references and reviews of the product? Are there testimonials or case histories?

- Is the information balanced? Are any exceptions or disclaimers noted?

- Does the information promise immediate or guaranteed results for little or no effort? These claims should raise suspicions.

- Does the information include words like "breakthrough," "miracle" or "secret"? Does the product claim to be a "recent discovery" that cannot be found or obtained anywhere else? These claims should raise suspicions.

- Are results described in specific or broad terms? The broader the claims, the less likely they are to be true.

- Does the information attempt to use guilt or fear to sell the product? Are you asked to pay in advance? These tactics indicate a possible scam.

- If it sounds too good to be true, it probably is.

Ten Red Flags of Junk Science

1. Recommendations that promise a quick fix.

2. Dire warnings of danger from a single product or regimen.

3. Claims that sound too good to be true.

4. Simplistic conclusions drawn from a complex study.

5. Recommendations based on a single study.

6. Dramatic statements that are refuted by reputable scientific organizations.

7. Lists of "good" and "bad" foods.

8. Recommendations made to help sell a product.

9. Recommendations based on studies published without peer review.

10. Recommendations from studies that ignore individual or group differences.

References

1. "Position of the American Dietetic Association: Food and Nutrition Misinformation," American Dietetic Association. April 2006.

2. Bellows, L. and R. Moore. "Nutrition Misinformation: How to Identify Fraud and Misleading Claims," Colorado State University Extension. September 2013.

3. Hermann, Janice R. "Nutritional Misinformation," Oklahoma State University Cooperative Extension Service. n.d.

Part Six

Nutrition and Weight Control

Chapter 35

The Health Risks of Overweight and Obesity

Chapter Contents

411

Section 35.1

Health Problems Associated with Weighing Too Much

This section includes text excerpted from "Do You Know Some of the Health Risks of Being Overweight?" National Institute of Diabetes and Digestive and Kidney Diseases (NIDDK), December 2012. Reviewed June 2016.

Do You Know Some of the Health Risks of Being Overweight?

Overweight and obesity may increase the risk of many health problems, including diabetes, heart disease, and certain cancers. If you are pregnant, excess weight may lead to short-and long-term health problems for you and your child.

How Can I Tell If I Weigh Too Much?

Gaining a few pounds during the year may not seem like a big deal. But these pounds can add up over time. How can you tell if your weight could increase your chances of developing health problems? Knowing two numbers may help you understand your risk: your body mass index (BMI) score and your waist size in inches.

Body Mass Index

The body mass index (BMI) is one way to tell whether you are at a normal weight, are overweight or have obesity. It measures your weight in relation to your height and provides a score to help place you in a category:

- Normal weight: BMI of 18.5 to 24.9

- Overweight: BMI of 25 to 29.9

- Obesity: BMI of 30 or higher

Waist Size

Another important number to know is your waist size in inches. Having too much fat around your waist may increase health risks even more than having fat in other parts of your body. Women with a waist size of more than 35 inches and men with a waist size of more than 40 inches may have higher chances of developing diseases related to obesity.

Know Your Health Numbers

Below are some numbers to aim for

Table 35.1. Know Your Health Numbers

Measure	Target
Target BMI	18.5-24.9
Waist Size	Men: less than 40 in. Women: less than 35 in.
Blood Pressure	120/80 mm Hg or less
LDL (bad cholesterol)	Less than 100 mg/dl
HDL (good cholesterol)	Men: more than 40 mg/dl Women: more than 50 mg/dl
Triglycerides	Less than 150 mg/dl
Blood sugar (fasting)	Less than 100 mg/dl

Type 2 Diabetes

Type 2 diabetes is a disease in which blood sugar levels are above normal. High blood sugar is a major cause of heart disease, kidney disease, stroke, amputation, and blindness. In 2009, diabetes was the seventh leading cause of death in the United States.

Type 2 diabetes is the most common type of diabetes. Family history and genes play a large role in type 2 diabetes. Other risk factors include a low activity level, poor diet, and excess body weight around the waist. In the United States, type 2 diabetes is more common among blacks, Latinos, and American Indians than among whites.

How Is Type 2 Diabetes Linked to Overweight?

About 80 percent of people with type 2 diabetes are overweight or obese. It isn't clear why people who are overweight are more likely to

413

develop this disease. It may be that being overweight causes cells to change, making them resistant to the hormone insulin. Insulin carries sugar from blood to the cells, where it is used for energy. When a person is insulin resistant, blood sugar cannot be taken up by the cells, resulting in high blood sugar. In addition, the cells that produce insulin must work extra hard to try to keep blood sugar normal. This may cause these cells to gradually fail.

How Can Weight Loss Help?

If you are at risk for type 2 diabetes, losing weight may help prevent or delay the onset of diabetes. If you have type 2 diabetes, losing weight and becoming more physically active can help you control your blood sugar levels and prevent or delay health problems. Losing weight and exercising more may also allow you to reduce the amount of diabetes medicine you take.

High Blood Pressure

Every time your heart beats, it pumps blood through your arteries to the rest of your body. Blood pressure is how hard your blood pushes against the walls of your arteries. High blood pressure (hypertension) usually has no symptoms, but it may cause serious problems, such as heart disease, stroke, and kidney failure.

A blood pressure of 120/80 mmHg (often referred to as "120 over 80") is considered normal. If the top number (systolic blood pressure) is consistently 140 or higher or the bottom number (diastolic blood pressure) is 90 or higher, you are considered to have high blood pressure.

How Is High Blood Pressure Linked to Overweight?

High blood pressure is linked to overweight and obesity in several ways. Having a large body size may increase blood pressure because your heart needs to pump harder to supply blood to all your cells. Excess fat may also damage your kidneys, which help regulate blood pressure.

How Can Weight Loss Help?

Weight loss that will get you close to the normal BMI range may greatly lower high blood pressure. Other helpful changes are to quit smoking, reduce salt, and get regular physical activity. However, if lifestyle changes aren't enough, your doctor may prescribe drugs to lower your blood pressure.

Heart Disease

Heart disease is a term used to describe several problems that may affect your heart. The most common type of problem happens when a blood vessel that carries blood to the heart becomes hard and narrow. This may keep the heart from getting all the blood it needs. Other problems may affect how well the heart pumps. If you have heart disease, you may suffer from a heart attack, heart failure, sudden cardiac death, angina (chest pain) or abnormal heart rhythm. Heart disease is the leading cause of death in the United States.

How Is Heart Disease Linked to Overweight?

People who are overweight or obese often have health problems that may increase the risk for heart disease. These health problems include high blood pressure, high cholesterol, and high blood sugar. In addition, excess weight may cause changes to your heart that make it work harder to send blood to all the cells in your body.

How Can Weight Loss Help?

Losing 5 to 10 percent of your weight may lower your chances of developing heart disease. If you weigh 200 pounds, this means losing as little as 10 pounds. Weight loss may improve blood pressure, cholesterol levels, and blood flow.

Stroke

A stroke happens when the flow of blood to a part of your brain stops, causing brain cells to die. The most common type of stroke, called ischemic stroke, occurs when a blood clot blocks an artery that carries blood to the brain. Another type of stroke, called hemorrhagic stroke, happens when a blood vessel in the brain bursts.

How Are Strokes Linked to Overweight?

Overweight and obesity are known to increase blood pressure. High blood pressure is the leading cause of strokes. Excess weight also increases your chances of developing other problems linked to strokes, including high cholesterol, high blood sugar, and heart disease.

How Can Weight Loss Help?

One of the most important things you can do to reduce your stroke risk is to keep your blood pressure under control. Losing weight may help you lower your blood pressure. It may also improve your cholesterol and blood sugar, which may then lower your risk for stroke.

Cancer

Cancer occurs when cells in one part of the body, such as the colon, grow abnormally or out of control. The cancerous cells sometimes spread to other parts of the body, such as the liver. Cancer is the second leading cause of death in the United States.

How Is Cancer Linked to Overweight?

Gaining weight as an adult increases the risk for several cancers, even if the weight gain doesn't result in overweight or obesity. It isn't known exactly how being overweight increases cancer risk. Fat cells may release hormones that affect cell growth, leading to cancer. Also, eating or physical activity habits that may lead to being overweight may also contribute to cancer risk.

How Can Weight Loss Help?

Avoiding weight gain may prevent a rise in cancer risk. Healthy eating and physical activity habits may lower cancer risk. Weight loss may also lower your risk, although studies have been inconclusive.

What Kinds of Cancers Are Linked to Overweight and Obesity?

Being overweight increases the risk of developing certain cancers, including the following:

- breast, after menopause
- colon and rectum
- endometrium (lining of the uterus)
- gallbladder
- kidney

Sleep Apnea

Sleep apnea is a condition in which a person has one or more pauses in breathing during sleep. A person who has sleep apnea may suffer from daytime sleepiness, difficulty focusing, and even heart failure.

How Is Sleep Apnea Linked to Overweight?

Obesity is the most important risk factor for sleep apnea. A person who is overweight may have more fat stored around his or her neck. This may make the airway smaller. A smaller airway can make breathing difficult or loud (because of snoring) or breathing may stop altogether for short periods of time. In addition, fat stored in the neck and throughout the body may produce substances that cause inflammation. Inflammation in the neck is a risk factor for sleep apnea.

How Can Weight Loss Help?

Weight loss usually improves sleep apnea. Weight loss may help to decrease neck size and lessen inflammation.

Osteoarthritis

Osteoarthritis is a common health problem that causes pain and stiffness in your joints. Osteoarthritis is often related to aging or to an injury, and most often affects the joints of the hands, knees, hips, and lower back.

How Is Osteoarthritis Linked to Overweight?

Being overweight is one of the risk factors for osteoarthritis, along with joint injury, older age, and genetic factors. Extra weight may place extra pressure on joints and cartilage (the hard but slippery tissue that covers the ends of your bones at a joint), causing them to wear away. In addition, people with more body fat may have higher blood levels of substances that cause inflammation. Inflamed joints may raise the risk for osteoarthritis.

How Can Weight Loss Help?

For those who are overweight or obese, losing weight may help reduce the risk of developing osteoarthritis. Weight loss of at least 5 percent of your body weight may decrease stress on your knees, hips, and lower back and lessen inflammation in your body.

Fatty Liver Disease

Fatty liver disease, also known as nonalcoholic steatohepatitis (NASH), occurs when fat builds up in the liver and causes injury.

Fatty liver disease may lead to severe liver damage, cirrhosis (scar tissue) or even liver failure.

Fatty liver disease usually produces mild or no symptoms. It is like alcoholic liver disease, but it isn't caused by alcohol and can occur in people who drink little or no alcohol.

How Is Fatty Liver Disease Linked to Overweight?

The cause of fatty liver disease is still not known. The disease most often affects people who are middle-aged, overweight or obese, and/or diabetic. Fatty liver disease may also affect children.

How Can Weight Loss Help?

Although there is no specific treatment for fatty liver disease, patients are generally advised to lose weight, eat a healthy diet, increase physical activity, and avoid drinking alcohol. If you have fatty liver disease, lowering your body weight to a healthy range may improve liver tests and reverse the disease to some extent.

Kidney Disease

Your kidneys are two bean-shaped organs that filter blood, removing extra water and waste products, which become urine. Your kidneys also help control blood pressure so that your body can stay healthy.

Kidney disease means that the kidneys are damaged and can't filter blood like they should. This damage can cause wastes to build up in the body. It can also cause other problems that can harm your health.

How Is Kidney Disease Linked to Overweight?

Obesity increases the risk of diabetes and high blood pressure, the most common causes of chronic kidney disease. Recent studies suggest that even in the absence of these risks, obesity itself may promote chronic kidney disease and quicken its progress.

How Can Weight Loss Help?

If you are in the early stages of chronic kidney disease, losing weight may slow the disease and keep your kidneys healthier longer. You should also choose foods with less salt (sodium), keep your blood pressure under control, and keep your blood glucose in the target range.

Pregnancy Problems

Overweight and obesity raise the risk of health problems for both mother and baby that may occur during pregnancy. Pregnant women who are overweight or obese may have an increased risk for

- developing gestational diabetes (high blood sugar during pregnancy);

- having preeclampsia (high blood pressure during pregnancy that can cause severe problems for both mother and baby if left untreated); and

- needing a C-section and, as a result, taking longer to recover after giving birth.

Babies of overweight or obese mothers are at an increased risk of being born too soon, being stillborn (dead in the womb after 20 weeks of pregnancy), and having neural tube defects (defects of the brain and spinal cord).

How Are Pregnancy Problems Linked to Overweight?

Pregnant women who are overweight are more likely to develop insulin resistance, high blood sugar, and high blood pressure. Overweight also increases the risks associated with surgery and anesthesia, and severe obesity increases surgery time and blood loss.

Gaining too much weight during pregnancy can have long-term effects for both mother and child. These effects include that the mother will have overweight or obesity after the child is born. Another risk is that the baby may gain too much weight later as a child or as an adult.

If you are pregnant, check Table 35.2 for general guidelines about weight gain. Talk to your healthcare provider about how much weight gain is right for you during pregnancy.

Table 35.2. Recommended amount of weight gain during pregnancy

Pre-pregnancy Weight	Amount to Gain
Underweight (BMI < 18.5)	28-40 lbs.
Normal Weight (BMI 18.5 - 24.9)	25-35 lbs.
Overweight (BMI 25 - 29.9)	15-25 lbs.
Obesity (BMI - 30+)	11-20 lbs.

How Can Weight Loss Help?

If you are overweight or obese and would like to become pregnant, talk to your healthcare provider about losing weight first. Reaching a normal weight before becoming pregnant may reduce your chances of developing weight-related problems. Pregnant women who are overweight or obese should speak with their healthcare provider about limiting weight gain and being physically active during pregnancy.

Losing excess weight after delivery may help women reduce their health risks. For example, if a woman developed gestational diabetes, losing weight may lower her risk of developing diabetes later in life.

How Can I Lower My Risk of Having Health Problems Related to Overweight and Obesity?

If you are considered to be overweight, losing as little as 5 percent of your body weight may lower your risk for several diseases, including heart disease and type 2 diabetes. If you weigh 200 pounds, this means losing 10 pounds. Slow and steady weight loss of 1/2 to 2 pounds per week, and not more than 3 pounds per week, is the safest way to lose weight.

Federal guidelines on physical activity recommend that you get at least 150 minutes a week of moderate aerobic activity (like biking or brisk walking). To lose weight or to maintain weight loss, you may need to be active for up to 300 minutes per week. You also need to do activities to strengthen muscles (like push-ups or sit-ups) at least twice a week.

Federal *Dietary Guidelines* and the MyPlate website recommend many tips for healthy eating that may also help you control your weight. Here are a few examples:

- Make half of your plate fruits and vegetables.

- Replace unrefined grains (white bread, pasta, white rice) with whole-grain options (whole wheat bread, brown rice, oatmeal).

- Enjoy lean sources of protein, such as lean meats, seafood, beans and peas, soy, nuts, and seeds.

For some people who have obesity and related health problems, bariatric (weight-loss) surgery may be an option. Bariatric surgery has been found to be effective in promoting weight loss and reducing the risk for many health problems.

Section 35.2

Portion Size and Obesity

This section includes text excerpted from "Larger Portion Sizes
Contribute to U.S. Obesity Problem," National Heart, Lung, and
Blood Institute (NHLBI), February 13, 2013.

Larger Portion Sizes Contribute to U.S. Obesity Problem

Food portions in America's restaurants have doubled or tripled
over the last 20 years, a key factor that is contributing to a potentially
devastating increase in obesity among children and adults. **We Can!**
(Ways to Enhance Children's Activities and Nutrition), a program
from the National Institutes of Health (NIH), offers parents tips to
help their families maintain a healthy weight.

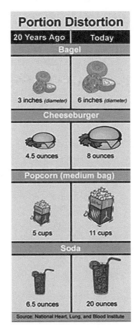

Figure 35.1. *Portion Distortion*

"Super-sized portions at restaurants have distorted what Americans consider a normal portion size, and that affects how much we eat at home as well," said Dr. Elizabeth G. Nabel, director of NIH's National Heart, Lung, and Blood Institute (NHLBI). "One way to keep calories in check is to keep food portions no larger than the size of your fist." Larger portions mean more calories, which can easily add up to extra weight.

Consider, for example, if you had today's portions of the following meals:

- **Breakfast**: a bagel (6 inches in diameter) and a 16-ounce coffee with sugar and milk.

- **Lunch**: two pieces of pepperoni pizza and a 20-ounce soda.

- **Dinner**: a chicken Caesar salad and a 20-ounce soda.

In one day, you would consume 1,595 more calories than if you had the same foods at typical portions served 20 years ago. Over the course of one year, if consumed daily, the larger portions could amount to more than 500,000 extra calories.

Controlling portion sizes and eating smarter can help you and your family avoid extra calories. Here are some tips from the NIH:

- Bring a healthy, low-calorie lunch to work and pack a healthy "brown bag" for your children.

- When eating out, order an appetizer instead of an entrée, share an entrée or eat half of a meal and bring the rest home.

- Cut high-calorie foods like cheese and chocolate into small pieces and eat fewer pieces.

- Substitute a salad for french fries.

- For snacks, serve fruits and vegetables instead of sweets.

Section 35.3

Weight Cycling

This section includes text excerpted from "Weight Cycling," National Institute of Diabetes and Digestive and Kidney Diseases (NIDDK), March 2006. Reviewed June 2016.

Weight cycling is the repeated loss and regain of body weight. This sometimes happens to people who go on weight-loss diets. A small cycle may include loss and regain of 5 to 10 lbs. In a large cycle, weight can change by 50 lbs or more.

Is Weight Cycling Harmful to My Health?

Experts are not sure if weight cycling leads to health problems. However, some studies suggest a link to high blood pressure, high cholesterol, gallbladder disease, and other problems. One study showed other problems may be linked to weight cycling as well. This study showed that women who weight cycle gain more weight over time than women who do not weight cycle. Binge eating (when a person eats a lot of food while feeling out of control) was also linked to women who weight cycle. The same study showed that women who weight cycle were also less likely to use physical activity to control their weight.

Weight cycling may affect your mental health too. People who weight cycle may feel depressed about their weight. However, weight cycling should not be a reason to "feel like a failure." If you feel down, try to focus on making changes in your eating and physical activity habits. Keeping a good attitude will help you stay focused.

If I Weight Cycle after a Diet, Will I Gain More Weight than I Had before the Diet? Will I Have Less Muscle?

Studies do not show that fat tissue increases after a weight cycle. Studies do not support decreases in muscle either. Many people simply regain the weight they lost while on the diet—they have the same amount of fat and muscle as they did before the weight cycle. Some people worry that weight cycling can put more fat around their stomach area. This is important since people who carry extra body weight around this area are more likely to develop type 2 diabetes. Studies show that people do not have more fat around their stomachs after a weight cycle. However, other studies suggest that women who are overweight and have a history of weight cycling have thicker layers of fat around their stomachs—compared to women who do not weight cycle. It is not clear how this relates to weight cycling.

How Can I Manage Weight and Avoid Weight Cycling?

Experts recommend different strategies for different people. The goal for everyone is to achieve a healthy weight. This can help prevent the health problems linked to weight cycling.

- People who are not overweight or obese, and have no health problems related to weight, should maintain a stable weight.

- People who are overweight or obese should try to achieve and maintain a modest weight loss. An initial goal of losing 10 percent of your body weight can help in your efforts to improve overall health.

If you need to lose weight, be ready to make lifelong changes. A healthy diet and physical activity are the keys to your efforts. Focus on making healthful food choices, such as eating more high-fiber foods like fruits and vegetables and cutting down on foods that are high in saturated or trans fats. Walking, jogging or other activities can help keep you active and feeling good.

If I Regain Lost Weight, Will It Be Even Harder to Lose It Again?

Losing weight after a weight cycle should not be harder. Studies show weight cycling does not affect how fast you burn food energy, which is called your "metabolic rate." This rate slows as we get older, but a healthy diet and regular physical activity can still help you achieve a healthy weight.

Is Staying Overweight Healthier than Weight Cycling?

This is a hard question to answer since experts are not sure whether weight cycling causes health problems. However, experts are sure that if you are overweight, losing weight is a good thing. Being overweight or obese is associated with the following health problems:

- high blood pressure

- heart disease

- stroke

- gallbladder disease

- fatty liver disease

- type 2 diabetes

- certain types of cancer

- arthritis

- breathing problems, such as sleep apnea (when breathing stops for short periods during sleep)

Not everyone who is overweight or obese has the same risk for these problems. Risk is affected by several factors: your gender, family history of disease, the amount of extra weight you have, and where fat is located on your body. You can improve your health with a modest weight loss. Losing just 10 percent of your body weight over 6 months will help.

Chapter 36

Childhood Obesity

Chapter Contents

Section 36.1

Understanding Childhood Obesity

This section contains text excerpted from documents published
by two public domain sources. Text under the headings marked
1 is excerpted from "Childhood Obesity Facts," Centers for
Disease Control and Prevention (CDC), August 27, 2015; Text
under the headings marked 2 is excerpted from "Childhood Obesity
Causes and Consequences," Centers for Disease Control and
Prevention (CDC), June 19, 2015.

Childhood Obesity Facts[1]

- Childhood obesity has more than doubled in children and qua-
drupled in adolescents in the past 30 years.

- The percentage of children aged 6–11 years in the United States
who were obese increased from 7% in 1980 to nearly 18% in
2012. Similarly, the percentage of adolescents aged 12–19 years
who were obese increased from 5% to nearly 21% over the same
period.

- In 2012, more than one third of children and adolescents were
overweight or obese.

- Overweight is defined as having excess body weight for a particular height from fat, muscle, bone, water or a combination of
these factors. Obesity is defined as having excess body fat.

- Overweight and obesity are the result of "caloric imbalance"—
too few calories expended for the amount of calories consumed—
and are affected by various genetic, behavioral, and environmental factors.

Childhood Obesity Causes and Consequences[2]

Childhood obesity is a complex health issue. It occurs when a child
is well above the normal or healthy weight for his or her age and
height. The main causes of excess weight in youth are similar to those
in adults, including individual causes such as behavior and genetics.

Behaviors can include dietary patterns, physical activity, inactivity, medication use, and other exposures. Additional contributing factors in our society include the food and physical activity environment, education and skills, and food marketing and promotion.

Behavior

Healthy behaviors include a healthy diet pattern and regular physical activity. Energy balance of the number of calories consumed from foods and beverages with the number of calories the body uses for activity plays a role in preventing excess weight gain. A healthy diet pattern follows the *Dietary Guidelines for Americans* which emphasizes eating whole grains, fruits, vegetables, lean protein, low-fat and fat-free dairy products and drinking water. The Physical Activity Guidelines for Americans recommends children do at least 60 minutes of physical activity every day.

Having a healthy diet pattern and regular physical activity is also important for long term health benefits and prevention of chronic diseases such as Type 2 diabetes and heart disease.

Community Environment

American society has become characterized by environments that promote increased consumption of less healthy food and physical inactivity. It can be difficult for children to make healthy food choices and get enough physical activity when they are exposed to environments in their home, child care center, school or community that are influenced by—

- **Advertising of less healthy foods.**

Nearly half of U.S. middle and high schools allow advertising of less healthy foods, which impacts students' ability to make healthy food choices. In addition, foods high in total calories, sugars, salt, and fat, and low in nutrients are highly advertised and marketed through media targeted to children and adolescents, while advertising for healthier foods is almost nonexistent in comparison.

- **Variation in licensure regulations among child care centers.**

More than 12 million children regularly spend time in child care arrangements outside the home. However, not all states use licensing regulations to ensure that child care facilities encourage more healthful eating and physical activity.

- **No safe and appealing place, in many communities, to play or be active.**

Many communities are built in ways that make it difficult or unsafe to be physically active. For some families, getting to parks and recreation centers may be difficult, and public transportation may not be available. For many children, safe routes for walking or biking to school or play may not exist. Half of the children in the United States do not have a park, community center, and sidewalk in their neighborhood. Only 27 states have policies directing community-scale design.

- **Limited access to healthy affordable foods.**

Some people have less access to stores and supermarkets that sell healthy, affordable food such as fruits and vegetables, especially in rural, minority, and lower-income neighborhoods. Supermarket access is associated with a reduced risk for obesity. Choosing healthy foods is difficult for parents who live in areas with an overabundance of food retailers that tend to sell less healthy food, such as convenience stores and fast food restaurants.

- **Greater availability of high-energy-dense foods and sugar sweetened beverages.**

High-energy-dense foods are ones that have a lot of calories in each bite. A recent study among children showed that a high-energy-dense diet is associated with a higher risk for excess body fat during childhood. Sugar sweetened beverages are the largest source of added sugar and an important contributor of calories in the diets of children in the United States. High consumption of sugar sweetened beverages, which have few, if any, nutrients, has been associated with obesity. On a typical day, 80% of youth drink sugar sweetened beverages.

- **Increasing portion sizes.**

Portion sizes of less healthy foods and beverages have increased over time in restaurants, grocery stores, and vending machines. Research shows that children eat more without realizing it if they are served larger portions. This can mean they are consuming a lot of extra calories, especially when eating high-calorie foods.

- **Lack of breastfeeding support.**

Breastfeeding protects against childhood overweight and obesity. However, in the United States, while 75% of mothers start out breastfeeding, only 13% of babies are exclusively breastfed at the end of 6 months. The success rate among mothers who want to breastfeed can be improved through active support from their families, friends, communities, clinicians, healthcare leaders, employers, and policymakers.

Consequences of Obesity

Health Risks Now

- Obesity during childhood can have a harmful effect on the body in a variety of ways. Children who are obese have a greater risk of—

- High blood pressure and high cholesterol, which are risk factors for cardiovascular disease (CVD). In one study, 70% of obese children had at least one CVD risk factor, and 39% had two or more.

- Increased risk of impaired glucose tolerance, insulin resistance and type 2 diabetes.

- Breathing problems, such as sleep apnea, and asthma.

- Joint problems and musculoskeletal discomfort.

- Fatty liver disease, gallstones, and gastro-esophageal reflux (i.e., heartburn).

- Psychological stress such as depression, behavioral problems, and issues in school.

- Low self-esteem and low self-reported quality of life.

- Impaired social, physical, and emotional functioning.

Health Risks Later

- Children who are obese are more likely to become obese adults. Adult obesity is associated with a number of serious health conditions including heart disease, diabetes, metabolic syndrome, and cancer.

- If children are obese, obesity and disease risk factors in adulthood are likely to be more severe.

Preventing Obesity[1]

- Healthy lifestyle habits, including healthy eating and physical activity, can lower the risk of becoming obese and developing related diseases.

- The dietary and physical activity behaviors of children and adolescents are influenced by many sectors of society, including families, communities, schools, child care settings, medical care providers, faith-based institutions, government agencies, the media, and the food and beverage industries and entertainment industries.

- Schools play a particularly critical role by establishing a safe and supportive environment with policies and practices that support healthy behaviors. Schools also provide opportunities for students to learn about and practice healthy eating and physical activity behaviors.

Section 36.2

Helping Your Overweight Child

This section includes text excerpted from "Helping Your Overweight Child," National Institute of Diabetes and Digestive and Kidney Diseases (NIDDK), June 2013.

Many young people struggle with excess weight. Almost 1 in 3 children ages 5 to 11 is considered to be overweight or obese. Weighing too much increases the chances that young people may develop some health problems—now and later in life. As a parent or other caregiver, you can do a lot to help your child reach and maintain a healthy weight. Healthy eating and physical activity habits are important for your child's well-being. You can take an active role to help your child—and your whole family—learn healthy habits that last a lifetime.

How Can I Tell If My Child Is Overweight?

Telling whether a child is overweight isn't always easy. Children grow at different rates at different times. Also, the amount of body fat changes with age and differs between girls and boys.

One way to determine a person's weight status is to calculate body mass index (BMI). The BMI measures a person's weight in relation to his or her height. The BMI of children is age-and sex-specific and known as the "BMI-for-age." BMI-for-age uses growth charts created by the Centers for Disease Control and Prevention in the year 2000.

A number called a percentile shows how your child's BMI compares with the BMI of others. For example, if your child's BMI is in the 90th percentile, this means that his or her BMI is greater than the BMI of 89 percent of children of the same age and sex. The main BMI-for-age categories are these:

- healthy weight: 5th to 84th percentile
- overweight: 85th to 94th percentile
- obese: 95th percentile or greater

Why Should I Be Concerned?

There are many reasons to care if your child is in the overweight or obese category. In the short run, he or she may develop joint pain and/ or breathing problems. These health issues may make it hard to keep up with friends. Some children may develop obesity-related health problems, such as diabetes, high blood pressure, and high cholesterol, because of excess weight.

Youth who weigh too much may become obese adults. This increases the chances that they may develop heart disease and certain cancers as adults.

If you are worried about your child's weight, talk to your healthcare provider. He or she can check your child's overall health and tell you if weight management may be helpful. Don't put your child on a weight-loss diet unless your healthcare provider tells you to.

How Can I Help My Child Develop Healthy Habits?

Parents and other caregivers can play an important role in helping children build healthy eating and physical activity habits that will last a lifetime.

To help your child develop healthy habits,

- be a positive role model. Children are good learners and they often mimic what they see. Choose healthy foods and active pas-times for yourself.

- involve the whole family in building healthy eating and physical activity habits. This benefits everyone and doesn't single out the child who is overweight.

433

What Tips May Help My Child Eat Better?

A healthy eating plan limits foods that lead to weight gain. Foods that should be limited include these:

- fats that are solid at room temperature (like butter and lard).

- foods that are high in calories, sugar, and salt like sugary drinks, chips, cookies, fries, and candy.

- refined grains (white flour, rice, and pasta).

Just like adults, children should replace unhealthy foods with a variety of healthy foods, including these:

- fruits, vegetables, nuts and seeds, and whole grains like brown rice.

- fat-free or low-fat milk and milk products or substitutes, like soy beverages that have added calcium and vitamin D.

- lean meats, poultry, seafood, beans and peas, soy products, and eggs.

The following changes may help your child eat healthier at home:

- Buy and serve more fruits and vegetables (fresh, frozen, canned or dried). Let your child choose them at the store. Use a new fruit to make smoothies.

- Buy fewer high-calorie foods like sugary drinks, chips, cookies, fries, and candy.

- Offer your child water or low-fat milk instead of fruit juice.

Other ways to support healthy eating habits include these:

- Make healthy choices easy. Put nutritious foods where they are easy to see and keep any high-calorie foods out of sight.

- Eat fast food less often. When you do visit a fast food restaurant, encourage your family to choose the healthier options, such as salads with low-fat dressing.

- Plan healthy meals and eat together as a family so you can explore a variety of foods together.

To help your child develop a healthy attitude toward food, try these ideas:

- Don't use food as a reward when encouraging kids to eat. Promising dessert to a child for eating vegetables, for example, sends the message that vegetables are less valuable than dessert.

- Explain the reasons for eating whatever it is you are serving. Don't make your child clean his or her plate.

- Limit eating to specific meal and snack times. At other times, the kitchen is "closed."

- Avoid large portions. Start with small servings and let your child ask for more if he or she is still hungry.

Keep healthy snack foods on hand. Try these:

- air-popped popcorn without butter.

- fresh, frozen, dried or canned fruit served plain or with low-fat yogurt.

- fresh vegetables, like baby carrots, cucumber, zucchini or tomatoes.

- low-sugar, whole-grain cereal with low-fat or fat-free milk or a milk substitute fortified with calcium and vitamin D.

What Tips May Help My Child Be More Active?

Kids need about 60 minutes of physical activity a day, but this doesn't have to happen all at once. Several short 10-or even 5-minute periods of activity throughout the day are just as good. If your children are not used to being active, encourage them to start with what they can do and build up to 60 minutes a day.

Here are some ways to help your child move every day:

- Set a good example. Show your child that you are physically active and that you have fun doing it.

- Encourage your child to join a sports team or class, such as basketball, dance or soccer at school or at your local community or recreation center.

- If your child feels uncomfortable participating in activities like sports, help him or her find physical activities that are fun and not competitive, such as dancing to music, playing tag, jumping rope or riding a bike.

- Be active together as a family. Assign active chores such as making the beds, sweeping/raking or vacuuming. Plan active outings such as a walk through a local park.

Kids spend a lot of time sitting down watching TV, playing video games or using the computer or hand-held devices like cell phones.

The following tips may help cut back on some of this inactive time:

- Limit Screen time to no more than 2 hours per day.

- Help your child find fun things to do like acting out favorite books or stories or doing a family art project.

- Encourage your child to get up and move during TV commercials and discourage snacking when sitting in front of a screen.

Fun Physical Activities

Activities that kids choose to do on their own are often best. Your child may enjoy trying the following:

- catching and throwing a ball

- climbing on a jungle gym or climbing wall

- dancing

- jumping rope

- playing hopscotch

- riding a bike

- shooting baskets

Where Can I Go for More Help?

If you have changed your family's eating and physical activity habits and your child has not reached a healthy weight, ask your healthcare provider about other options. He or she may be able to refer you to a weight-control specialist or program.

Here are some things a weight-control program should do:

- Include a variety of healthcare professionals on staff, including doctors, exercise physiologists, psychiatrists or psychologists, and registered dietitians.

- Evaluate your child's weight, growth, and health before enrolling him or her in the program. The program should also monitor these factors while your child is enrolled.

- Adapt to the specific age and abilities of your child. Programs for 4-year-olds should be different from those for 10-year-olds.

- Help your family keep up healthy eating and physical activity behaviors after the program ends.

Be Supportive

Throughout any process or program that you undertake to address your child's weight, be supportive. Help your child set specific goals and track his or her progress. Reward successes with praise and hugs. Be positive.

Tell your child that he or she is loved, special, and important. Children's feelings about themselves are often based on how they think their parents and other caregivers feel about them.

Listen to your child's concerns about his or her weight. Overweight children probably know better than anyone else that they have a weight problem. They need support, understanding, and encouragement from caring adults.

Chapter 37

Healthy Weight Loss

Chapter Contents

Section 37.1

Assessing Your Weight and Finding a Balance

This section contains text excerpted from the following sources: Text in this section begins with excerpts from "Assessing Your Weight," Centers for Disease Control and Prevention (CDC), May 15, 2015; Text under the heading "The Caloric Balance Equation" is excerpted from "Finding a Balance," Centers for Disease Control and Prevention (CDC), May 15, 2015.

A high amount of body fat can lead to weight-related diseases and other health issues and being underweight can also put one at risk for health issues. BMI (body mass index) and waist circumference are two measures that can be used as screening tools to estimate weight status in relation to potential disease risk. However, BMI and waist circumference are not diagnostic tools for disease risks. A trained healthcare provider should perform other health assessments in order to evaluate disease risk and diagnose disease status.

How to Measure and Interpret Weight Status

Adult Body Mass Index or BMI

Body mass index (BMI) is a person's weight in kilograms divided by the square of height in meters. A high BMI can be an indicator of high body fatness and having a low BMI can be an indicator of having too low body fatness. BMI can be used as a screening tool but is not diagnostic of the body fatness or health of an individual.

- **If your BMI is less than 18.5,** it falls within the underweight range.

- **If your BMI is 18.5 to 24.9,** it falls within the normal or Healthy Weight range.

- **If your BMI is 25.0 to 29.9,** it falls within the overweight range.

- **If your BMI is 30.0 or higher,** it falls within the obese range.

Weight that is higher than what is considered as a healthy weight for a given height is described as overweight or obese. Weight that is lower than what is considered as healthy for a given height is described as underweight.

At an individual level, BMI can be used as a screening tool but is not diagnostic of the body fatness or health of an individual. A trained healthcare provider should perform appropriate health assessments in order to evaluate an individual's health status and risks.

Adult Body Mass Index or BMI

Height and weight must be measured in order to calculate BMI. It is most accurate to measure height in meters and weight in kilograms. However, the BMI formula has been adapted for height measured in inches and weight measured in pounds. These measurements can be taken in a healthcare provider's office or at home using a tape measure and scale.

Waist Circumference

Another way to estimate your potential disease risk is to measure your waist circumference. Excessive abdominal fat may be serious because it places you at greater risk for developing obesity-related conditions, such as Type 2 Diabetes, high blood pressure, and coronary artery disease. Your waistline may be telling you that you have a higher risk of developing obesity-related conditions if you are:

- A man whose waist circumference is more than 40 inches

- A non-pregnant woman whose waist circumference is more than 35 inches

Waist circumference can be used as a screening tool but is not diagnostic of the body fatness or health of an individual. A trained healthcare provider should perform appropriate health assessments in order to evaluate an individual's health status and risks.

How to Measure Your Waist Circumference?

To correctly measure waist circumference:

- Stand and place a tape measure around your middle, just above your hipbones.

- Make sure tape is horizontal around the waist.

- Keep the tape snug around the waist, but not compressing the skin.

- Measure your waist just after you breathe out.

The Caloric Balance Equation

When it comes to maintaining a healthy weight for a lifetime, the bottom line is–**calories count**! Weight management is all about balance—balancing the number of calories you consume with the number of calories your body uses or "burns off."

- A *calorie* is defined as a unit of energy supplied by food. A calorie is a calorie regardless of its source. Whether you're eating carbohydrates, fats, sugars or proteins, all of them contain calories.

- *Caloric balance* is like a scale. To remain in balance and maintain your body weight, the calories consumed (from foods) must be balanced by the calories used (in normal body functions, daily activities, and exercise).

Table 37.1. The Caloric Balance Status

If you are...	Your caloric balance status is...
Maintaining your weight	"**in balance**." You are eating roughly the same number of calories that your body is using. Your weight will remain stable.
Gaining weight	"**in caloric excess**." You are eating more calories than your body is using. You will store these extra calories as fat and you'll gain weight.
Losing weight	"**in caloric deficit**." You are eating fewer calories than you are using. Your body is pulling from its fat storage cells for energy, so your weight is **decreasing**.

Am I in Caloric Balance?

If you are maintaining your current body weight, you are in caloric balance. If you need to gain weight or to lose weight, you'll need to tip the balance scale in one direction or another to achieve your goal.

If you need to tip the balance scale in the direction of losing weight, keep in mind that it takes approximately 3,500 calories below your calorie needs to lose a pound of body fat. To lose about 1 to 2 pounds per week, you'll need to reduce your caloric intake by 500–1000 calories per day.

To learn how many calories you are currently eating, begin writing down the foods you eat and the beverages you drink each day. By writing down what you eat and drink, you become more aware of everything you are putting in your mouth. Also, begin writing down the physical activity you do each day and the length of time you do it. Here are simple paper and pencil tools to assist you:

- Food Diary

- Physical Activity Diary

Physical activities (both daily activities and exercise) help tip the balance scale by increasing the calories you expend each day.

Section 37.2

Eating for a Healthy Weight

This section includes text excerpted from "Healthy Eating for a Healthy Weight," Centers for Disease Control and P revention (CDC), November 9, 2015.

A healthy lifestyle involves many choices. Among them, choosing a balanced diet or healthy eating plan. So how do you choose a healthy eating plan? Let's begin by defining what a healthy eating plan is.

According to the *Dietary Guidelines for Americans*, a healthy eating plan:

- Emphasizes fruits, vegetables, whole grains, and fat-free or low-fat milk and milk products

- Includes lean meats, poultry, fish, beans, eggs, and nuts

- Is low in saturated fats, trans fats, cholesterol, salt (sodium), and added sugars

- Stays within your daily calorie needs

Eat Healthy and Enjoy It!

A healthy eating plan that helps you manage your weight includes a variety of foods you may not have considered. If "healthy eating" makes you think about the foods you can't have, try refocusing on all the new foods you can eat—

- **Fresh, Frozen or Canned Fruits?** don't think just apples or bananas. All fresh, frozen or canned fruits are great choices. Be sure to try some "exotic" fruits, too. How about a mango? Or a juicy pineapple or kiwi fruit! When your favorite fresh fruits aren't in season, try a frozen, canned or dried variety of a fresh fruit you enjoy. One caution about canned fruits is that they may contain added sugars or syrups. Be sure and choose canned varieties of fruit packed in water or in their own juice.

- **Fresh, Frozen or Canned Vegetables?** try something new. You may find that you love grilled vegetables or steamed vegetables with an herb you haven't tried like rosemary. You can sauté (pan fry) vegetables in a non-stick pan with a small amount of cooking spray. Or try frozen or canned vegetables for a quick side dish—just microwave and serve. When trying canned vegetables, look for vegetables without added salt, butter or cream sauces. Commit to going to the produce department and trying a new vegetable each week.

- **Calcium-rich foods?** you may automatically think of a glass of low-fat or fat-free milk when someone says "eat more dairy products." But what about low-fat and fat-free yogurts without added sugars? These come in a wide variety of flavors and can be a great dessert substitute for those with a sweet tooth.

- **A new twist on an old favorite**? if your favorite recipe calls for frying fish or breaded chicken, try healthier variations using baking or grilling. Maybe even try a recipe that uses dry beans in place of higher-fat meats. Ask around or search the internet and magazines for recipes with fewer calories, you might be surprised to find you have a new favorite dish!

Do I Have to Give up My Favorite Comfort Food?

No! Healthy eating is all about balance. You can enjoy your favorite foods even if they are high in calories, fat or added sugars. The key is eating them only once in a while, and balancing them out with healthier foods and more physical activity.

Some general tips for comfort foods:

• Eat them less often. If you normally eat these foods every day, cut back to once a week or once a month. You'll be cutting your calories because you're not having the food as often.

• Eat smaller amounts. If your favorite higher-calorie food is a chocolate bar, have a smaller size or only half a bar.

• Try a lower-calorie version. Use lower-calorie ingredients or prepare food differently. For example, if your macaroni and cheese recipe uses whole milk, butter, and full-fat cheese, try remaking it with nonfat milk, less butter, light cream cheese, fresh spinach and tomatoes. Just remember to not increase your portion size.

The point is, you can figure out how to include almost any food in your healthy eating plan in a way that still helps you lose weight or maintain a healthy weight.

Section 37.3

Mindful Eating

This section includes text excerpted from "Mindful Eating," U.S. Department of Veterans Affairs (VA), November 20, 2013.

What Is Mindfulness?

Mindfulness means being fully aware of what is going on within and around you at each moment. Mindfulness can be applied to many aspects of life. Being mindful of your eating may help with weight management. Being mindful involves being aware of yourself and your surroundings physically, emotionally, and mentally. It means paying attention to each changing moment.

What Is Mindful Eating?

Mindful eating takes the concept of mindfulness and applies it to why, when, where, what, and how you eat. This means being aware of both the physical and emotional feelings connected to eating.

- **Observe your body**. Notice hunger and fullness signals that guide you to start and stop eating

- **Do not judge yourself** or your reaction to food

- **Notice your reaction to food**. What do you like, what don't you like?

- **Savor your food.** While eating, notice all of the colors, smells, flavors, and textures of the food.

Mindfulness may help you to avoid overeating. First bites may be the most satisfying, and additional bites may not be as pleasurable. This can help with portion control.

Be Aware. Ask Yourself, "Am I..."

- Physically hungry? (on a scale from "1" to "10")

- Eating quickly or slowly?

- Dining in-the-moment–Am I mindlessly munching or noticing each bite?

- Multi-tasking or truly focused on this meal or snack?

- Feeling my stomach rumbling?

- Bored, stressed, tired, anxious, angry, sad, etc.?

Here Are Some Tips:

- Take a breath and ask yourself, "Am I truly hungry?" before you reach for food.

- Begin practicing mindfulness. Start by eating one meal a day in a slower, more aware manner.

- Focus on eating. Avoid doing other activities while you eat (working, talking on the phone, watching TV, driving, reading, etc.).

- Set a timer for 20 minutes and take the whole time to eat the meal.

- Eat silently for 5 minutes (think about what it took to produce that meal, from the sun and water, to the farmer, to the grocer, to the cook).

- Slow down. Eat with your non-dominant hand or try using chopsticks.

Section 37.4

How to Cut Calories from Your Diet?

This section includes text excerpted from "Cutting Calories," Centers for Disease Control and Prevention (CDC), May 15, 2015.

Once you start looking, you can find ways to cut calories for your meals, snacks, and even beverages. Here are some examples to get you started.

Eat More, Weigh Less?

Eating fewer calories doesn't necessarily mean eating less food. To be able to cut calories without eating less and feeling hungry, you need to replace some higher calorie foods with foods that are lower in calories *and* fill you up. In general, these foods contain a lot of water and are high in fiber.

Rethink Your Drink

Most people try to reduce their calorie intake by focusing on food, but another way to cut calories may be to change what you drink. You may find that you're consuming quite a few calories just in the beverages you have each day. Find out how you can make better drink choices to reduce your calorie intake.

How to Use Fruits and Vegetables to Help Manage Your Weight

Learn about fruits and vegetables and their role in your weight management plan. Tips to cut calories by substituting fruits and vegetables are included with meal-by-meal examples. You will also find snack ideas that are 100 calories or less. With these helpful tips, you will soon be on your way to adding more fruits and vegetables into your healthy eating plan.

Ideas for Every Meal

Table 37.2. Ideas for Every Meal

Breakfast	Substitution	Calories Reduced by
Top your cereal with low fat or fat-free milk instead of 2% or whole milk.	1 cup of fat-free milk instead of 1 cup of whole milk	63
Use a non-stick pan and cooking spray (rather than butter) to scramble or fry eggs	1 spray of cooking spray instead of 1 pat of butter	34
Choose reduced-calorie margarine spread for toast rather than butter or stick margarine.	2 pats of reduced calorie margarine instead of 2 pats of butter	36
Lunch	**Substitution**	**Calories Reduced by**
Add more vegetables such as cucumbers, lettuce, tomato, and onions to a sandwich instead of extra meat or cheese.	2 slices of tomatoes, ¼ cup of sliced cucumbers, and 2 slices of onions instead of an extra slice (3/4 ounce) of cheese and 2 slices (1 ounce) of ham	154
Accompany a sandwich with salad or fruit instead of chips or French fries.	½ cup diced raw pineapple instead of 1 ounce bag of potato chips	118
Choose vegetable-based broth soups rather than cream- or meat-based soups.	1 cup of vegetable soup instead of 1 cup cream of chicken soup	45

Table 37.2. Continued

Breakfast	Substitution	Calories Reduced by
When eating a salad, dip your fork into dressing instead of pouring lots of dressing on the salad.	½ TBSP of regular ranch salad dressing instead of 2 TBSP of regular ranch dressing	109
When eating out, substitute a broth-based soup or a green lettuce salad for French fries or chips as a side dish	A side salad with a packet of low-fat vinaigrette dressing instead of a medium order of French fries	270
Dinner	**Substitution**	**Calories Reduced by**
Have steamed or grilled vegetables rather than those sautéed in butter or oil. Try lemon juice and herbs to flavor the vegetables. You can also sauté with non-stick cooking spray.	½ cup steamed broccoli instead of ½ cup broccoli sautéed in 1/2 TBSP of vegetable oil.	62
Modify recipes to reduce the amount of fat and calories. For example, when making lasagna, use part-skim ricotta cheese instead of whole-milk ricotta cheese. Substitute shredded vegetables, such as carrots, zucchini, and spinach for some of the ground meat in lasagna.	1 cup of part-skim ricotta cheese instead of 1 cup whole milk ricotta cheese	89
When eating out, have a cocktail or dessert instead of both during the same eating occasion.	Choosing one or the other saves you calories. A 12-ounce beer has about 153 calories. A slice of apple pie (1/6 of a 8" pie) has 277 calories.	153 if you have the apple pie without the drink 277 if you have a drink and no pie.
When having pizza, choose vegetables as toppings and just a light sprinkling of cheese instead of fatty meats.	One slice of a cheese pizza instead of one slice of a meat and cheese pizza	60
Snacks	**Substitution**	**Calories Reduced by**

Table 37.2. Continued

Breakfast	Substitution	Calories Reduced by
Choose air-popped popcorn instead of oil-popped popcorn and dry-roasted instead of oil-roasted nuts.	3 cups of air-popped popcorn instead of 3 cups of oil-popped popcorn	73
Avoid the vending machine by packing your own healthful snacks to bring to work. For example, consider vegetable sticks, fresh fruit, low fat or nonfat yogurt without added sugars or a small handful of dry-roasted nuts.	An eight-ounce container of no sugar added nonfat yogurt instead of a package of 6 peanut butter crackers	82
Choose sparkling water instead of sweetened drinks or alcoholic beverages.	A bottle of carbonated water instead of a 12-ounce can of soda with sugar	136
Instead of cookies or other sweet snacks, have some fruit for a snack.	One large orange instead of 3 chocolate sandwich cookies	54

Section 37.5

Avoiding Portion Size Pitfalls

This section includes text excerpted from "How to Avoid Portion Size Pitfalls to Help Manage Your Weight," Centers for Disease Control and Prevention (CDC), August 18, 2015.

How to Avoid Portion Size Pitfalls to Help Manage Your Weight

When eating at many restaurants, it's hard to miss that portion sizes have gotten larger in the last few years. The trend has also spilled over into the grocery store and vending machines, where a bagel has become a BAGEL and an "individual" bag of chips can easily feed more than one. Research shows that people unintentionally consume more calories when faced with larger portions. This can mean significant excess calorie intake, especially when eating high-calorie foods. Here are some tips to help you avoid some common portion-size pitfalls.

Portion control when eating out. Many restaurants serve more food than one person needs at one meal. Take control of the amount of food that ends up on your plate by splitting an entrée with a friend. Or, ask the wait person for a "to-go" box and wrap up half your meal as soon as it's brought to the table.

Portion control when eating in. To minimize the temptation of second and third helpings when eating at home, serve the food on individual plates, instead of putting the serving dishes on the table. Keeping the excess food out of reach may discourage overeating.

Portion control in front of the TV. When eating or snacking in front of the TV, put the amount that you plan to eat into a bowl or container instead of eating straight from the package. It's easy to overeat when your attention is focused on something else.

Go ahead, spoil your dinner. We learned as children not to snack before a meal for fear of "spoiling our dinner." Well, it's time to forget that old rule. If you feel hungry between meals, eat a healthy snack, like a piece of fruit or small salad, to avoid overeating during your next meal.

Be aware of large packages. For some reason, the larger the package, the more people consume from it without realizing it. To minimize this effect:

- Divide up the contents of one large package into several smaller containers to help avoid over-consumption.

- Don't eat straight from the package. Instead, serve the food in a small bowl or container.

Out of sight, out of mind. People tend to consume more when they have easy access to food. Make your home a "portion friendly zone."

- Replace the candy dish with a fruit bowl.

- Store especially tempting foods, like cookies, chips or ice cream, out of immediate eyesight, like on a high shelf or at the back of the freezer. Move the healthier food to the front at eye level.

- When buying in bulk, store the excess in a place that's not convenient to get to, such as a high cabinet or at the back of the pantry.

Section 37.6

Improving Your Eating Habits

This section includes text excerpted from "Improving Your Eating Habits," Centers for Disease Control and Prevention (CDC), May 15, 2015.

Improving Your Eating Habits

When it comes to eating, we have strong habits. Some are good ("I always eat breakfast"), and some are not so good ("I always clean my plate"). Although many of our eating habits were established during childhood, it doesn't mean it's too late to change them.

Making sudden, radical changes to eating habits such as eating nothing but cabbage soup, can lead to short term weight loss. However, such radical changes are neither healthy nor a good idea, and won't be successful in the long run. Permanently improving your eating habits requires a thoughtful approach in which you Reflect, Replace, and Reinforce.

- **REFLECT** on all of your specific eating habits, both bad and good; and, your common triggers for unhealthy eating.

- **REPLACE** your unhealthy eating habits with healthier ones.

- **REINFORCE** your new, healthier eating habits.

Reflect, Replace, Reinforce: A Process for Improving Your Eating Habits

1. **Create a list of your eating habits**. Keeping a food diary for a few days, in which you write down everything you eat and

the time of day you ate it, will help you uncover your habits. For example, you might discover that you always seek a sweet snack to get you through the mid-afternoon energy slump. It's good to note how you were feeling when you decided to eat, especially if you were eating when not hungry. Were you tired? Stressed out?

2. **Highlight the habits** on your list that may be leading you to overeat. Common eating habits that can lead to weight gain are:

    - Eating too fast

    - Always cleaning your plate

    - Eating when not hungry

    - Eating while standing up (may lead to eating mindlessly or too quickly)

    - Always eating dessert

    - Skipping meals (or maybe just breakfast)

3. **Look at the unhealthy eating habits** you've highlighted. Be sure you've identified all the triggers that cause you to engage in those habits. Identify a few you'd like to work on improving first. Don't forget to pat yourself on the back for the things you're doing right. Maybe you almost always eat fruit for dessert or you drink low-fat or fat-free milk. These are good habits! Recognizing your successes will help encourage you to make more changes.

4. **Create a list of "cues"** by reviewing your food diary to become more aware of when and where you're "triggered" to eat for reasons other than hunger. Note how you are typically feeling at those times. Often an environmental "cue" or a particular emotional state, is what encourages eating for non-hunger reasons. Common triggers for eating when not hungry are:

    - Opening up the cabinet and seeing your favorite snack food.

    - Sitting at home watching television.

    - Before or after a stressful meeting or situation at work.

    - Coming home after work and having no idea what's for dinner.

    - Having someone offer you a dish they made "just for you!"

- Walking past a candy dish on the counter.

- Sitting in the break room beside the vending machine.

- Seeing a plate of doughnuts at the morning staff meeting.

- Swinging through your favorite drive-through every morning.

- Feeling bored or tired and thinking food might offer a pick-me-up.

   i. Circle the "cues" on your list that you face on a daily or weekly basis. Going home for the Thanksgiving holiday may be a trigger for you to overeat, and eventually, you want to have a plan for as many eating cues as you can. But for now, focus on the ones you face more often.

   ii. Ask yourself these questions for each "cue" you've circled:

   1. Is there anything I can do to avoid the cue or situation? This option works best for cues that don't involve others. For example, could you choose a different route to work to avoid stopping at a fast food restaurant on the way? Is there another place in the break room where you can sit so you're not next to the vending machine?

   2. For things I can't avoid, can I do something differently that would be healthier? Obviously, you can't avoid all situations that trigger your unhealthy eating habits, like staff meetings at work. In these situations, evaluate your options. Could you suggest or bring healthier snacks or beverages? Could you offer to take notes to distract your attention? Could you sit farther away from the food so it won't be as easy to grab something? Could you plan ahead and eat a healthy snack before the meeting?

   iii. Replace unhealthy habits with new, healthy ones. For example, in reflecting upon your eating habits, you may realize that you eat too fast when you eat alone. So, make a commitment to share a lunch each week with a colleague or have a neighbor over for dinner one night a week. Other strategies might include putting your fork down between bites or minimizing other distractions (i.e. watching the news during dinner) that might keep you from paying attention to how quickly—and how much—you're eating.

iv. **Reinforce your new, healthy habits and be patient with yourself**. Habits take time to develop. It doesn't happen overnight. When you do find yourself engaging in an unhealthy habit, stop as quickly as possible and ask yourself: Why do I do this? When did I start doing this? What changes do I need to make? Be careful not to berate yourself or think that one mistake "blows" a whole day's worth of healthy habits. You can do it! It just takes one day at a time!

Chapter 38

Weight Loss and Nutrition Myths

Weight-Loss and Nutrition Myths

"Lose 30 pounds in 30 days!"
"Eat as much as you want and still lose weight!"
"Try the thigh buster and lose inches fast!"
Have you heard these claims before? A large number of diets and tools are available, but their quality may vary. It can be hard to know what to believe.

Weight-Loss and Diet Myths

Myth: Fad diets will help me lose weight and keep it off.

Fact: Fad diets are not the best way to lose weight and keep it off. These diets often promise quick weight loss if you strictly reduce what you eat or avoid some types of foods. Some of these diets may help you lose weight at first. But these diets are hard to follow. Most people quickly get tired of them and regain any lost weight.

Fad diets may be unhealthy. They may not provide all of the nutrients your body needs. Also, losing more than 3 pounds a week after the first few weeks may increase your chances of developing gallstones (solid matter in the gallbladder that can cause pain). Being on a diet of fewer than 800 calories a day for a long time may lead to serious heart problems.

This chapter includes text excerpted from "Weight-Loss and Nutrition Myths," National Institute of Diabetes and Digestive and Kidney Diseases (NIDDK), October 2014.

TIP: Research suggests that safe weight loss involves combining a reduced-calorie diet with physical activity to lose 1/2 to 2 pounds a week (after the first few weeks of weight loss). Make healthy food choices. Eat small portions. Build exercise into your daily life. Combined, these habits may be a healthy way to lose weight and keep it off. These habits may also lower your chances of developing heart disease, high blood pressure, and type 2 diabetes.

Myth: Grain products such as bread, pasta, and rice are fattening. I should avoid them when trying to lose weight.

Fact: A grain product is any food made from wheat, rice, oats, cornmeal, barley or another cereal grain. Grains are divided into two subgroups, whole grains and refined grains. Whole grains contain the entire grain kernel—the bran, germ, and endosperm. Examples include brown rice and whole-wheat bread, cereal, and pasta. Refined grains have been milled, a process that removes the bran and germ. This is done to give grains a finer texture and improve their shelf life, but it also removes dietary fiber, iron, and many B vitamins.

People who eat whole grains as part of a healthy diet may lower their chances of developing some chronic diseases. Government dietary guidelines advise making half your grains whole grains. For example, choose 100 percent whole-wheat bread instead of white bread, and brown rice instead of white rice.

TIP: To lose weight, reduce the number of calories you take in and increase the amount of physical activity you do each day. Create and follow a healthy eating plan that replaces less healthy options with a mix of fruits, veggies, whole grains, protein foods, and low-fat dairy.

Meal Myths

Myth: Some people can eat whatever they want and still lose weight.

Fact: To lose weight, you need to burn more calories than you eat and drink. Some people may seem to get away with eating any kind of food they want and still lose weight. But those people, like everyone, must use more energy than they take in through food and drink to lose weight.

A number of factors such as your age, genes, medicines, and lifestyle habits may affect your weight. If you would like to lose weight, speak with your healthcare provider about factors that may affect your weight. Together, you may be able to create a plan to help you reach your weight and health goals.

Eat the rainbow!

When making half of your plate fruits and veggies, choose foods with vibrant colors that are packed with fiber, minerals, and vitamins.

Red: bell peppers, cherries, cranberries, onions, red beets, strawberries, tomatoes, watermelon

Green: avocado, broccoli, cabbage, cucumber, dark lettuce, grapes, honeydew, kale, kiwi, spinach, zucchini

Orange and yellow: apricots, bananas, carrots, mangoes, oranges, peaches, squash, sweet potatoes

Blue and purple: blackberries, blueberries, grapes, plums, purple cabbage, purple carrots, purple potatoes

TIP: When trying to lose weight, you can still eat your favorite foods as part of a healthy eating plan. But you must watch the **total number of calories** that you eat. Reduce your portion sizes. Find ways to limit the calories in your favorite foods. For example, you can bake foods rather than frying them. Use low-fat milk in place of cream. Make half of your plate fruits and veggies.

Myth: "Low-fat" or "fat-free" means no calories.

Fact: A serving of low-fat or fat-free food may be lower in calories than a serving of the full-fat product. But many processed low-fat or fat-free foods have just as many calories as the full-fat versions of the same foods—or even more calories. These foods may contain added flour, salt, starch or sugar to improve flavor and texture after fat is removed. These items add calories.

TIP: Read the Nutrition Facts label on a food package to find out how many calories are in a serving. Check the serving size, too—it may be less than you are used to eating.

Myth: Fast foods are always an unhealthy choice. You should not eat them when dieting.

Fact: Many fast foods are unhealthy and may affect weight gain. However, if you do eat fast food, choose menu options with care. Both

459

at home and away, choose healthy foods that are nutrient rich, low in calories, and small in portion size.

TIP: To choose healthy, low-calorie options, check the nutrition facts. These are often offered on the menu or on restaurant websites. And know that the nutrition facts often do not include sauces and extras. Try these tips:

- Avoid "value" combo meals, which tend to have more calories than you need in one meal.

- Choose fresh fruit items or nonfat yogurt for dessert.

- Limit your use of toppings that are high in fat and calories, such as bacon, cheese, regular mayonnaise, salad dressings, and tartar sauce.

- Pick steamed or baked items over fried ones.

- Sip on water or fat-free milk instead of soda.

Myth: If I skip meals, I can lose weight.

Fact: Skipping meals may make you feel hungrier and lead you to eat more than you normally would at your next meal. In particular, studies show a link between skipping breakfast and obesity. People who skip breakfast tend to be heavier than people who eat a healthy breakfast.

TIP: Choose meals and snacks that include a variety of healthy foods. Try these examples:

- For a quick breakfast, make oatmeal with low-fat milk, topped with fresh berries. Or eat a slice of whole-wheat toast with fruit spread.

- Pack a healthy lunch each night, so you won't be tempted to rush out of the house in the morning without one.

- For healthy nibbles, pack a small low-fat yogurt, a couple of whole-wheat crackers with peanut butter or veggies with hummus.

Myth: Eating healthy food costs too much.

Fact: Eating better does not have to cost a lot of money. Many people think that fresh foods are healthier than canned or frozen ones. For example, some people think that spinach is better for you raw than frozen or canned. However, canned or frozen fruits and veggies provide as many nutrients as fresh ones, at a lower cost. Healthy options include low-salt canned veggies and fruit canned in its own juice or water-packed. Remember to rinse canned veggies to remove excess salt. Also, some canned seafood, like tuna, is easy to keep on the shelf, healthy, and low-cost. And canned, dried or frozen beans, lentils, and peas are also healthy sources of protein that are easy on the wallet.

TIP: Check the nutrition facts on canned, dried, and frozen items. Look for items that are high in calcium, fiber, potassium, protein, and vitamin D. Also check for items that are low in added sugars, saturated fat, and sodium.

Food Myths

Myth: Eating meat is bad for my health and makes it harder to lose weight.

Fact: Eating lean meat in small amounts can be part of a healthy plan to lose weight. Chicken, fish, pork, and red meat contain some cholesterol and saturated fat. But they also contain healthy nutrients like iron, protein, and zinc.

TIP: Choose cuts of meat that are lower in fat, and trim off all the fat you can see. Meats that are lower in fat include chicken breast, pork loin and beef round steak, flank steak, and extra lean ground beef. Also, watch portion size. Try to eat meat or poultry in portions of 3 ounces or less. Three ounces is about the size of a deck of cards.

Myth: Dairy products are fattening and unhealthy.

Fact: Fat-free and low-fat cheese, milk, and yogurt are just as healthy as whole-milk dairy products, and they are lower in fat and calories. Dairy products offer protein to build muscles and help organs work well, and calcium to strengthen bones. Most milk and some yogurts have extra vitamin D added to help your body use calcium. Most Americans don't get enough calcium and vitamin D. Dairy is an easy way to get more of these nutrients.

TIP: Based on Government guidelines, you should try to have 3 cups a day of fat-free or low-fat milk or milk products. This can include soy beverages fortified with vitamins. If you can't digest lactose (the sugar found in dairy products), choose lactose-free or low-lactose dairy products or other foods and beverages that have calcium and vitamin D:

calcium: soy-based beverages or tofu made with calcium sulfate; canned salmon; dark leafy greens like collards or kale

vitamin D: cereals or soy-based beverages

Myth: "Going vegetarian" will help me lose weight and be healthier.

Fact: Research shows that people who follow a vegetarian eating plan, on average, eat fewer calories and less fat than non-vegetarians. Some research has found that vegetarian-style eating patterns are associated with lower levels of obesity, lower blood pressure, and a reduced risk of heart disease.

Vegetarians also tend to have lower body mass index (BMI) scores than people with other eating plans. (The BMI measures body fat based on a person's height in relation to weight). But vegetarians—like others—can make food choices that impact weight gain, like eating large amounts of foods that are high in fat or calories or low in nutrients.

The types of vegetarian diets eaten in the United States can vary widely. Vegans do not consume any animal products, while lacto-ovo vegetarians eat milk and eggs along with plant foods. Some people have eating patterns that are mainly vegetarian but may include small amounts of meat, poultry or seafood.

TIP: If you choose to follow a vegetarian eating plan, be sure you get enough of the nutrients that others usually take in from animal products such as cheese, eggs, meat, and milk. Nutrients that may be lacking in a vegetarian diet are listed in the sidebar, along with foods and beverages that may help you meet your body's needs for these nutrients.

Table 38.1. Nutrient and Common Sources

Nutrient	Common Sources
Calcium	dairy products, soy beverages with added calcium, tofu made with calcium sulfate, collard greens, kale, broccoli
Iron	cashews, spinach, lentils, chickpeas, bread or cereal with added iron
Protein	eggs, dairy products, beans, peas, nuts, seeds, tofu, tempeh, soy-based burgers

Table 38.1. Continued

Nutrient	Common Sources
Vitamin B12	eggs, dairy products, fortified cereal or soy beverages, tempeh, miso (tempeh and miso are foods made from soybeans)
Vitamin D	foods and beverages with added vitamin D, including milk, soy beverages or cereal
Zinc	whole grains (check the ingredients list on product labels for the words "whole" or "whole grain" before the grain ingredient's name), nuts, tofu, leafy greens (spinach, cabbage, lettuce)

Chapter 39

Diet Medications and Supplements

Chapter Contents

Section 39.1

Dietary Supplements for Weight Loss

This section includes text excerpted from "Dietary
Supplements for Weight Loss: Fact Sheet for Consumers,"
Office on Dietary Supplements (ODS), National Institutes
of Health (NIH), February 17, 2016.

What Are Weight-Loss Dietary Supplements and What Do They Do?

The proven ways to lose weight are by eating healthful foods, cutting calories, and being physically active. But making these lifestyle changes isn't easy, so you might wonder if taking a dietary supplement that's promoted for weight loss might help.

This section describes what's known about the safety and effectiveness of many ingredients that are commonly used in weight-loss dietary supplements. Sellers of these supplements might claim that their products help you lose weight by blocking the absorption of fat or carbohydrates, curbing your appetite or speeding up your metabolism. But there's little scientific evidence that weight-loss supplements actually work. Many are expensive, some can interact or interfere with medications, and a few might be harmful.

If you're thinking about taking a dietary supplement to lose weight, talk with your healthcare provider. This is especially important if you have high blood pressure, diabetes, heart disease or other medical conditions.

What Are the Ingredients in Weight-Loss Dietary Supplements?

Weight-loss supplements contain many ingredients—like herbs, fiber, and minerals—in different amounts and in many combinations. Sold in forms such as capsules, tablets, liquids, and powders, some products have dozens of ingredients.

Common ingredients in weight-loss supplements are described below in alphabetical order. You'll learn what's known about whether each ingredient works and is safe. Figuring out whether these ingredients really help you lose weight safely is complicated, though. Most products contain more than one ingredient, and ingredients can work differently when they're mixed together.

You may be surprised to learn that makers of weight-loss supplements rarely carry out studies in people to find out whether their product really works and is safe. And when studies are done, they usually involve only small numbers of people taking the supplement for just a few weeks or months. To know whether a weight-loss supplement can really help people lose weight safely and keep it off, larger groups of people need to be studied for a longer time.

How Are Weight-Loss Dietary Supplements Regulated?

The U.S. Food and Drug Administration (FDA) regulates weight-loss supplements differently from prescription or over-the-counter drugs. As with other dietary supplements, the FDA does not test or approve weight loss supplements before they are sold. Manufacturers are responsible for making sure that their supplements are safe and that the label claims are truthful and not misleading.

When the FDA finds an unsafe dietary supplement, it may remove the supplement from the market or ask the supplement maker to recall it. The FDA and the Federal Trade Commission may also take action against companies that make false weight-loss claims about their supplements; add pharmaceutical drugs to their supplements; or claim that their supplements can diagnose, treat, cure or prevent a disease.

Can Weight-Loss Dietary Supplements Be Harmful?

Weight-loss supplements, like all dietary supplements, can have harmful side effects and might interact with prescription and over-the-counter medications. Almost all weight-loss supplements have several ingredients that have not been tested in combination with one another, and their combined effects are unknown.

Tell your healthcare providers about any weight-loss supplements or other supplements you take. This information will help them work with you to prevent supplement-drug interactions, harmful side effects, and other risks.

Interactions with Medications

Like most dietary supplements, some weight-loss supplements may interact or interfere with other medicines or supplements you take. For example, caffeine's effect may be stronger if you take it with other stimulants (such as bitter orange), and chitosan might increase the blood-thinning effects of warfarin (Coumadin®) to dangerous levels. If you take dietary supplements and medications on a regular basis, be sure to talk about this with your healthcare provider.

Fraudulent and Adulterated Products

Be very cautious when you see weight-loss supplements with tempting claims, such as "magic diet pill," "melt away fat," and "lose weight without diet or exercise." If the claim sounds too good to be true, it probably is. These products may not help you lose weight-and they could be dangerous.

Weight-loss products, marketed as dietary supplements, are sometimes adulterated with prescription drug ingredients or controlled substances. Because U.S. law doesn't allow these ingredients to be in dietary supplements, they won't be listed on the product label and they could harm you.

Weight-loss supplements can be sold without being tested or approved by the U.S. Food and Drug Administration (FDA). Once a supplement that's suspected of causing serious health problems is on the market, the FDA can recall that product.

Choosing a Sensible Approach to Weight Loss

Weight-loss supplements can be expensive, and they might not work. The best way to lose weight and keep it off is to follow a healthy eating plan, reduce calories, and exercise regularly under the guidance of your healthcare provider.

As a bonus, lifestyle changes that help you lose weight might also improve your mood and energy level and lower your risk of heart disease, diabetes, and some types of cancer.

Section 39.2

Beware of Miracle Weight Loss Products

This section includes text excerpted from "Beware of Products
Promising Miracle Weight Loss," U.S. Food and Drug
Administration (FDA), January 5, 2015.

"This year, I'm going to lose some weight."

If you find yourself making this common New Year's resolution,
know this: many so-called "miracle" weight loss supplements and foods
(including teas and coffees) don't live up to their claims. Worse, they
can cause serious harm, say FDA regulators. The agency has found
hundreds of products that are marketed as dietary supplements but
actually contain hidden active ingredients (components that make a
medicine effective against a specific illness) contained in prescription
drugs, unsafe ingredients that were in drugs that have been removed
from the market or compounds that have not been adequately studied
in humans.

"When the product contains a drug or other ingredient which is
not listed as an ingredient we become especially concerned about the
safety of the product," says James P. Smith, M.D., an acting deputy
director in FDA's Office of Drug Evaluation.

Tainted Products

For example, FDA has found weight-loss products tainted with
the prescription drug ingredient sibutramine. This ingredient was in
an FDA-approved drug called Meridia, which was removed from the
market in October 2010 because it caused heart problems and strokes.

"We've also found weight-loss products marketed as supplements
that contain dangerous concoctions of hidden ingredients including
active ingredients contained in approved seizure medications, blood
pressure medications, and antidepressants," says a senior regulatory
manager at FDA. Most recently, FDA has found a number of products
marketed as dietary supplements containing fluoxetine, the active
ingredient found in Prozac, a prescription drug marketed for the treatment of depression and other conditions. Another product contained

triamterene, a powerful diuretic (sometimes known as "water pills") that can have serious side-effects and should only be used under the supervision of a healthcare professional.

Many of these tainted products are imported, sold online, and heavily promoted on social media sites. Some can also be found on store shelves.

And if you're about to take what you think of as "natural" dietary supplements, such as bee pollen or Garcinia cambogia, you should be aware that FDA has found some of these products also contain hidden active ingredients contained in prescription drugs.

"The only natural way to lose weight is to burn more calories than you take in," says James P. Smith, M.D. That means a combination of healthful eating and physical activity.

Dietary Supplements Are Not FDA-Approved

Under the Federal Food, Drug and Cosmetics Act (as amended by the Dietary Supplement Health and Education Act of 1994), dietary supplement firms do not need FDA approval prior to marketing their products. It is the company's responsibility to make sure its products are safe and that any claims made about such products are true.

But just because you see a supplement product on a store shelf does not mean it is safe, Humbert says. FDA has received numerous reports of harm associated with the use of weight loss products, including increased blood pressure, heart palpitations (a pounding or racing heart), stroke, seizure and death. When safety issues are suspected, FDA must investigate and, when warranted, take steps to have these products removed from the market.

FDA has issued over 30 public notifications and recalled 7 tainted weight loss products in 2014. The agency also has issued warning letters, seized products, and criminally prosecuted people responsible for marketing these illegal diet products. In addition, FDA maintains an online list of tainted weight-loss products.

To help people with long-term weight management, FDA has approved prescription drugs such as Belviq, Qsymia, and Contrave, but these products are intended for people at least 18 years of age who:

- have a body mass index (BMI, a standard measure of body fat) of 30 or greater (considered obese); or

- have a BMI of 27 or greater (considered overweight) and have at least one other weight-related health condition.

Moreover, if you are going to embark on any type of weight control campaign, you should talk to your healthcare professional about it first, Smith says.

Know the Warning Signs

Look for potential warning signs of tainted products, such as:

- promises of a quick fix, for example, "lose 10 pounds in one week."

- use of the words "guaranteed" or "scientific breakthrough."

- products marketed in a foreign language.

- products marketed through mass e-mails.

- products marketed as herbal alternatives to an FDA-approved drug or as having effects similar to prescription drugs.

Section 39.3

Bee Pollen Weight Loss Product Scams

This section includes text excerpted from "Some Bee Pollen Weight Loss Products Are a Dangerous Scam," U.S. Food and Drug Administration (FDA), June 19, 2014.

Products labeled to contain bee pollen that promise to help you lose weight or reshape your body could actually harm you, warns the U.S. Food and Drug Administration (FDA).

Bee pollen is the pollen that bees collect from flowers; it is the food that nourishes bee larvae. But it's not a miracle ingredient, says Gary Coody, R.Ph., FDA's national health fraud coordinator.

Some bee pollen products marketed for weight loss have been found to contain hidden and potentially dangerous ingredients that may be harmful for people who have conditions such as irregular heartbeat, high blood pressure and bipolar disorders (a brain disorder that causes unusual shifts in mood), says Coody.

FDA recently warned consumers to immediately stop using one of these products—Zi Xiu Tang Bee Pollen—because it contains at least one potentially harmful ingredient that is not listed on the product's label.

Zi Xiu Tang is just one of several bee pollen products that the FDA has found to contain undeclared sibutramine and/or phenolphthalein. Others include Ultimate Formula, Fat Zero, Bella Vi Amp'd Up, Insane Amp'd Up, Slim Trim U, Infinity, Perfect Body Solution, Asset Extreme, Asset Extreme Plus, Asset Bold and Asset Bee Pollen. All these products marketed for weight loss included bee pollen in the list of ingredients.

The agency has received from consumers and healthcare professionals more than 50 adverse event reports associated with the use of tainted bee pollen weight loss products. The reports include at least one death, serious cardiac issues, chest pain, heart palpitations, tachycardia (increased heart rate), increased blood pressure, seizures, suicidal thoughts, anxiety, insomnia and diarrhea.

In addition, many bee pollen weight loss products are marketed as dietary supplements with claims to treat or prevent a variety of diseases and signs or symptoms of disease, including obesity, allergies, high blood pressure and high cholesterol. By law, dietary supplements may not claim to treat or prevent a disease.

"When people buy these tainted bee pollen weight loss products, they are unknowingly taking one or more hidden drugs that have been banned from the market," Coody warns.

The case of Zi Xiu Tang Bee Pollen illustrates the potential dangers posed by unscrupulous promoters of quick health fixes.

A Dangerous Concoction

FDA labs have analyzed 15 different Zi Xiu Tang Bee Pollen samples from various distributors with a variety of expiration dates and lot numbers. All products tested, including those that claim to be "genuine" and "anti-counterfeit," had undeclared drug ingredients: sibutramine and/or phenolphthalein.

Sibutramine is a controlled substance that was removed from the market in October 2010 after clinical data indicated that it posed an increased risk of heart attack and stroke. Sibutramine substantially increases the blood pressure and/or pulse in some people and can be risky for patients with a history of coronary artery disease, congestive heart failure, heart arrhythmias or stroke, says Jason Humbert, a senior regulatory manager with FDA's Office of Regulatory Affairs.

Phenolphthalein, a laxative and a suspected cancer-causing agent, isn't approved in the United States. FDA has classified phenolphthalein as not generally recognized as safe and effective.

"They will tell you you're going to get thirsty and need to drink more water. They won't tell you that's a side effect of sibutramine," Coody says of the vendors of tainted supplements. "They'll tell you that you may not feel well because you're detoxifying your body. Well, you're not feeling well because of the side effects of sibutramine."

The product conveys an image of authenticity, fitness and health, Coody says. "These folks are very savvy in how they market the product. They are going to make you think that it's not only exotic but also all natural," he adds.

FDA is also investigating other bee pollen weight loss products suspected to contain hidden drugs. "But we cannot test every product," Coody says.

An Elaborate Marketing Scheme

Zi Xiu Tang Bee Pollen is sold in health stores, fitness centers and spas. It's even touted by some healthcare practitioners.

Manufacturers and distributors of Zi Xiu Tang have created an anti-counterfeit system to persuade consumers that their product is "authentic" and that not all bee pollen products are the same ("That theirs is the real thing–the good stuff," Humbert says). The ruse includes a 16-digit code on the package that consumers can use to go online and "validate" whether the product is "genuine" or counterfeit.

There are also legitimate-looking websites and a huge social media presence, especially on Facebook and YouTube, to market the product. "It's a very elaborate and sophisticated scheme," says Humbert. "It preys on people's weaknesses. They want the product to work."

Zi Xiu Tang Bee Pollen was placed on Import Alert to prevent it from being shipped into the United States. But the product is still entering the country illegally, Coody says. FDA is investigating and may issue additional warning letters or take enforcement action, such as issuing an administrative detention order against products with undeclared drugs, bringing a seizure action in federal court or seeking an injunction or criminal prosecution against the firm or responsible individuals.

Chapter 40

Popular Fad Diets

Introduction to Popular Fad Diets

The many popular diets and diet plans on the market today can be confusing and overwhelming for consumers to navigate. People who want to lose weight are bombarded with advertisements for various diets all claiming to provide the secret to rapid weight loss with little or no effort. Some of these diets eliminate or restrict various foods, while others focus on including only certain foods. A diet can be considered a fad if it promises to deliver drastic weight loss in a short amount of time, without exercise, and if it is based on an unbalanced approach to nutrition. Many popular fad diets can be organized by type: high protein, low carbohydrate, fasting, food-specific, liquid only, and so on.

High-Protein Diets

High-protein diets promote an eating plan based largely on foods containing protein, usually meat, eggs, cheese, and other dairy products. The theory behind high-protein diets is that the body must work harder to digest protein, and in doing so, more calories are burned. Studies have found that diets high in protein can cause certain health problems, as the body works to process excess protein. High-protein diets can cause rapid initial weight loss as the body eliminates water while processing extra protein. Typically, any weight lost on a high-protein diet will be regained.

"Popular Fad Diets," © 2016 Omnigraphics. Reviewed June 2016.

Low-Carbohydrate Diets

The main premise of low-carbohydrate diets is the severe restriction of calories from carbohydrates (sugar). Most low-carbohydrate diets suggest replacing foods high in carbohydrates with foods high in protein. In this way, low-carbohydrate diets are similar to high-protein diets. A low-carbohydrate diet is often high in fat. A high-fat diet causes a condition known as ketosis, which can act as an appetite suppressant. The theory of low-carbohydrate diets is that the suppressed appetite will result in the dieter consuming fewer calories overall. Studies of low-carbohydrate diets have shown that dieters are at risk for health problems including kidney malfunction and heart disease. Many people who follow a low-carbohydrate diet report feeling sluggish and tired, and typically any weight that is lost will be regained.

Detoxifying Diets

Detoxifying diets are often high-fiber diets, and sometimes include increased consumption of fats and oils. The theory of this type of detoxification is that the fiber helps the dieter to feel full, therefore consuming fewer calories throughout the day. It is also believed that a high-fiber diet will cleanse the digestive system through the elimination of more solid waste. Side effects of a high-fiber detoxifying diet often include gastrointestinal distress, bloating, cramps, and dehydration. Studies have shown no permanent weight loss from this type of detoxifying diet.

Fasting Diets

Fasting diets require dieters to consume nothing but clear liquids for a short period of time, typically one to five days. This is believed to help rid the body of toxins. Fasting can result in temporary weight loss due to consuming far fewer calories than normal, though the weight generally returns once the fast is ended. Fasting produces a host of side effects, including dizziness, lethargy, and feeling weak or tired.

Food-Specific Diets

Food-specific diets recommend consumption of a single type of food, such as grapefruit, cabbage or protein shakes. These diets are based on the theory that certain foods have special properties that promote weight-loss. Food-specific diets do not provide the range of vitamins, minerals, and other nutrients needed to support bodily functions. If maintained over an extended period of time, the side effects of food-specific diets can be serious.

Popular Diet Plans

The Atkins Diet

The Atkins Diet is a low-carbohydrate, high-protein diet created by Dr. Robert Atkins, an American cardiologist. The main premise of the Atkins Diet is that eating too many carbohydrates causes obesity and other health problems. A diet that is low in carbohydrates produces metabolic activity that results in less hunger and also in weight loss. The Atkins Diet is structured in four phases: induction; weight loss; pre-maintenance; lifetime maintenance. Dieters move through the four phases at their own pace. Early phases of the Atkins Diet allow consumption of seafood, poultry, meat, eggs, cheese, salad vegetables, oils, butter, and cream. Later phases allow consumption of foods such as nuts, fruits, wine, beans, whole grains, and other vegetables. The Atkins Diet recommends avoidance of certain foods such as fruit, bread, most grains, starchy vegetables, and dairy products other than cheese, cream, and butter. The Atkins Diet may help people feel full longer, and may result in weight loss as long as the diet in continued. Side effects may result from consuming low amounts of fiber and certain vitamins and minerals, while consuming larger amounts of saturated fat, cholesterol, and red meat.

The Zone Diet

The Zone Diet was created by Dr. Barry Spears and is based on the genetic evolution of humans. The main premise of the Zone Diet is that humans should maintain a diet similar to that of our ancient hunter-gatherer ancestors. The Zone Diet focuses on lean protein, natural carbohydrates (fruit) and natural fiber (vegetables) while avoiding or eliminating processed carbohydrates such as grains and products made from grains. The Zone Diet recommends a food plan that is made up of 40 percent natural carbohydrates. 30 percent fat, and 30 percent protein. The emphasis is on food choices, not amount of calories. This percentage should apply to every meal and snack that is eaten. Close evaluation of the Zone Diet has revealed that at its core, the Zone Diet is a very low-calorie eating plan that is lacking in certain nutrients, vitamins, and minerals.

Weight Watchers

Weight Watchers was founded by Jean Nidetch in 1963. The Weight Watchers program focuses on weight loss through diet, exercise, and the use of support networks. Members are given the option of joining a group or following the program online. In either case, educational materials and support are available to assist members. The Weight Watchers support network is considered a critical aspect of the program, as it is believed that dieters need constant positive reinforcement in order to achieve and maintain long-term weight loss. The Weight Watchers program is structured in two phases: weight loss and maintenance. During weight loss, dieters work to lose weight slowly, with the goal of one to two pounds per week. Once the goal weight has been attained, dieters move into the maintenance phase, during which they gradually adjust their food intake until they are neither losing nor gaining weight. In general, Weight Watchers is viewed as providing a healthy approach to dieting.

Ornish Lifestyle Medicine

The Ornish Lifestyle Medicine program was created by Dr. Dean Ornish. The main premise of the program is that foods are neither good nor bad, but some are healthier than others. The Ornish diet focuses on fruits, vegetables, whole grains, legumes, soy products, nonfat dairy, natural egg whites, and fats that contain omega three fatty acids. The Ornish diet is plant-based; meat, poultry, and fish are excluded. Portion control is recommended, but caloric intake is not restricted unless a person is trying to lose weight. The program recommends small, frequent meals spread out throughout the day to support constant energy and avoid hunger. The consumption of caffeine is discouraged though allowed in small amounts. The Ornish program recommends exercise and low-dose multivitamin supplements. In general, the Ornish program is viewed as a healthy diet.

Diet Safety

Fad diets may produce initial weight loss results, but the potential for undesirable side effects should not be ignored. The human body needs simple carbohydrates (glucose) for energy and brain function. Low-carbohydrate and high-protein diets are not nutritionally balanced enough to meet the needs of children and some adults, particularly women who are pregnant, plan to become pregnant, or are nursing a baby. If maintained for an extended period of time, high-protein, low-carbohydrate diets can result in health problems such as heart disease, kidney problems, and certain cancers.

Weight loss is achieved by eating fewer calories than are consumed by physical activity. Because most fad diets require people to consumer very few calories, these diets can result in weight loss. However, because most fad diets are not nutritionally balanced and cannot be maintained for long periods of time, people usually find that any weight lost is regained once they stop following the diet and return to their old eating habits. The most effective weight-loss strategies are those that include a healthy, balanced diet combined with exercise.

References

1. "Diet Fads vs. Diet Truths," January 2004.

2. Nordqvist, Christian. "The Eight Most Popular Diets Today," Medical News Today. October 1, 2015.

3. "Nutrition Fact Sheet," Alaska Department of State Health Services, Nutrition Services Section. 2005.

Chapter 41

Consuming Foods Marketed as Low Fat or Diet

Chapter Contents

Section 41.1

Fat Replacers

This section includes text excerpted from "Response to Consumer Demand for Reduced-Fat Foods; Multi-Functional Fat Replacers," U.S. Department of Agriculture (USDA), December 2010. Reviewed June 2016.

As one of nutritional and functional components of diets, fat delivers pleasing taste and flavor as well as what food scientists call 'mouth-feel' in foods, thus providing positive sensory attributes. However, a number of studies have documented that excessive consumption of foods high in fat leads to health problems including obesity and heart disease. Thus, the food industry is facing the challenge of searching for new alternatives for fat in foods without any quality loss. Typically, fat can be replaced in foods by modifying the food formulation with carbo-hydrate-, protein-, and lipid-based ingredients. Even though a variety of fat replacers have been developed, there are unfortunately no ideal fat replacers which completely function like conventional fat. How-ever, more recent development of food processing technology allows multi-functional fat replacers with unique qualities to be created and used in the most appropriated product applications. Consumers can therefore benefit from the use of multi-functional fat replacers with health-enhancing effects and keep enjoying food products with reduced content of fat and calorie.

Classification of Fat Replacers

It is well recognized that fat plays critical functional roles in foods by providing tender texture, glossy appearance, good flavor, emulsify-ing property, and so on. Thus fat gives positive sensory and functional properties when incorporated into food formulations and its contribu-tion to physiological benefits is also well-documented. Therefore the removal of fat in food formulations can cause undesirable changes in food quality attributes. Fat replacers indicate food ingredients that can take the place of all or some of the fat in foods and yet give sim-ilar organoleptic properties to the foods. In general, they serve two purposes which are the reduction of fat and calorie contents since fat has energy values of 9 kcal/g. Depending on their chemical structure, fat replacers are classified into lipid-, protein-, and carbohydrate-based fat replacers.

Furthermore, another terms of fat replacers which are fat substitutes and fat mimetics (also called analogs and mimics), have been widely used. Fat substitutes indicate any ingredients of which chemical structure and physical property are similar to those of triglycerides. Therefore, most of fat substitutes indicates lipid-based fat replacers and can be used by replacing fat on an equal weight basis. On the other hand, carbohydrate-and protein-based fat replacers belong to fat mimetics which have similar organoleptic/physical characteristics to fat. Fat in foods may not be replaced with fat mimetics on a one-to-one basis.

Reduction of Fat and Calorie

From a conceptual point of view, fat replacement is the reduction in fat-constituted calories by using food ingredients with less calories than conventional fat. Therefore, one of the strategies to develop fat replacers is to explore reduced-calorie compounds from non-lipid-based sources (such as carbohydrates and proteins) or manipulate the composition of fatty acids for lipid-based fat replacers (such as structured lipid). Since most of fat replacers from carbohydrate or protein sources have less energy (i.e. generally 4 kcal/g). the energy density of the foods can be readily reduced. As previously mentioned, a diet high in fat leads to undesirable health problems such as obesity, high blood pressure, and heart disease. Hence, the reduced content of fat and calorie derived from the use of fat replacers is a nutritional approach to prevent chronic diseases, thus providing beneficial health effects.

Physiological Benefits

Healthy innovation is most widespread in the global food industry. Hence, when developing or discovering fat replacers, another factor to be considered is health-functional property derived from their physiological activities. In this aspect, carbohydrate-based fat replacers (especially from dietary fibers) impart various health benefits to the consumers when incorporated into food formulations at appropriate levels. Thus, fiber-based ingredients are becoming increasingly important as health-promoting functional materials. For example, microcrystalline cellulose, which is non-digestible and has zero-calories, has been used as a fat replacer for meat products, ice cream, salad dressing, and so on.

Also, food applications have benefited from the use of methylcellulose gums such as hydroxypropyl methylcellulose (HPMC) which is regarded as a soluble dietary fiber. Specially, the linkage of □-glucan and its physiological effects has been suggested by a number of in vitro and in vivo studies, demonstrating that □-glucan is effective in reducing cholesterol level, controlling blood glucose level, and reducing the risk of colon cancer.

Extension to Diverse Reduced-Fat Foods

Fat replacers have been widely used in two food categories which are baked and dairy products. It would be because they belong to the representative groups containing high contents of fat and calories. Also, it is readily easy and convenient to modify their formulations without any significant quality loss. Thus, a number of studies on fat replacement in foods have been used mainly in baked or dairy products as a model system for fat replacement. However, the type of foods where fat is replaced has been recently diversified with increasing consumer demand for variety. For example, cocoa butter in chocolate was recently replaced with □-glucan-rich hydrocolloids.

In addition, fried foods are one of the representative foods with high amount of oil and calorie which is thought to contribute to health problems like overweight and obesity. Even though fat replacement is not necessary in fried foods, the role of ingredients which reduce the oil uptake of fried foods is in good agreement with that of fat replacers in terms of reducing the content of fat (or oil) and calorie. When □-glucan-rich flour from barley was evaluated as an oil barrier. it was found to absorb almost about half as much oil during frying than wheat batters.

Section 41.2

Fat-Free versus Regular Calorie Consumption

This section includes text excerpted from "Fat-Free versus Regular Calorie Comparison," National Heart, Lung, and Blood Institute (NHLBI), July 9, 2010. Reviewed June 2016.

Fats and Calories

A calorie is a calorie is a calorie, whether it comes from fat or carbohydrate. Anything eaten in excess can lead to weight gain. You can lose weight by eating fewer calories and by increasing your physical activity. Reducing the amount of fat and saturated fat that you eat is one easy way to limit your overall calorie intake. However, eating fat-free or reduced-fat foods isn't always the answer to weight loss. This is especially true when you eat more of the reduced-fat food than you would of the regular item. The following list of foods and their reduced-fat varieties will show you that just because a product is fat-free, it doesn't mean that it is "calorie-free." And, calories do count!

Table 41.1. Fat-Free Versus Regular Calorie Comparison

Fat-Free or Reduced-Fat	Calories	Regular	Calories
Reduced-fat peanut butter, 2 Tbsp	187	Regular peanut butter, 2 Tbsp	191
Reduced-fat chocolate chip cookies, 3 cookies (30 g)	118	Regular chocolate chip cookies, 3 cookies (30 g)	142
Fat-free fig cookies, 2 cookies (30 g)	102	Regular fig cookies, 2 cookies (30 g)	111
Fat-free vanilla frozen yogurt (<1% fat), ½ C	100	Regular whole milk vanilla frozen yogurt (3–4% fat), ½ C	104

Table 41.1. Continued

Fat-Free or Reduced-Fat	Calories	Regular	Calories
Light vanilla ice cream (7% fat), ½ C	111	Regular vanilla ice cream, (11% fat), ½ C	133
Fat-free caramel topping, 2 Tbsp	103	Caramel topping, homemade with butter, 2 Tbsp	103
Low-fat granola cereal, approx. ½ C (55 g)	213	Regular granola cereal, approx. ½ C (55 g)	257
Low-fat blueberry muffin, 1 small (2½ inch)	131	Regular blueberry muffin, 1 small (2½ inch)	138
Baked tortilla chips, 1 oz	113	Regular tortilla chips, 1 oz	143
Low-fat cereal bar, 1 bar (1.3 oz)	130	Regular cereal bar, 1 bar (1.3 oz)	140

Part Seven

Nutrition for People with Other Medical Concerns

Chapter 42

Nutrition and Diabetes

Chapter Contents

Section 42.1

What People with Diabetes Need to Know about Eating

This section includes text excerpted from "Eat Right!" Centers for Disease Control and Prevention (CDC), April 15, 2016.

Learning how to eat right is an important part of controlling your diabetes. This section will provide tips on healthy eating, weight control, recipes and special diets. Remember, eating healthy is not just for people with diabetes.

What Healthy Food Choices Should I Make?

Eat smaller portions. Learn what a serving size is for different foods and how many servings you need in a meal.

Eat less fat. Choose fewer high-fat foods and use less fat for cooking. You especially want to limit foods that are high in saturated fats or trans fat, such as:

- Fatty cuts of meat.

- Fried Foods.

- Whole milk and dairy products made from whole milk

- Cakes, candy, cookies, crackers, and pies.

- Salad dressings.

- Lard, shortening, stick margarine, and nondairy creamers.

What Should I Eat More Of?

Eat more fiber by eating more whole-grain foods. Whole grains can be found in:

- Breakfast cereals made with 100% whole grains.

- Oatmeal.

- Whole grain rice.

- Whole-wheat bread, bagels, pita bread, and tortillas.

Eat a variety of fruits and vegetables every day. Choose fresh, frozen, canned or dried fruit and 100% fruit juices most of the time. Eat plenty of veggies like these:

- Dark green veggies (e.g., broccoli, spinach, brussels sprouts).

- Orange veggies (e.g., carrots, sweet potatoes, pumpkin, winter squash).

- Beans and peas (e.g., black beans, garbanzo beans, kidney beans, pinto beans, split peas, lentils).

What Should I Eat Less Of?

Eat fewer foods that are high in sugar, such as:

- Fruit-flavored drinks.
- Sodas.
- Tea or coffee sweetened with sugar.

Use less salt in cooking and at the table. Eat fewer foods that are high in salt, such as:

- Canned and package soups.
- Canned vegetables.
- Pickles.
- Processed meats.

Where Can I Learn about Making a Diabetes Meal Plan?

- Contact a registered dietitian to make a meal plan just for you.
- Visit the Academy of Nutrition and Dietetics, formerly the American Dietetic Association Website to find a nutrition professional that can help you develop a healthy meal plan (www. eatright.org).
- Visit the American Association of Diabetes Educators to find a diabetes educator (www.diabeteseducator.org).
- Visit the American Diabetes Association Website for more information on carbohydrate counting and the exchange method (www.diabetes.org)

Section 42.2

Nutrition Tips to Prevent Type 2 Diabetes

This section includes text excerpted from "Choose More Than 50 Ways to Prevent Type 2 Diabetes," National Institute of Diabetes and Digestive and Kidney Diseases (NIDDK), September 2014.

50 Ways to Prevent Type 2 Diabetes

Reduce Portion Sizes

Portion size is the amount of food you eat, such as 1 cup of fruit or 6 ounces of meat. If you are trying to eat smaller portions, eat a half of a bagel instead of a whole bagel or have a 3-ounce hamburger instead of a 6-ounce hamburger. Three ounces is about the size of your fist or a deck of cards.

Put Less on Your Plate

1. Drink a large glass of water 10 minutes before your meal so you feel less hungry.

2. Keep meat, chicken, turkey, and fish portions to about 3 ounces.

3. Share one dessert.

Eat a Small Meal

4. Use teaspoons, salad forks or child-size forks, spoons, and knives to help you take smaller bites and eat less.

5. Make less food look like more by serving your meal on a salad or breakfast plate.

6. Eat slowly. It takes 20 minutes for your stomach to send a signal to your brain that you are full.

7. Listen to music while you eat instead of watching TV (people tend to eat more while watching TV).

How Much Should I Eat?

Try filling your plate like this:

- 1/4 protein
- 1/4 grains
- 1/2 vegetables and fruit
- dairy (low-fat or skim milk)

Move More Each Day

Find ways to be more active each day. Try to be active for at least 30 minutes, 5 days a week. Walking is a great way to get started and you can do it almost anywhere at any time. Bike riding, swimming, and dancing are also good ways to move more.

If you are looking for a safe place to be active, contact your local parks department or health department to ask about walking maps, community centers, and nearby parks.

Dance It Away

8. Show your kids the dances you used to do when you were their age.

9. Turn up the music and jam while doing household chores.

10. Work out with a video that shows you how to get active.

Let's Go

11. Deliver a message in person to a co-worker instead of sending an e-mail.

12. Take the stairs to your office. Or take the stairs as far as you can, and then take the elevator the rest of the way.

13. March in place while you watch TV.

14. Choose a place to walk that is safe, such as your local mall.

15. Get off of the bus one stop early and walk the rest of the way home or to work if it is safe.

Make Healthy Food Choices

Find ways to make healthy food choices. This can help you manage your weight and lower your chances of getting type 2 diabetes.

Choose to eat more vegetables, fruits, and whole grains. Cut back on high-fat foods like whole milk, cheeses, and fried foods. This will help you reduce the amount of fat and calories you take in each day.

Snack on a Veggie

16. Buy a mix of vegetables when you go food shopping.

17. Choose veggie toppings like spinach, broccoli, and peppers for your pizza.

18. Try eating foods from other countries. Many of these dishes have more vegetables, whole grains, and beans.

19. Buy frozen and low-salt (sodium) canned vegetables. They may cost less and keep longer than fresh ones.

20. Serve your favorite vegetable and a salad with low-fat macaroni and cheese.

Cook with Care

21. Stir fry, broil or bake with non-stick spray or low-salt broth. Cook with less oil and butter.

22. Try not to snack while cooking or cleaning the kitchen.

23. Cook with smaller amounts of cured meats (smoked turkey and turkey bacon). They are high in salt.

Cook in Style

24. Cook with a mix of spices instead of salt.

25. Try different recipes for baking or broiling meat, chicken, and fish.

26. Choose foods with little or no added sugar to reduce calories.

27. Choose brown rice instead of white rice.

Eat Healthy on the Go

28. Have a big vegetable salad with low-calorie salad dressing when eating out. Share your main dish with a friend or have the other half wrapped to go.

29. Make healthy choices at fast food restaurants. Try grilled chicken (with skin removed) instead of a cheeseburger.

30. Skip the fries and chips and choose a salad.

31. Order a fruit salad instead of ice cream or cake.

Rethink Your Drink

32. Find a water bottle you really like (from a church or club event, favorite sports team, etc.) and drink water from it every day.

33. Peel and eat an orange instead of drinking orange juice.

34. If you drink whole milk, try changing to 2% milk. It has less fat than whole milk. Once you get used to 2% milk, try 1% or fat-free (skim) milk. This will help you reduce the amount of fat and calories you take in each day.

35. Drink water instead of juice and regular soda.

Eat Smart

36. Make at least half of your grains whole grains, such as whole grain breads and cereals, brown rice, and quinoa.

37. Use whole grain bread for toast and sandwiches.

38. Keep a healthy snack with you, such as fresh fruit, a handful of nuts, and whole grain crackers.

39. Slow down at snack time. Eating a bag of low-fat popcorn takes longer than eating a candy bar.

40. Share a bowl of fruit with family and friends.

41. Eat a healthy snack or meal before shopping for food. Do not shop on an empty stomach.

42. Shop at your local farmer's market for fresh, local food.

Keep Track

43. Make a list of food you need to buy before you go to the store.

44. Keep a written record of what you eat for a week. It can help you see when you tend to overeat or eat foods high in fat or calories.

Read the Label

45. Compare food labels on packages.

46. Choose foods lower in saturated fats, trans fats, cholesterol, calories, salt, and added sugars.

Take Care of Your Mind, Body, and Soul

You Can Exhale

47. Take time to change the way you eat and get active. Try one new food or activity a week.

48. Find ways to relax. Try deep breathing, taking a walk or listening to your favorite music.

49. Pamper yourself. Read a book, take a long bath or meditate.

50. Think before you eat. Try not to eat when you are bored, upset or unhappy.

Section 42.3

Diabetes and Carbohydrate Counting

This section includes text excerpted from "What I Need
to Know about Carbohydrate Counting and Diabetes,"
National Institute of Diabetes and Digestive and Kidney
Diseases (NIDDK), December 2013.

What Is Carbohydrate Counting?

Carbohydrate counting, also called carb counting, is a meal planning tool for people with type 1 or type 2 diabetes. Carbohydrate counting involves keeping track of the amount of carbohydrate in the foods you eat each day.

Carbohydrates are one of the main **nutrients** found in food and drinks. Protein and fat are the other main nutrients. Carbohydrates include sugars, starches, and fiber. Carbohydrate counting can help you control your blood glucose, also called blood sugar, levels because carbohydrates affect your blood **glucose** more than other nutrients.

Healthy carbohydrates, such as whole grains, fruits, and vegetables, are an important part of a healthy eating plan because they can provide both energy and nutrients, such as vitamins and minerals, and fiber. Fiber can help you prevent **constipation**, lower your **cholesterol** levels, and control your weight.

Unhealthy carbohydrates are often food and drinks with added sugars. Although unhealthy carbohydrates can also provide energy, they have little to no nutrients.

The amount of carbohydrate in foods is measured in grams. To count grams of carbohydrate in foods you eat, you'll need to

- know which foods contain carbohydrates;

- learn to estimate the number of grams of carbohydrate in the foods you eat; and

- add up the number of grams of carbohydrate from each food you eat to get your total for the day.

Your doctor can refer you to a **dietitian** or diabetes educator who can help you develop a healthy eating plan based on carbohydrate counting.

Which Foods Contain Carbohydrates?

The following foods items contain carbohydrates.

- grains, such as bread, noodles, pasta, crackers, cereals, and rice.

- fruits, such as apples, bananas, berries, mangoes, melons, and oranges.

- dairy products, such as milk and yogurt.

- legumes, including dried beans, lentils, and peas.

- snack foods and sweets, such as cakes, cookies, candy, and other desserts.

- juices, soft drinks, fruit drinks, sports drinks, and energy drinks that contain sugars.

- vegetables, especially "starchy" vegetables such as potatoes, corn, and peas.

Potatoes, peas, and corn are called starchy vegetables because they are high in starch. These vegetables have more carbohydrates per serving than nonstarchy vegetables.

Examples of nonstarchy vegetables are asparagus, broccoli, carrots, celery, green beans, lettuce and other salad greens, peppers, spinach, tomatoes, and zucchini.

Foods that do not contain carbohydrates include meat, fish, and poultry; most types of cheese; nuts; and oils and other fats.

What Happens When I Eat Foods Containing Carbohydrates?

When you eat foods containing carbohydrates, your digestive system breaks down the sugars and starches into glucose. Glucose is one of the simplest forms of sugar. Glucose then enters your bloodstream from your digestive tract and raises your blood glucose levels. The hormone **insulin**, which comes from the **pancreas** or from insulin shots, helps cells throughout your body absorb glucose and use it for energy. Once glucose moves out of the blood into cells, your blood glucose levels go back down.

How Can Carbohydrate Counting Help Me?

Carbohydrate counting can help keep your blood glucose levels close to normal. Keeping your blood glucose levels as close to normal as possible may help you.

- stay healthy longer.
- prevent or delay diabetes problems such as kidney disease, blindness, nerve damage, and blood vessel disease that can lead to heart attacks, strokes, and **amputations**—surgery to remove a body part.
- feel better and more energetic.

You may also need to take diabetes medicines or have insulin shots to control your blood glucose levels. Discuss your blood glucose targets with your doctor. Targets are numbers you aim for. To meet your targets, you will need to balance your carbohydrate intake with physical activity and diabetes medicines or insulin shots.

How Can I Tell Whether Carbohydrate Counting Is Working for Me?

Checking your blood glucose levels can help you tell whether carbohydrate counting is working for you. You can check your blood glucose levels using a glucose meter.

You should also have an A1C blood test at least twice a year. The A1C test reflects the average amount of glucose in your blood during the past 3 months.

If your blood glucose levels are too high, you may need to make changes in your eating plan or other lifestyle changes. For example, you may need to make wiser food choices, be more physically active or make changes to your diabetes medicines. Talk with your doctor about what changes you need to make to control your blood glucose levels.

If you use an insulin pump or take more than one daily insulin shot, ask your doctor how to adjust your insulin when you eat something that isn't in your usual eating plan.

Can I Use Carbohydrate Counting If I Am Pregnant?

You can use carbohydrate counting to help control your blood glucose levels when you are pregnant. Meeting your blood glucose targets during pregnancy is important for your and your baby's health. High blood glucose during pregnancy can harm the baby and increase the baby's chances of having type 2 diabetes later in life.

Women diagnosed with **gestational** diabetes—a type of diabetes that develops only during pregnancy—can also use carbohydrate counting to help control their blood glucose levels.

Talk with your doctor about using carbohydrate counting to help meet your blood glucose targets during your pregnancy.

Chapter 43

Nutrition and Heart Disease

Chapter Contents

Section 43.1

Eating for a Healthy Heart

This section includes text excerpted from "Heart-Healthy Eating,"
Office on Women's Health (OWH), U.S. Department of Health and
Human Services (HHS), June 30, 2014.

Heart-healthy eating is an important way to lower your risk for
heart disease and stroke. Heart disease is the number one cause of
death for American women. Stroke is the number three cause of death.
To get the most benefit for your heart, you should choose more fruits,
vegetables and foods with whole grains and healthy proteins. You also
should eat less food with added sugar, calories, and unhealthy fats.

What Foods Should I Eat to Help Lower My Risk for Heart Disease and Stroke?

You should choose these foods most of the time:

- **Fruits and vegetables.** At least half of your plate should be
  fruits and vegetables.

- **Grains**. At least half of your grains should be whole grains.

- **Fat-free or low-fat dairy products**. These include milk, calcium-fortified soy drinks (soy milk), cheese, yogurt, and other milk
  products.

- **Seafoods, skinless poultry, lean meats, beans, egg, and
  unsalted nuts.**

What Foods Should I Limit to Lower My Risk of Heart Disease and Stroke?

You should limit:

- **Saturated fats**. These fats are found in foods such as pizza, ice
  cream, fried chicken, many cakes and cookies, bacon, and hamburgers. Check the Nutrition Facts label for saturated fat. Less
  than 10% of your daily calories should be from saturated fats.

- **Trans fat**. These fats are found mainly in commercially pre-pared baked goods, snack foods, fried foods, and margarine. The U.S. Food and Drug Administration (FDA) is taking action to remove artificial trans fats from our food supply because of their risk to heart health. Check the Nutrition Facts label and choose foods with no trans fats as much as possible.

- **Cholesterol**. Cholesterol is found in foods made from animals, such as bacon, whole milk, cheese made from whole milk, ice cream, full-fat frozen yogurt, and eggs. Fruits and vegetables do not contain cholesterol. You should eat less than 300 milligrams of cholesterol per day. Check the Nutrition Facts label for choles-terol. Foods with 20% or more of the "Daily Value" of cholesterol are high in cholesterol.

- **Sodium**. Sodium is found in salt, but most of the sodium we eat is not from the salt that we add while cooking or at the table. Most of our sodium comes from breads and rolls, cold cuts, pizza, hot dogs, cheese, pasta dishes, and condiments (like ketchup and mustard). Limit your daily sodium to less than 2,300 milligrams (equal to a teaspoon), unless your doctor says something else. Check the nutrition facts label for sodium. Foods with 20% or more of the "Daily value" of sodium are high in sodium.

- **Added sugars**. Foods like fruit and dairy products naturally contain sugar. But you should limit foods that contain added sugars. These foods include sodas, sports drinks, cakes, candy, and ice cream. Check the Nutrition Facts label for added sugars and limit how much food you eat with added sugars.

What Tools Can Help Me Choose Foods That Are Good for My Heart?

The following resources can help you choose heart-healthy foods.

- **ChooseMyPlate** (choosemyplate.gov). This resource is based on the *Dietary Guidelines for Americans*. You can use the Super-Tracker tool to create a personal daily food plan based on your goals.

- **Dietary Approaches to Stop Hypertension (DASH) eating plan** (www.nhlbi.nih.gov/health/ health-topics/topics/dash/). The DASH diet is for people with hypertension to help them lower their blood pressure. But it can also be used to help prevent heart disease.

- **Therapeutic Lifestyle Changes** (TLC) diet (www.nhlbi.nih. gov/health/public/heart/chol/ chol_tlc.pdf). The TLC diet helps people with unhealthy cholesterol levels.

Section 43.2

The DASH Eating Plan

This section includes text excerpted from "Description of the DASH Eating Plan," National Heart, Lung, and Blood Institute (NHLBI), September 16, 2015.

DASH is a flexible and balanced eating plan that helps creates a heart-healthy eating style for life.

The DASH eating plan requires no special foods and instead provides daily and weekly nutritional goals. This plan recommends:

- Eating vegetables, fruits, and whole grains.

- Including fat-free or low-fat dairy products, fish, poultry, beans, nuts, and vegetable oils.

- Limiting foods that are high in saturated fat, such as fatty meats, full-fat dairy products, and tropical oils such as coconut, palm kernel, and palm oils.

- Limiting sugar-sweetened beverages and sweets.

Based on these recommendations, the following table shows examples of daily and weekly servings that meet DASH eating plan targets for a 2,000-calorie-a-day diet.

When following the DASH eating plan, it is important to choose foods that are:

- Low in saturated and trans fats.

- Rich in potassium, calcium, magnesium, fiber, and protein.

- Lower in sodium.

Table 43.1. Daily and Weekly DASH Eating Plan Goals for a 2,000-Calorie-A-Day Diet

Food Group	Daily Servings
Grains	6–8
Meats, poultry, and fish	6 or less
Vegetables	4–5
Fruit	4–5
Low-fat or fat-free dairy products	2–3
Fats and oils	2–3
Sodium	2,300 mg*
Weekly Servings	
Nuts, seeds, dry beans, and peas	4–5
Sweets	5 or less

1,500 milligrams (mg) sodium lowers blood pressure even further than 2,300 mg sodium daily.

Following the DASH Eating Plan

The Dietary Approaches to Stop Hypertension (DASH) eating plan is easy to follow using common foods available in your grocery store. The plan includes daily servings from different food groups. The number of servings you should have depends on your daily calorie (energy) needs.

To figure out your calorie needs, you need to consider your age and physical activity level. If you want to maintain your current weight, you should eat only as many calories as you burn by being physically active. This is called energy balance.

If you need to lose weight, you should eat fewer calories than you burn or increase your activity level to burn more calories than you eat.

Consider your physical activity level. Are you sedentary, moderately active or active?

- Sedentary means that you do only light physical activity as part of your typical daily routine.

- Moderately active means that you do physical activity equal to walking about 1.5 to 3 miles a day at 3 to 4 miles per hour, plus light physical activity.

- Active means that you do physical activity equal to walking more than 3 miles per day at 3 to 4 miles per hour, plus light physical activity.

Use the chart below to estimate your daily calorie needs.

Table 43.2. Daily Calorie Needs for Women

Age (years)	Calories Needed for Sedentary Activity Level	Calories Needed for Moderately Active Activity Level	Calories Needed for Active Activity Level
19–30	2000	2,000–2,200	2400
31–50	1800	2000	2200
51	1600	1800	2,000–2,200

Table 43.3. Daily Calorie Needs for Men

Age (years)	Calories Needed for Sedentary Activity Level	Calories Needed for Moderately Active Activity Level	Calories Needed for Active Activity Level
19–30	2400	2,600–2,800	3000
31–50	2200	2,400–2,600	2,800–3,000
51	2000	2,200–2,400	2,400–2,800

After figuring out your daily calorie needs, go to the table below and find the closest calorie level to yours. This table estimates the number of servings from each food group that you should have. Serving quantities are per day, unless otherwise noted.

Table 43.4. DASH Eating Plan—Number of Food Servings by Calorie Level

Food Group	1,200 Cal.	1,400 Cal.	1,600 Cal.	1,800 Cal.	2,000 Cal.	2,600 Cal.	3,100 Cal.
Grains[a]	4–5	5–6	6	6	6–8	10–11	12–13
Vegetables	3–4	3–4	3–4	4–5	4–5	5–6	6
Fruits	3–4	4	4	4–5	4–5	5–6	6
Fat-free or low-fat dairy products[b]	2–3	2–3	2–3	2–3	2–3	3	3–4
Lean meats, poultry, and fish	3 or less	3–4 or less	3–4 or less	6 or less	6 or less	6 or less	6–9
Nuts, seeds, and legumes	3 per week	3 per week	3–4 per week	4 per week	4–5 per week	1	1

Table 43.4. Continued

Food Group	1,200 Cal.	1,400 Cal.	1,600 Cal.	1,800 Cal.	2,000 Cal.	2,600 Cal.	3,100 Cal.
Fats and oils[c]	1	1	2	2–3	2–3	3	4
Sweets and added sugars	3 or less per week	3 or less per week	3 or less per week	5 or less per week	5 or less per week	≤2	≤2
Maximum sodium limit[d]	2,300 mg/day	2,300 mg/day	2,300 mg/day	2,300 mg/day	2,300 mg/day	2,300 mg/day	2,300 mg/day

a. Whole grains are recommended for most grain servings as a good source of fiber and nutrients.

b. For lactose intolerance, try either lactase enzyme pills with dairy products or lactose-free or lactose-reduced milk.

c. Fat content changes the serving amount for fats and oils. For example, 1 Tbsp regular salad dressing = one serving; 1 Tbsp low-fat dressing = one-half serving; 1 Tbsp fat-free dressing = zero servings.

d. The DASH eating plan has a sodium limit of either 2,300 mg or 1,500 mg per day.

Table 43.5. DASH Eating Plan—Serving Sizes, Examples, and Significance

Food Group	Serving Sizes	Examples and Notes	Significance of Each Food Group to the DASH Eating Plan
Grains[a]	1 slice bread 1 oz dry cereal[b] ½ cup cooked rice, pasta or cereal[b]	Whole-wheat bread and rolls, whole-wheat pasta, English muffin, pita bread, bagel, cereals, grits, oatmeal, brown rice, unsalted pretzels and popcorn	Major sources of energy and fiber
Vegetables	1 cup raw leafy vegetable ½ cup cut-up raw or cooked vegetable ½ cup vegetable juice	Broccoli, carrots, collards, green beans, green peas, kale, lima beans, potatoes, spinach, squash, sweet potatoes, tomatoes	Rich sources of potassium, magnesium, and fiber

Table 43.5. Continued

Food Group	Serving Sizes	Examples and Notes	Significance of Each Food Group to the DASH Eating Plan
Fruits	1 medium fruit ¼ cup dried fruit ½ cup fresh, frozen or canned fruit ½ cup fruit juice	Apples, apricots, bananas, dates, grapes, oranges, grapefruit, grapefruit juice, mangoes, melons, peaches, pineapples, raisins, strawberries, tangerines	Important sources of potassium, magnesium, and fiber
Fat-free or low-fat dairy products[c]	1 cup milk or yogurt 1½ oz cheese	Fat-free milk or buttermilk; fat-free, low-fat or reduced-fat cheese; fat-free/low-fat regular or frozen yogurt	Major sources of calcium and protein
Lean meats, poultry, and fish	1 oz cooked meats, poultry or fish 1 egg	Select only lean; trim away visible fats; broil, roast or poach; remove skin from poultry	Rich sources of protein and magnesium
Nuts, seeds, and legumes	1/3 cup or 1½ oz nuts 2 Tbsp peanut butter 2 Tbsp or ½ oz seeds ½ cup cooked legumes (dried beans, peas)	Almonds, filberts, mixed nuts, peanuts, walnuts, sunflower seeds, peanut butter, kidney beans, lentils, split peas	Rich sources of energy, magnesium, protein, and fiber
Fats and oils[d]	1 tsp soft margarine 1 tsp vegetable oil 1 Tbsp mayonnaise 2 Tbsp salad dressing	Soft margarine, vegetable oil (canola, corn, olive, safflower), low-fat mayonnaise, light salad dressing	The DASH study had 27% of calories as fat, including fat in or added to foods
Sweets and added sugars	1 Tbsp sugar 1 Tbsp jelly or jam ½ cup sorbet, gelatin dessert 1 cup lemonade	Fruit-flavored gelatin, fruit punch, hard candy, jelly, maple syrup, sorbet and ices, sugar	Sweets should be low in fat

a. Whole grains are recommended for most grain servings as a good source of fiber and nutrients.

b. Serving sizes vary between ½ cup and 1¼ cups, depending on cereal type. Check the product's Nutrition Facts label.

c. For lactose intolerance, try either lactase enzyme pills with dairy products or lactose-free or lactose-reduced milk.

d. Fat content changes the serving amount for fats and oils. For example, 1 Tbsp regular salad dressing=one serving; 1 Tbsp low-fat dressing=one-half serving; 1 Tbsp fat-free dressing=zero servings.

The DASH Eating Plan as Part of a Heart-Healthy Lifestyle

The DASH eating plan is just one key part of a heart-healthy life-style, and combining it with other lifestyle changes such as physical activity can help you control your blood pressure and LDL-cholesterol for life.

To help prevent and control high blood pressure:

- Be physically active.

- Maintain a healthy weight.

- Limit alcohol intake.

- Manage and cope with stress.

Other lifestyle changes can improve your overall health, such as:

- If you smoke, quit.

- Get plenty of sleep.

To help make lifelong lifestyle changes, try making one change at a time and add another when you feel that you have successfully adopted the earlier changes. When you practice several healthy lifestyle habits, you are more likely to achieve and maintain healthy blood pressure and cholesterol levels.

Living with the DASH Eating Plan

Understanding the DASH eating plan will help you start and follow this plan for life.

Controlling Daily Sodium and Calories

To benefit from the proven DASH eating plan, it is important to limit daily sodium levels to 2,300 mg or 1,500 mg if desired, and to consume the appropriate amount of calories to maintain a healthy weight or lose weight if needed.

Ways to Control Sodium Levels

The key to lowering your sodium intake is to make healthier food choices when you're shopping, cooking, and eating out.

Table 43.6. Tips for Lowering Sodium When Shopping, Cooking, and Eating Out

Shopping	Cooking	Eating Out
• Read food labels, and choose items that are lower in sodium and salt, particularly for convenience foods and condiments.* • Choose fresh poultry, fish, and lean meats instead of cured food such as bacon and ham. • Choose fresh or frozen versus canned fruits and vegetables. • Avoid food with added salt, such as pickles, pickled vegetables, olives, and sauerkraut. • Avoid instant or flavored rice and pasta.	• Don't add salt when cooking rice, pasta, and hot cereals. • Flavor your foods with salt-free seasoning blends, fresh or dried herbs and spices, or fresh lemon or lime juice. • Rinse canned foods or foods soaked in brine before using to remove the sodium. • Use less table salt to flavor food.	• Ask that foods be prepared without added salt or MSG, commonly used in Asian foods. • Avoid choosing menu items that have salty ingredients such as bacon, pickles, olives, and cheese. • Avoid choosing menu items that include foods that are pickled, cured, smoked, or made with soy sauce or broth. • Choose fruit or vegetables as a side dish, instead of chips or fries.

Examples of convenience foods are frozen dinners, prepackaged foods, and soups; examples of condiments are mustard, ketchup, soy sauce, barbecue sauce, and salad dressings.

Most of the sodium Americans eat comes from processed and prepared foods, such as breads, cold cuts, pizza, poultry, soups, sandwiches and burgers, cheese, pasta and meat dishes, and salty snacks. Therefore, healthier choices when shopping and eating out are particularly important.

Ways to Control Calories

To benefit from the DASH eating plan, it is important to consume the appropriate amount of calories to maintain a healthy weight. To help, read nutrition labels on food, and plan for success with DASH eating plan sample menus and other heart-healthy recipes.

The DASH eating plan can be used to help you lose weight. To lose weight, follow the DASH eating plan and try to reduce your total daily calories gradually. Find out your daily calorie needs or goals with the Body Weight Planner and calorie chart. Talk with your doctor before beginning any diet or eating plan.

General tips for reducing daily calories include:

- Eat smaller portions more frequently throughout the day.

- Reduce the amount of meat that you eat while increasing the amount of fruits, vegetables, whole grains or dry beans.

- Substitute low-calorie foods, such as when snacking (choose fruits or vegetables instead of sweets and desserts) or drinking (choose water instead of soda or juice), when possible.

Increasing Daily Potassium

The DASH eating plan is designed to be rich in potassium, with a target of 4,700 mg potassium daily, to enhance the effects of reducing sodium on blood pressure. The following are examples of potassium-rich foods

Table 43.7. Sample Foods and Potassium Levels

Food	Potassium (mg)
Potato, 1 small	738
Plain yogurt, nonfat or low-fat, 8 ounces	530–570
Sweet potato, 1 medium	542
Orange juice, fresh, 1 cup	496
Lima beans, ½ cup	478
Soybeans, cooked, ½ cup	443
Banana, 1 medium	422
Fish (cod, halibut, rockfish, trout, tuna), 3 ounces	200–400
Tomato sauce, ½ cup	405
Prunes, stewed, ½ cup	398
Skim milk, 1 cup	382
Apricots, ¼ cup	378
Pinto beans, cooked, ½ cup	373
Pork tenderloin, 3 ounces	371
Lentils, cooked, ½ cup	365
Kidney beans, cooked, ½ cup	360
Split peas, cooked, ½ cup	360
Almonds, roasted, 1/3 cup	310

Section 43.3

Tips to Control Your Cholesterol

This section includes text excerpted from "Tips to Control Your
Cholesterol," National Heart, Lung, and Blood Institute (NHLBI),
December 2013.

High cholesterol and triglyceride levels can lead to heart disease.
Talk to your doctor about your risk for heart disease. Have your cholesterol checked and follow these simple changes to keep your cholesterol
at normal levels.

Are You at Risk?

Understanding your cholesterol numbers helps you to know if you
are at risk for heart disease. The way to find out is through a lipid
panel, which is a blood test.

Use this chart to learn what a lipid panel measures and what the
numbers mean.

Table 43.8. Are You at Risk?

A Lipid Panel Is a Blood Test That Measures:	Here Is What Your Cholesterol Numbers Mean:
Total Cholesterol Cholesterol is a soft, waxy, fat-like substance found in the body. Your body uses cholesterol to produce hormones and some vitamins.	• **Less than 200 mg/dL:** Desirable • **200-239 mg/dL:** Borderline high depending on your other risk factors, you may be at a higher risk for heart disease. • **240 mg/dL or higher:** High You are at a higher risk for clogged arteries and a heart attack.
LDL "Bad Cholesterol" LDL carries cholesterol to your blood vessels, clogging them like rust in a pipe. Remember the L in LDL for "Lousy," and the "Lower" it is, the better.	• **Less than 100 mg/dL:** Desirable • **100–129 mg/dL:** Near desirable • **130–159 mg/dL:** Borderline high • **160 mg/dL or more:** High

Table 43.8. Continued

A Lipid Panel Is a Blood Test That Measures:	Here Is What Your Cholesterol Numbers Mean:
HDL "Good Cholesterol" HDL helps clean fat and cholesterol from your blood vessels. Just remember the H in HDL for "Healthy", and the "Higher" it is, the better.	**Keep this above 40 mg/dL**
Triglycerides Triglycerides are another type of fat in the blood. When you eat too many calories, drink alcohol or smoke, your body makes more triglycerides. When your triglycerides are high, it puts you at increased risk for heart disease.	**Keep this below 150 mg/dL**

Be a Smart Shopper

Choose foods lower in saturated fat, trans fat, and cholesterol. Here are some shopping ideas:

Table 43.9. Be A Smart Shopper

Choose:	Instead Of:
Chicken breast or drumstick (skin removed before cooking)	Chicken wing or thigh (skin on while cooking)
Pork—ears, neck bone, feet, ham hocks, round, sirloin, loin	Pork—hog maws, lunch meat, vienna sausage, bacon, ribs
Egg whites	Egg yolks
Skim or 1% milk	Whole milk
Vegetable oil (such as canola, safflower or sesame)	Lard, butter, shortening

Modify How You Cook

Trim the fat from meat, and remove the skin and fat from chicken and turkey before cooking. Cook ground meat, drain the fat, and rinse with hot tap water. This removes half the fat. Cool soups, and remove the layer of fat that rises to the top. Bake, steam, broil or grill food instead of frying. Use oils low in saturated fat, such as canola, safflower, and sesame oil.

Make Healthy Choices

Choose fresh vegetables and fruits instead of high-fat foods like chips or fries. Use fat-free or low-fat salad dressing, mayonnaise or sour cream. Use small amounts of tub margarine instead of butter.

Chapter 44

Lactose Intolerance

What Is Lactose Intolerance?

Lactose intolerance is a condition in which people have digestive symptoms—such as bloating, diarrhea, and gas—after eating or drinking milk or milk products.

Lactase deficiency and lactose malabsorption may lead to lactose intolerance:

- **Lactase deficiency**. In people who have a lactase deficiency, the small intestine produces low levels of lactase and cannot digest much lactose.

- **Lactose malabsorption**. Lactase deficiency may cause lactose malabsorption. In lactose malabsorption, undigested lactose passes to the colon. The colon, part of the large intestine, absorbs water from stool and changes it from a liquid to a solid form. In the colon, bacteria break down undigested lactose and create fluid and gas. Not all people with lactase deficiency and lactose malabsorption have digestive symptoms.

People have lactose intolerance when lactase deficiency and lactose malabsorption cause digestive symptoms. Most people with lactose intolerance can eat or drink some amount of lactose without having digestive symptoms. Individuals vary in the amount of lactose they can tolerate.

This chapter includes text excerpted from "Lactose Intolerance," National Institute of Diabetes and Digestive and Kidney Diseases (NIDDK), June 2014.

People sometimes confuse lactose intolerance with a milk allergy. While lactose intolerance is a digestive system disorder, a milk allergy is a reaction by the body's immune system to one or more milk proteins. An allergic reaction to milk can be life threatening even if the person eats or drinks only a small amount of milk or milk product. A milk allergy most commonly occurs in the first year of life, while lactose intolerance occurs more often during adolescence or adulthood.

Four Types of Lactase Deficiency May Lead to Lactose Intolerance

1. **Primary lactase deficiency**, also called lactase nonpersistence, is the most common type of lactase deficiency. In people with this condition, lactase production declines over time. This decline often begins at about age 2; however, the decline may begin later. Children who have lactase deficiency may not experience symptoms of lactose intolerance until late adolescence or adulthood. Researchers have discovered that some people inherit genes from their parents that may cause a primary lactase deficiency.

2. **Secondary lactase deficiency** results from injury to the small intestine. Infection, diseases or other problems may injure the small intestine. Treating the underlying cause usually improves the lactose tolerance.

3. **Developmental lactase deficiency** may occur in infants born prematurely. This condition usually lasts for only a short time after they are born.

4. **Congenital lactase deficiency** is an extremely rare disorder in which the small intestine produces little or no lactase enzyme from birth. Genes inherited from parents cause this disorder.

What Are the Symptoms of Lactose Intolerance?

The following are the common symptoms of lactose intolerance.

*   abdominal bloating, a feeling of fullness or swelling in the abdomen

*   abdominal pain

*   diarrhea

- gas

- nausea

Symptoms occur 30 minutes to 2 hours after consuming milk or milk products. Symptoms range from mild to severe based on the amount of lactose the person ate or drank and the amount a person can tolerate.

How Does Lactose Intolerance Affect Health?

In addition to causing unpleasant symptoms, lactose intolerance may affect people's health if it keeps them from consuming enough essential nutrients, such as calcium and vitamin D. People with lactose intolerance may not get enough calcium if they do not eat calcium-rich foods or do not take a dietary supplement that contains calcium. Milk and milk products are major sources of calcium and other nutrients in the diet. Calcium is essential at all ages for the growth and maintenance of bones. A shortage of calcium intake in children and adults may lead to bones that are less dense and can easily fracture later in life, a condition called osteoporosis.

How Is Lactose Intolerance Diagnosed?

A healthcare provider makes a diagnosis of lactose intolerance based on

- medical, family, and diet history, including a review of symptoms

- a physical exam

- medical tests

Medical, family, and diet history. A healthcare provider will take a medical, family, and diet history to help diagnose lactose intolerance. During this discussion, the healthcare provider will review a patient's symptoms. However, basing a diagnosis on symptoms alone may be misleading because digestive symptoms can occur for many reasons other than lactose intolerance. For example, other conditions such as irritable bowel syndrome, celiac disease, inflammatory bowel disease or small bowel bacterial overgrowth can cause digestive symptoms.

Physical exam. A physical exam may help diagnose lactose intolerance or rule out other conditions that cause digestive symptoms. During a physical exam, a healthcare provider usually

- checks for abdominal bloating

- uses a stethoscope to listen to sounds within the abdomen

- taps on the abdomen to check for tenderness or pain

A healthcare provider may recommend eliminating all milk and milk products from a person's diet for a short time to see if the symptoms resolve. Symptoms that go away when a person eliminates lactose from his or her diet may confirm the diagnosis of lactose intolerance.

Medical tests. A healthcare provider may order special tests to provide more information. Healthcare providers commonly use two tests to measure how well a person digests lactose:

- **Hydrogen breath test**. This test measures the amount of hydrogen in a person's breath. Normally, only a small amount of hydrogen is detectable in the breath when a person eats or drinks and digests lactose. However, undigested lactose produces high levels of hydrogen. For this test, the patient drinks a beverage that contains a known amount of lactose. A healthcare provider asks the patient to breathe into a balloon-type container that measures breath hydrogen level. In most cases, a healthcare provider performs this test at a hospital, on an outpatient basis. Smoking and some foods and medications may affect the accuracy of the results. A healthcare provider will tell the patient what foods or medications to avoid before the test.

- **Stool acidity test**. Undigested lactose creates lactic acid and other fatty acids that a stool acidity test can detect in a stool sample. Healthcare providers sometimes use this test to check acidity in the stools of infants and young children. A child may also have glucose in his or her stool as a result of undigested lactose. The healthcare provider will give the child's parent or caretaker a container for collecting the stool specimen. The parent or caretaker returns the sample to the healthcare provider, who sends it to a lab for analysis.

How Much Lactose Can a Person with Lactose Intolerance Have?

Most people with lactose intolerance can tolerate some amount of lactose in their diet and do not need to avoid milk or milk products completely. Avoiding milk and milk products altogether may cause people to take in less calcium and vitamin D than they need.

Individuals vary in the amount of lactose they can tolerate. A variety of factors—including how much lactase the small intestine produces—can affect how much lactose an individual can tolerate. For example, one person may have severe symptoms after drinking a small amount of milk, while another person can drink a large amount without having symptoms. Other people can easily eat yogurt and hard cheeses such as cheddar and Swiss, while they are not able to eat or drink other milk products without having digestive symptoms.

Research suggests that adults and adolescents with lactose malabsorption could eat or drink at least 12 grams of lactose in one sitting without symptoms or with only minor symptoms. This amount is the amount of lactose in 1 cup of milk. People with lactose malabsorption may be able to eat or drink more lactose if they eat it or drink it with meals or in small amounts throughout the day.

How Is Lactose Intolerance Managed?

Many people can manage the symptoms of lactose intolerance by changing their diet. Some people may only need to limit the amount of lactose they eat or drink. Others may need to avoid lactose altogether. Using lactase products can help some people manage their symptoms.

For people with secondary lactase deficiency, treating the underlying cause improves lactose tolerance. In infants with developmental lactase deficiency, the ability to digest lactose improves as the infants mature. People with primary and congenital lactase deficiency cannot change their body's ability to produce lactase.

Eating, Diet, and Nutrition

People may find it helpful to talk with a healthcare provider or a registered dietitian about a dietary plan. A dietary plan can help people manage the symptoms of lactose intolerance and make sure they get enough nutrients. Parents, caretakers, child care providers, and others who serve food to children with lactose intolerance should follow the dietary plan recommended by the child's healthcare provider or registered dietitian.

Milk and milk products. Gradually introducing small amounts of milk or milk products may help some people adapt to them with fewer symptoms. Often, people can better tolerate milk or milk products by having them with meals, such as having milk with cereal or having cheese with crackers. People with lactose intolerance are generally

519

more likely to tolerate hard cheeses, such as cheddar or Swiss, than a glass of milk. A 1.5-ounce serving of low-fat hard cheese has less than 1 gram of lactose, while a 1-cup serving of low-fat milk has about 11 to 13 grams of lactose. However, people with lactose intolerance are also more likely to tolerate yogurt than milk, even though yogurt and milk have similar amounts of lactose.

Lactose-free and lactose-reduced milk and milk products. Lactose-free and lactose-reduced milk and milk products are available at most supermarkets and are identical nutritionally to regular milk and milk products. Manufacturers treat lactose-free milk with the lactase enzyme. This enzyme breaks down the lactose in the milk. Lactose-free milk remains fresh for about the same length of time or, if it is ultra-pasteurized, longer than regular milk. Lactose-free milk may have a slightly sweeter taste than regular milk.

Lactase products. People can use lactase tablets and drops when they eat or drink milk products. The lactase enzyme digests the lactose in the food and therefore reduces the chances of developing digestive symptoms. People should check with a healthcare provider before using these products because some groups, such as young children and pregnant and breastfeeding women, may not be able to use them.

What Products Contain Lactose?

Lactose is present in many food products and in some medications.

Food Products

Lactose is in all milk and milk products. Manufacturers also often add milk and milk products to boxed, canned, frozen, packaged, and prepared foods. People who have digestive symptoms after consuming a small quantity of lactose should be aware of the many food products that may contain even small amounts of lactose, such as

- bread and other baked goods
- waffles, pancakes, biscuits, cookies, and the mixes to make them
- processed breakfast foods such as doughnuts, frozen waffles and pancakes, toaster pastries, and sweet rolls
- processed breakfast cereals
- instant potatoes, soups, and breakfast drinks

- potato chips, corn chips, and other processed snacks
- processed meats such as bacon, sausage, hot dogs, and lunch meats
- margarine
- salad dressings
- liquid and powdered milk-based meal replacements
- protein powders and bars
- candies
- nondairy liquid and powdered coffee creamers
- nondairy whipped toppings

People can check the ingredients on food labels to find possible sources of lactose in food products. If a food label includes any of the following words, the product contains lactose:

- milk
- lactose
- whey
- curds
- milk by-products
- dry milk solids
- nonfat dry milk powder

Medications

Some medications also contain lactose, including prescription medications such as birth control pills and over-the-counter medications such as products to treat stomach acid and gas. These medications most often cause symptoms in people with severe lactose intolerance. People with lactose intolerance who take medications that contain lactose should speak with their healthcare provider about other options.

Chapter 45

Food Allergies

Chapter Contents

Section 45.1

About Food Allergies

This section includes text excerpted from "Food
Allergies: What You Need to Know," U.S. Food and
Drug Administration (FDA), May 24, 2016.

Each year, millions of Americans have allergic reactions to food.
Although most food allergies cause relatively mild and minor symptoms,some food allergies can cause severe reactions, and may even be
life-threatening.

There is no cure for food allergies. Strict avoidance of food allergens—and early recognition and management of allergic reactions to
food—are important measures to prevent serious health consequences.

FDA's Role

Labeling

To help Americans avoid the health risks posed by food allergens,
Congress passed the **Food Allergen Labeling and consumer Protection Act of 2004 (FALCPA)**. The law applies to all foods whose
labeling is regulated by U.S. Food and Drug Administration (FDA),
both domestic and imported. (FDA regulates the labeling of all foods,
except for poultry, most meats, certain egg products, and most alcoholic beverages.)

- Before FALCPA, the labels of foods made from two or more
  ingredients were required to list all **ingredients** by their common or usual names. The names of some ingredients, however,
  do not clearly identify their food source.

- Now, the law requires that labels must clearly identify the **food
  source names** of all ingredients that are—or contain any protein derived from—the eight most common **food allergens**,
  which FALCPA defines as "**major food allergens.**"

As a result, food labels help allergic consumers to identify offending
foods or ingredients so they can more easily avoid them.

Food Allergies

What to Do If Symptoms Occur

The appearance of symptoms after eating food may be a sign of a food allergy. The food(s) that caused these symptoms should be avoided, and the affected person, should contact a doctor or healthcare provider for appropriate testing and evaluation.

- Persons found to have a food allergy should be taught to **read labels** and **avoid the offending foods**. They should also be taught, in case of accidental ingestion, to **recognize the early symptoms** of an allergic reaction, and be properly educated on—and armed with—appropriate treatment measures.

- Persons with a known food allergy who begin experiencing symptoms while or after, eating a food should **initiate treatment immediately**, and go to a **nearby emergency** room if symptoms progress.

Severe Food Allergies Can Be Life-Threatening

Following ingestion of a food allergen(s), a person with food allergies can experience a severe, life-threatening allergic reaction called **anaphylaxis**.

This Can Lead To:

- constricted airways in the lungs.
- severe lowering of blood pressure and shock (**"anaphylactic shock"**).
- suffocation by swelling of the throat.

Each Year in the United States It Is Estimated That Anaphylaxis to Food Results In:

- 30,000 emergency room visits
- 2,000 hospitalizations
- 150 deaths

Prompt administration of epinephrine by autoinjector (e.g., Epipen) during early symptoms of anaphylaxis may help prevent these serious consequences.

What Are Major Food Allergens?

While more than 160 foods can cause allergic reactions in people with food allergies, the law identifies the eight most common allergenic foods. These foods account for 90 percent of food allergic reactions, and are the food sources from which many other ingredients are derived.

The eight foods identified by the law are:

1. Milk

2. Eggs

3. Fish (e.g., bass, flounder, cod)

4. Crustacean shellfish (e.g., crab, lobster, shrimp)

5. Tree nuts (e.g., almonds, walnuts, pecans)

6. Peanuts

7. Wheat

8. Soybeans

These eight foods, and any ingredient that contains protein derived from one or more of them, are designated as "major food allergens" by FALCPA.

How Major Food Allergens Are Listed

The law requires that food labels identify the food source names of all major food allergens used to make the food. This requirement is met if the common or usual name of an ingredient (e.g., buttermilk) that is a major food allergen already identifies that allergen food source name (i.e., milk). Otherwise, the allergen food source name must be declared at least once on the food label in one of two ways.

The name of the food source of a major food allergen must appear:

1. In parentheses following the name of the ingredient.

   Examples: "lecithin (soy)," "flour (wheat)," and "whey (milk)"

   –OR–

2. Immediately after or next to the list of ingredients in a "contains" statement

   Example: "Contains Wheat, Milk, and Soy."

Know the Symptoms

Symptoms of food allergies typically appear from within a few minutes to two hours after a person has eaten the food to which he or she is allergic.

Allergic reactions can include:

- hives
- flushed skin or rash
- tingling or itchy sensation in the mouth
- face, tongue or lip swelling
- vomiting and/or diarrhea
- abdominal cramps
- coughing or wheezing
- dizziness and/or lightheadedness
- swelling of the throat and vocal cords
- difficulty breathing
- loss of consciousness

Food Allergen "Advisory" Labeling

FALCPA's labeling requirements do not apply to the potential or unintentional presence of major food allergens in foods resulting from "cross-contact" situations during manufacturing, e.g., because of shared equipment or processing lines. In the context of food allergens, "cross-contact" occurs when a residue or trace amount of an allergenic food becomes incorporated into another food not intended to contain it. FDA guidance for the food industry states that food allergen advisory statements, e.g., "may contain [allergen]" or "produced in a facility that also uses [allergen]" should not be used as a substitute for adhering to current good manufacturing practices and must be truthful and not misleading. FDA is considering ways to best manage the use of these types of statements by manufacturers to better inform consumers.

Allergy Alert: Mild Symptoms Can Become More Severe

Initially mild symptoms that occur after ingesting a food allergen are not always a measure of mild severity. In fact, if not treated promptly, these symptoms can become more serious in a very short amount of time, and could lead to **anaphylaxis**.

Section 45.2

Reading Food Labels for Allergen Content

This section includes text excerpted from "Have Food Allergies? Read the Label," U.S. Food and Drug Administration (FDA), May 20, 2016.

Since 2006, it has been much easier for people allergic to certain foods to avoid packaged products that contain them, says Rhonda Kane, a registered dietitian and consumer safety officer at the U.S. Food and Drug Administration (FDA).

This is because a federal law requires that the labels of most packaged foods marketed in the United States disclose—in simple-to-understand terms—when they are made with a "major food allergen."

The law allows manufacturers a choice in how they identify the specific "food source names," such as "milk," "cod," "shrimp," or "walnuts," of the major food allergens on the label. They must be declared either in:

- the ingredient list, such as "casein (milk)" or "nonfat dry milk," or

- a separate "Contains" statement, such as "Contains milk," placed immediately after or next to the ingredient list.

"So first look for the 'Contains' statement and if your allergen is listed, put the product back on the shelf," says Kane. "If there is no 'Contains' statement, it's very important to read the entire ingredient list to see if your allergen is present. If you see its name even once, it's back to the shelf for that food too."

There are many different ingredients that contain the same major food allergen, but sometimes the ingredients' names do not indicate their specific food sources. For example, casein, sodium caseinate, and whey are all milk proteins. Although the same allergen can be present in multiple ingredients, its "food source name" (for example, milk) must appear in the ingredient list just once to comply with labeling requirements.

"Contains" and "May Contain" Have Different Meanings

If a "Contains" statement appears on a food label, it must include the food source names of all major food allergens used as ingredients. For example, if "whey," "egg yolks," and a "natural flavor" that contained peanut proteins are listed as ingredients, the "Contains" statement must identify the words "milk," "egg," and "peanuts."

Some manufacturers voluntarily include a "may contain" statement on their labels when there is a chance that a food allergen could be present. A manufacturer might use the same equipment to make different products. Even after cleaning this equipment, a small amount of an allergen (such as peanuts) that was used to make one product (such as cookies) may become part of another product (such as crackers). In this case, the cracker label might state "may contain peanuts."

Be aware that the "may contain" statement is voluntary, says Kane. "You still need to read the ingredient list to see if the product contains your allergen."

When in Doubt, Leave It Out

Manufacturers can change their products' ingredients at any time, so Kane says it's a good idea to check the ingredient list when you buy the product—even if you have eaten it before and didn't have an allergic reaction.

"If you're unsure about whether a food contains any ingredient to which you are sensitive, don't buy the product or check with the manufacturer first to ask what it contains," says Kane. "We all want convenience, but it's not worth playing Russian roulette with your life or that of someone under your care."

Chapter 46

Celiac Disease and a Gluten-Free Diet

What Is Celiac Disease?

Celiac disease is an immune disorder in which people cannot tolerate gluten because it damages the inner lining of their small intestine and prevents it from absorbing nutrients. The small intestine is the tube shaped organ between the stomach and large intestine. Gluten is a protein found in wheat, rye, and barley and occasionally in some products such as vitamin and nutrient supplements, lip balms, and certain medications.

The immune system is the body's natural defense system and normally protects the body from infection. However, when a person has celiac disease, gluten causes the immune system to react in a way that can cause intestinal inflammation—irritation or swelling—and long-lasting damage.

When people with celiac disease eat foods or use products containing gluten, their immune system responds by damaging or destroying villi—the tiny, fingerlike projections on the inner lining of the small intestine. Villi normally absorb nutrients from food and pass the nutrients through the walls of the small intestine and into the bloodstream. Without healthy villi, people can become malnourished, no matter how much food they eat.

This chapter includes text excerpted from "Celiac Disease," National Institute of Diabetes and Digestive and Kidney Diseases (NIDDK), June 2015.

What Causes Celiac Disease?

Researchers do not know the exact cause of celiac disease. Celiac disease sometimes runs in families. In 50 percent of people who have celiac disease, a family member, when screened, also has the disease.

A person's chances of developing celiac disease increase when his or her genes—traits passed from parent to child—have variants or changes. In celiac disease, certain gene variants and other factors, such as a person's exposure to things in his or her environment, can lead to celiac disease.

For most people, eating something with gluten is harmless. For others, an exposure to gluten can cause or trigger, celiac disease to become active. Sometimes surgery, pregnancy, childbirth, a viral infection or severe emotional stress can also trigger celiac disease symptoms.

How Common Is Celiac Disease and Who Is Affected?

As many as 1 in 141 Americans has celiac disease, although most remain undiagnosed. Celiac disease affects children and adults in all parts of the world and is more common in Caucasians and females.

Celiac disease is also more common among people with certain genetic diseases, including Down syndrome and Turner syndrome–a condition that affects girls' development.

What Are the Signs and Symptoms of Celiac Disease?

A person may experience digestive signs and symptoms or symptoms in other parts of the body. Digestive signs and symptoms are more common in children including

- abdominal bloating
- chronic diarrhea
- constipation
- gas
- pale, foul-smelling or fatty stool
- stomach pain
- nausea
- vomiting

Being unable to absorb nutrients during the years when nutrition is critical to a child's normal growth and development can lead to other health problems, such as

- failure to thrive in infants
- slowed growth and short stature

- weight loss
- irritability or change in mood
- delayed puberty
- dental enamel defects of permanent teeth

Adults are less likely to have digestive signs and symptoms and may instead have one or more of the following:

- anemia
- bone or joint pain
- canker sores inside the mouth
- depression or anxiety
- dermatitis herpetiformis, an itchy, blistering skin rash
- fatigue or feeling tired
- infertility or recurrent miscarriage
- missed menstrual periods
- seizures
- tingling numbness in the hands and feet
- weak and brittle bones or osteoporosis
- headaches

Intestinal inflammation can cause other symptoms, such as

- feeling tired for long periods of time
- abdominal pain and bloating
- ulcers
- blockages in the intestine

Celiac disease can produce an autoimmune reaction or a self-directed immune reaction, in which a person's immune system attacks healthy cells in the body. This reaction can spread outside of the gastrointestinal tract to affect other areas of the body, including

- spleen
- skin
- nervous system
- bones
- joints

Recognizing celiac disease can be difficult because some of its symptoms are similar to those of other diseases and conditions. Celiac disease can be confused with

- irritable bowel syndrome (IBS)
- iron-deficiency anemia caused by menstrual blood loss
- lactose intolerance
- inflammatory bowel disease
- diverticulitis
- intestinal infections
- chronic fatigue syndrome

As a result, celiac disease has long been underdiagnosed or misdiagnosed. As healthcare providers become more aware of the many varied symptoms of the disease and reliable blood tests become more available, diagnosis rates are increasing, particularly for adults.

How Is Celiac Disease Diagnosed?

A healthcare provider diagnoses celiac disease with

- a medical and family history
- a physical exam
- blood tests
- an intestinal biopsy
- a skin biopsy

Medical and Family History

Taking a medical and family history may help a healthcare provider diagnose celiac disease. He or she will ask the patient or caregiver to provide a medical and family history, specifically if anyone in the patient's family has a history of celiac disease.

Physical Exam

A physical exam may help diagnose celiac disease. During a physical exam, a healthcare provider usually

- examines the patient's body for malnutrition or a rash.

- uses a stethoscope to listen to sounds within the abdomen.

- taps on the patient's abdomen checking for bloating and pain.

Blood Tests

A blood test involves drawing blood at a healthcare provider's office or a commercial facility and sending the sample to a lab for analysis. A blood test can show the presence of antibodies that are common in celiac disease.

If blood test results are negative and a healthcare provider still suspects celiac disease, he or she may order additional blood tests, which can affect test results.

Before the blood tests, patients should continue to eat a diet that includes foods with gluten, such as breads and pastas. If a patient stops eating foods with gluten before being tested, the results may be negative for celiac disease even if the disease is present.

Intestinal Biopsy

If blood tests suggest that a patient has celiac disease, a healthcare provider will perform a biopsy of the patient's small intestine to confirm the diagnosis. A biopsy is a procedure that involves taking a piece of tissue for examination with a microscope. A healthcare provider performs the biopsy in an outpatient center or a hospital. He or she will give the patient light sedation and a local anesthetic. Some patients may receive general anesthesia.

During the biopsy, a healthcare provider removes tiny pieces of tissue from the patient's small intestine using an endoscope—a small, flexible camera with a light. The healthcare provider carefully feeds the endoscope down the patient's esophagus and into the stomach and small intestine. A small camera mounted on the endoscope transmits a video image to a monitor, allowing close examination of the intestinal lining. The healthcare provider then takes the samples using tiny tools that he or she passes through the endoscope. A pathologist—a doctor who specializes in examining tissues to diagnose diseases—examines the tissue in a lab. The test can show damage to the villi in the small intestine.

Skin Biopsy

When a healthcare provider suspects that a patient has dermatitis herpetiformis, he or she will perform a skin biopsy. A skin biopsy is a procedure that involves removing tiny pieces of skin tissue for examination with a microscope. A healthcare provider performs the biopsy in an outpatient center or a hospital. The patient receives a local anesthetic; however, in some cases, the patient will require general anesthesia.

A pathologist examines the skin tissue in a lab and checks the tissue for antibodies that are common in celiac disease. If the skin tissue tests positive for the antibodies, a healthcare provider will perform blood tests to confirm celiac disease. If the skin biopsy and blood tests both suggest celiac disease, the patient may not need an intestinal biopsy for diagnosis.

Genetic Tests

In some cases, a healthcare provider will order genetic blood tests to confirm or rule out a diagnosis of celiac disease. Most people with celiac disease have gene pairs that contain at least one of the human leukocyte antigen (HLA) gene variants. However, these variants are also common in people without celiac disease, so their presence alone cannot diagnose celiac disease.

If a biopsy and other blood tests do not give a clear diagnosis of celiac disease, a healthcare provider may test a patient for HLA gene variants. If the gene variants are not present, celiac disease is unlikely.

Did You Know That Medications and Nonfood Products May Contain Gluten?

Medications, supplements, and other products may also contain lecithin, a hidden source of gluten. People with celiac disease should ask a pharmacist about the ingredients in

- prescription and over-the-counter medications;
- vitamins and mineral supplements; and
- herbal and nutritional supplements.

Other products can be ingested or transferred from a person's hands to his or her mouth. Reading product labels can help people avoid gluten exposure. If a product's label does not list its ingredients, the manufacturer should provide a list upon request.

Products that can contain gluten include

- lipstick, lip gloss, and lip balm
- cosmetics

- skin and hair products

- toothpaste and mouthwash

- glue on stamps and envelopes

- children's modeling dough, such as Play-Doh

Eating, Diet, and Nutrition

Eating, diet, and nutrition play a significant role in treating celiac disease. People with the disease should maintain a gluten-free diet by avoiding products that contain gluten. In other words, a person with celiac disease should not eat most grains, pasta, and cereal, and many processed foods.

People with celiac disease can eat a well balanced diet with a variety of foods. They can use potato, rice, soy, amaranth, quinoa, buckwheat or bean flour instead of wheat flour. They can buy gluten-free bread, pasta, and other products from stores or order products from special food companies. Meanwhile, "plain"—meaning no additives or seasonings—meat, fish, rice, fruits, and vegetables do not contain gluten, so people with celiac disease can eat these foods.

In the past, healthcare providers and dietitians advised people with celiac disease to avoid eating oats. Evidence suggests that most people with the disease can safely eat small amounts of oats, as long as the oats are not contaminated with wheat gluten during processing. People with celiac disease should talk with their healthcare team when deciding whether to include oats in their diet.

Eating out and shopping can be a challenge. Newly diagnosed people and their families may find support groups helpful as they adjust to a new approach to eating. People with celiac disease should

- read food labels—especially canned, frozen, and processed foods—for ingredients that contain gluten.

- avoid ingredients such as hydrolyzed vegetable protein, also called lecithin or soy lecithin.

- ask restaurant servers and chefs about ingredients and food preparation inquire whether a gluten-free menu is available.

- ask a dinner or party host about gluten free options before attending a social gathering.

Foods that are packaged as gluten-free tend to cost more than the same foods containing gluten. People following a gluten-free diet may find that naturally gluten-free foods are less expensive. With practice, looking for gluten can become second nature

The Gluten-Free Diet

The Academy of Nutrition and Dietetics has published recommendations for a gluten free diet. The following chart illustrates these recommendations. This list is not complete, so people with celiac disease should discuss gluten-free food choices with a dietitian or healthcare professional who specializes in celiac disease. People with celiac disease should always read food ingredient lists carefully to make sure the food does not contain gluten.

Table 46.1. Gluten-Free Foods and Foods That Contain Gluten

Foods and Ingredients That Contain Gluten	
barley rye triticale (a cross between wheat and rye) wheat, including including einkorn, emmer, spelt, kamut wheat starch, wheat bran, wheat germ, cracked wheat, hydrolyzed wheat protein	brewer's yeast dextrin malt (unless a gluten-free source is named, such as corn malt) modified food starch oats (not labeled gluten-free) starch

Other Wheat Products That Contain Gluten		
bromated flour durum flour enriched flour farina	graham flour phosphated flour plain flour	self-rising flour semolina white flour

Processed Foods That May Contain Wheat, Barley or Rye*		
bouillon cubes brown rice syrup candy chewing gum chips/potato chips cold cuts, hot dogs, salami, sausage	communion wafers french fries gravies imitation fish matzo and matzo meal rice mixes	sauces seasoned tortilla chips self-basting turkey soups soy sauce vegetables in sauce

*Most of these foods can be found gluten-free. When in doubt, check with the food manufacturer.

Food Products and Ingredients Made from Barley*		
ale beer malt malt beverages	malted milk malt extract malt syrup malt vinegar	other fermented beverages porter stout

Table 46.1. Continued

People should only consume these foods if they are labeled gluten-free—such as sorghum-based beer—or they list a grain source other than barley, wheat or rye—such as corn malt.			
Foods That Do Not Contain Gluten			
amaranth	legumes	quinoa	tapioca
arrowroot	lentils	rice	tef (or teff)
buckwheat	millet	sago	wild rice
cassava	nuts	seeds	yucca
corn	oats (labeled gluten-	sorghum	
flax	free)	soy	
	potatoes		

Food Labeling Requirements

On August 2, 2013, the U.S. Food and Drug Administration (FDA) published a new regulation defining the term "gluten free" for voluntary food labeling. This federal definition standardizes the meaning of "gluten-free" foods regulated by the FDA. Foods regulated by the U.S. Department of Agriculture (USDA), including meat and egg products, are not subject to this regulation. The regulation requires that any food with the term "gluten-free" on the label must meet all of the requirements of the definition, including that the food should contain fewer than 20 parts per million of gluten. The FDA rule also requires foods with the claims "no gluten," "free of gluten," and "without gluten" to meet the definition for "gluten-free."

If a food that is labeled "gluten-free" includes "wheat" on the ingredients list or "contains wheat" after the list, the following statement must be included on the label: "The wheat has been processed to allow this food to meet the FDA requirements for gluten-free food." If this statement is included, people with celiac disease may consume foods labeled "gluten-free."

Chapter 47

Eating Disorders

What Are Eating Disorders?

There is a commonly held view that eating disorders are a lifestyle choice. Eating disorders are actually serious and often fatal illnesses that cause severe disturbances to a person's eating behaviors. Obsessions with food, body weight, and shape may also signal an eating disorder. Common eating disorders include anorexia nervosa, bulimia nervosa, and binge eating disorder.

What Are the Signs and Symptoms?

Anorexia Nervosa

People with anorexia nervosa may see themselves as overweight, even when they are dangerously underweight. People with anorexia nervosa typically weigh themselves repeatedly, severely restrict the amount of food they eat, and eat very small quantities of only certain foods. Anorexia nervosa has the highest mortality rate of any mental disorder. While many young women and men with this disorder die from complications associated with starvation, others die of suicide. In women, suicide is much more common in those with anorexia than with most other mental disorders.

This chapter includes text excerpted from "Eating Disorders," National Institute of Mental Health (NIMH), February 2016.

Symptoms include:

- Extremely restricted eating

- Extreme thinness (emaciation)

- A relentless pursuit of thinness and unwillingness to maintain a normal or healthy weight

- Intense fear of gaining weight

- Distorted body image, a self-esteem that is heavily influenced by perceptions of body weight and shape or a denial of the seriousness of low body weight.

Other symptoms may develop over time, including:

- Thinning of the bones (osteopenia or osteoporosis)

- Mild anemia and muscle wasting and weakness

- Brittle hair and nails

- Dry and yellowish skin

- Growth of fine hair all over the body (lanugo)

- Severe constipation

- Low blood pressure, slowed breathing and pulse

- Damage to the structure and function of the heart

- Brain damage

- Multiorgan failure

- Drop in internal body temperature, causing a person to feel cold all the time

- Lethargy, sluggishness or feeling tired all the time

- Infertility

Bulimia Nervosa

People with bulimia nervosa have recurrent and frequent episodes of eating unusually large amounts of food and feeling a lack of control over these episodes. This binge eating is followed by behavior that compensates for the overeating such as forced vomiting, excessive use of laxatives or diuretics, fasting, excessive exercise or a combination of these behaviors. Unlike anorexia nervosa, people with bulimia nervosa usually maintain what is considered a healthy or relatively normal weight.

Symptoms include:

- Chronically inflamed and sore throat

- Swollen salivary glands in the neck and jaw area

- Worn tooth enamel and increasingly sensitive and decaying teeth as a result of exposure to stomach acid

- Acid reflux disorder and other gastrointestinal problems

- Intestinal distress and irritation from laxative abuse

- Severe dehydration from purging of fluids

- Electrolyte imbalance (too low or too high levels of sodium, calcium, potassium and other minerals) which can lead to stroke or heart attack

Binge Eating Disorder

People with binge eating disorder lose control over his or her eating. Unlike bulimia nervosa, periods of binge eating are not followed by purging, excessive exercise or fasting. As a result, people with binge eating disorder often are overweight or obese. Binge eating disorder is the most common eating disorder in the US.

Symptoms include:

- Eating unusually large amounts of food in a specific amount of time

- Eating even when you're full or not hungry

- Eating fast during binge episodes

- Eating until you're uncomfortably full

- Eating alone or in secret to avoid embarrassment

- Feeling distressed, ashamed or guilty about your eating

- Frequently dieting, possibly without weight loss

What Are the Risk Factors of Eating Disorders?

Eating disorders frequently appear during the teen years or young adulthood but may also develop during childhood or later in life. These disorders affect both genders, although rates among women are 2½ times greater than among men. Like women who have eating disorders, men also have a distorted sense of body image. For example, men may have muscle dysmorphia, a type of disorder marked by an extreme concern with becoming more muscular.

Researchers are finding that eating disorders are caused by a complex interaction of genetic, biological, behavioral, psychological, and social factors. Researchers are using the latest technology and science to better understand eating disorders.

One approach involves the study of human genes. Eating disorders run in families. Researchers are working to identify DNA variations that are linked to the increased risk of developing eating disorders.

Brain imaging studies are also providing a better understanding of eating disorders. For example, researchers have found differences in patterns of brain activity in women with eating disorders in comparison with healthy women. This kind of research can help guide the development of new means of diagnosis and treatment of eating disorders.

What Are the Treatments and Therapies Available for Eating Disorders?

Adequate nutrition, reducing excessive exercise, and stopping purging behaviors are the foundations of treatment. Treatment plans are tailored to individual needs and may include one or more of the following:

- Individual, group, and/or family psychotherapy
- Medical care and monitoring
- Nutritional counseling
- Medications

Psychotherapies

Psychotherapies such as a family-based therapy called the Maudsley approach, where parents of adolescents with anorexia nervosa assume responsibility for feeding their child, appear to be very effective in helping people gain weight and improve eating habits and moods

To reduce or eliminate binge eating and purging behaviors, people may undergo cognitive behavioral therapy (CBT), which is another type of psychotherapy that helps a person learn how to identify distorted or unhelpful thinking patterns and recognize and change inaccurate beliefs

Medications

Evidence also suggests that medications such as antidepressants, antipsychotics or mood stabilizers approved by the U.S. Food and Drug Administration (FDA) may also be helpful for treating eating disorders and other co-occurring illnesses such as anxiety or depression. Check the FDA's website for the latest information on warnings, patient medication guides or newly approved medications.

Chapter 48

Cancer and Nutrition

Chapter Contents

Section 48.1

Nutrition in Cancer Care

This section includes text excerpted from "Overview of Nutrition in Cancer Care," National Cancer Institute (NCI), January 8, 2016.

Good Nutrition Is Important for Cancer Patients

Several randomized controlled trials, some including only small numbers of patients, have investigated whether taking antioxidant supplements during cancer treatment alters the effectiveness or reduces the toxicity of specific therapies. Although these trials had mixed results, some found that people who took antioxidant supplements during cancer therapy had worse outcomes, especially if they were smokers.

Additional large randomized controlled trials are needed to provide clear scientific evidence about the potential benefits or harms of taking antioxidant supplements during cancer treatment. Until more is known about the effects of antioxidant supplements in cancer patients, these supplements should be used with caution. Cancer patients should inform their doctors about their use of any dietary supplement.

Healthy Eating Habits Are Important during Cancer Treatment

Nutrition therapy is used to help cancer patients get the nutrients they need to keep up their body weight and strength, keep body tissue healthy, and fight infection. Eating habits that are good for cancer patients can be very different from the usual healthy eating guidelines.

Healthy eating habits and good nutrition can help patients deal with the effects of cancer and its treatment. Some cancer treatments work better when the patient is well nourished and gets enough calories and protein in the diet. Patients who are well nourished may have a better prognosis (chance of recovery) and quality of life.

Cancer Can Change the Way the Body Uses Food

Some tumors make chemicals that change the way the body uses certain nutrients. The body's use of protein, carbohydrates, and fat may be affected, especially by tumors of the stomach or intestines. A patient may seem to be eating enough, but the body may not be able to absorb all the nutrients from the food.

Cancer and Cancer Treatments May Affect Nutrition

For many patients, the effects of cancer and cancer treatments make it hard to eat well. Cancer treatments that affect nutrition include:

- Surgery
- Chemotherapy
- Radiation therapy
- Immunotherapy
- Stem cell transplant

When the head, neck, esophagus, stomach or intestines are affected by the cancer treatment, it is very hard to take in enough nutrients to stay healthy.

The side effects of cancer and cancer treatment that can affect eating include:

- Anorexia (loss of appetite)
- Mouth sores
- Dry mouth
- Trouble swallowing
- Nausea
- Vomiting
- Diarrhea
- Constipation
- Pain
- Depression
- Anxiety

Cancer and cancer treatments may affect taste, smell, appetite, and the ability to eat enough food or absorb the nutrients from food. This can cause malnutrition (a condition caused by a lack of key nutrients). Malnutrition can cause the patient to be weak, tired, and unable to fight infections or get through cancer treatment. Malnutrition may be made worse if the cancer grows or spreads. Eating too little protein and calories is a very common problem for cancer patients. Having enough protein and calories is important for healing, fighting infection, and having enough energy.

Anorexia and Cachexia Are Common Causes of Malnutrition in Cancer Patients

Anorexia (the loss of appetite or desire to eat) is a common symptom in people with cancer. Anorexia may occur early in the disease or later, if the cancer grows or spreads. Some patients already have anorexia when they are diagnosed with cancer. Almost all patients who have advanced cancer will have anorexia. Anorexia is the most common cause of malnutrition in cancer patients.

Cachexia is a condition marked by a loss of appetite, weight loss, muscle loss, and general weakness. It is common in patients with tumors of the lung, pancreas, and upper gastrointestinal tract. It is important to watch for and treat cachexia early in cancer treatment because it is hard to correct.

Cancer patients may have anorexia and cachexia at the same time. Weight loss can be caused by eating fewer calories, using more calories or both.

It Is Important to Treat Weight Loss Caused by Cancer and Its Treatment

It is important that cancer symptoms and side effects that affect eating and cause weight loss are treated early. Both nutrition therapy and medicine can help the patient stay at a healthy weight. Medicine may be used for the following:

- To help increase appetite

- To help digest food

- To help the muscles of the stomach and intestines contract (to keep food moving along)

- To prevent or treat nausea and vomiting

- To prevent or treat diarrhea

- To prevent or treat constipation

- To prevent and treat mouth problems (such as dry mouth, infection, pain, and sores)

- To prevent and treat pain

Section 48.2

Nutrition and Cancer Prevention

This section includes text excerpted from "Nutrition
in Cancer Care (PDQ®)–Patient Version," National
Cancer Institute (NCI), January 8, 2016.

Following Certain Dietary Guidelines May Help Prevent Cancer

The American Cancer Society and the American Institute for Cancer Research both have dietary guidelines that may help prevent cancer. Their guidelines are a lot alike and include the following:

- Eat a plant-based diet with a large variety of fruits and vegetables.
- Eat foods low in fat.
- Eat foods low in salt.
- Get to and stay at a healthy weight.
- Be active for 30 minutes on most days of the week.
- Drink few alcoholic drinks or don't drink at all.
- Prepare and store food safely.
- Do not use tobacco in any form.

The Effect of Soy on Breast Cancer and Breast Cancer Prevention Is Being Studied

Study results include the following:

- Some studies show that eating soy may decrease the risk of having breast cancer.
- Taking soy supplements in the form of powders or pills has not been shown to prevent breast cancer.
- Adding soy foods to the diet after being diagnosed with breast cancer has not been shown to keep the breast cancer from coming back.

551

Soy has substances in it that act like estrogen in the body. Studies were done to find out how soy affects breast cancer in patients who have tumors that need estrogen to grow. Some studies have shown that soy foods are safe for women with breast cancer when eaten in moderate amounts as part of a healthy diet.

If you are a breast cancer survivor be sure to check the most up-to-date information when deciding whether to include soy in your diet.

Section 48.3

Antioxidants and Cancer Prevention

This section includes text excerpted from "Antioxidants and Cancer Prevention," National Cancer Institute (NCI), January 16, 2014.

What Are Antioxidants?

Antioxidants are chemicals that interact with and neutralize free radicals, thus preventing them from causing damage. Antioxidants are also known as "free radical scavengers."

The body makes some of the antioxidants it uses to neutralize free radicals. These antioxidants are called endogenous antioxidants. However, the body relies on external (exogenous) sources, primarily the diet, to obtain the rest of the antioxidants it needs. These exogenous antioxidants are commonly called dietary antioxidants. Fruits, vegetables, and grains are rich sources of dietary antioxidants. Some dietary antioxidants are also available as dietary supplements.

Examples of dietary antioxidants include beta-carotene, lycopene, and vitamins A, C, and E (alpha-tocopherol). The mineral element selenium is often thought to be a dietary antioxidant, but the antioxidant effects of selenium are most likely due to the antioxidant activity of proteins that have this element as an essential component (i.e., selenium-containing proteins), and not to selenium itself.

Can Antioxidant Supplements Help Prevent Cancer?

In laboratory and animal studies, the presence of increased levels of exogenous antioxidants has been shown to prevent the types of free radical damage that have been associated with cancer development. Therefore, researchers have investigated whether taking dietary antioxidant supplements can help lower the risk of developing or dying from cancer in humans.

Many observational studies, including case–control studies and cohort studies, have been conducted to investigate whether the use of dietary antioxidant supplements is associated with reduced risks of cancer in humans. Overall, these studies have yielded mixed results. Because observational studies cannot adequately control for biases that might influence study outcomes, the results of any individual observational study must be viewed with caution.

Randomized controlled clinical trials, however, lack most of the biases that limit the reliability of observational studies. Therefore, randomized trials are considered to provide the strongest and most reliable evidence of the benefit and/or harm of a health-related intervention. To date, nine randomized controlled trials of dietary antioxidant supplements for cancer prevention have been conducted worldwide. Overall, the nine randomized controlled clinical trials did not provide evidence that dietary antioxidant supplements are beneficial in primary cancer prevention. In addition, a systematic review of the available evidence regarding the use of vitamin and mineral supplements for the prevention of chronic diseases, including cancer, conducted for the United States Preventive Services Task Force (USPSTF) likewise found no clear evidence of benefit in preventing cancer.

It is possible, however, that the lack of benefit in clinical studies can be explained by differences in the effects of the tested antioxidants when they are consumed as purified chemicals as opposed to when they are consumed in foods, which contain complex mixtures of antioxidants, vitamins, and minerals. Therefore, acquiring a more complete understanding of the antioxidant content of individual foods, how the various antioxidants and other substances in foods interact with one another, and factors that influence the uptake and distribution of food-derived antioxidants in the body are active areas of ongoing cancer prevention research.

Should People Already Diagnosed with Cancer Take Antioxidant Supplements?

Several randomized controlled trials, some including only small numbers of patients, have investigated whether taking antioxidant supplements during cancer treatment alters the effectiveness or reduces the toxicity of specific therapies. Although these trials had mixed results, some found that people who took antioxidant supplements during cancer therapy had worse outcomes, especially if they were smokers.

Additional large randomized controlled trials are needed to provide clear scientific evidence about the potential benefits or harms of taking antioxidant supplements during cancer treatment. Until more is known about the effects of antioxidant supplements in cancer patients, these supplements should be used with caution. Cancer patients should inform their doctors about their use of any dietary supplement.

Chapter 49

Nutrition and Oral Health

Nutritional Deficiencies and Oral Health

The oral tissues can also reflect nutritional status and exposure to risk factors such as tobacco. The tongue appears smooth in pernicious anemia. Group B vitamin deficiency is associated with oral mucositis and ulcers, glossitis, and burning sensations of the tongue. Scurvy, caused by severe vitamin C deficiency, is associated with gingival swelling, bleeding, ulceration, and tooth loosening. Lack of vitamin D in utero or infancy impairs tooth development. Enamel hypoplasia may result from high levels of fluoride or from disturbances in calcium and phosphate metabolism, which can occur in hypoparathyroidism, gastroenteritis, and celiac disease.

How to Reverse the Tooth Decay Process and Avoid a Cavities

You probably know that a dental cavity is a hole in a tooth. But did you know that a cavity is the result of the tooth decay process that

---

This chapter contains text excerpted from the following sources: Text under the heading "Nutritional Deficiencies and Oral Health" is excerpted from "Linkages with General Health," National Institute of Dental and Craniofacial Research (NIDCR), March 07, 2014; Text beginning with the heading "What's inside Our Mouths?" is excerpted from "The Tooth Decay Process: How to Reverse It and Avoid a Cavity," National Institute of Dental and Craniofacial Research (NIDCR), National Institutes of Health (NIH), May 2013.

happens over time? Did you know that you can interrupt and even reverse this process to avoid a cavity?

This chapter explains how the tooth decay process starts and how it can be stopped or even reversed to keep your child from getting cavities.

What's inside Our Mouths?

Our mouths are full of bacteria. Hundreds of different types live on our teeth, gums, tongue, and other places in our mouths. Some bacteria are helpful. But some can be harmful such as those that play a role in the tooth decay process.

Tooth decay is the result of an infection with certain types of bacteria that use sugars in food to make acids. Over time, these acids can make a cavity in the tooth.

What Goes on inside Our Mouths All Day?

Throughout the day, a tug of war takes place inside our mouths.

On one team are dental plaque—a sticky, colorless film of bacteria—plus foods and drinks that contain sugar or starch (such as milk, bread, cookies, candy, soda, juice, and many others). Whenever we eat or drink something that contains sugar or starch, the bacteria use them to produce acids. These acids begin to eat away at the tooth's hard outer surface or enamel.

On the other team are the minerals in our saliva (such as calcium and phosphate) plus fluoride from toothpaste, water, and other sources. This team helps enamel repair itself by replacing minerals lost during an "acid attack."

Our teeth go through this natural process of losing minerals and regaining minerals all day long.

How Does a Cavity Develop?

When a tooth is exposed to acid frequently—for example, if you eat or drink often, especially foods or drinks containing sugar and starches—the repeated cycles of acid attacks cause the enamel to continue to lose minerals. A white spot may appear where minerals have been lost. This is a sign of early decay.

Tooth decay can be stopped or reversed at this point. Enamel can repair itself by using minerals from saliva, and fluoride from toothpaste or other sources.

But if the tooth decay process continues, more minerals are lost. Over time, the enamel is weakened and destroyed, forming a cavity. A cavity is permanent damage that a dentist has to repair with a filling.

How Can We Help Teeth Win the Tug of War and Avoid a Cavity?

Fluoride is a mineral that can prevent tooth decay from progressing. It can even reverse or stop, early tooth decay.

Fluoride works to protect teeth. It . . .

- prevents mineral loss in tooth enamel and replaces lost minerals.

- reduces the ability of bacteria to make acid.

You can get fluoride by:

- Drinking fluoridated water from a community water supply; about 74 percent of Americans served by a community water supply system receive fluoridated water.

- Brushing with a fluoride toothpaste.

If your dentist thinks you need more fluoride to keep your teeth healthy, he or she may—

- Apply a fluoride gel or varnish to tooth surfaces.

- Prescribe fluoride tablets.

- Recommend using a fluoride mouth rinse.

About Bottled Water

Most bottled water does not contain enough fluoride to prevent tooth decay. If your child drinks only bottled water, talk with a dentist or doctor about whether your child needs additional fluoride in the form of a tablet, varnish or gel.

Keep an Eye on How Often Your Child Eats, as Well as What She Eats

Your child's diet is important in preventing a cavity.

Remember . . . every time we eat or drink something that contains sugar or starches, bacteria in our mouth use the sugar and starch to produce acids. These acids begin to eat away at the tooth's enamel.

Our saliva can help fight off this acid attack. But if we eat frequently throughout the day—especially foods and drinks containing sugar and starches—the repeated acid attacks will win the tug of war, causing the tooth to lose minerals and eventually develop a cavity.

That's why it's important to keep an eye on how often your children eat as well as what they eat.

Tooth-Friendly Tips

- Limit between-meal snacks. This reduces the number of acid attacks on teeth and gives teeth a chance to repair themselves.

- Save candy, cookies, soda, and other sugary drinks for special occasions

- Limit fruit juice. Follow the Daily Juice Recommendations external link from the American Academy of Pediatrics.

- Make sure your child doesn't eat or drink anything with sugar in it after bedtime tooth brushing. Saliva flow decreases during sleep. Without enough saliva, teeth are less able to repair themselves after an acid attack.

Make Sure Your Child Brushes

Brushing with fluoride toothpaste is important for preventing cavities.

Here's what you should know about brushing:

- Have your child brush two times per day

- Supervise young children when they brush—

- For children aged 2 to 6, you put the toothpaste on the brush. Use only a pea-sized amount of fluoride toothpaste.

- Encourage your child to spit out the toothpaste rather than swallow it. Children under 6 tend to swallow much of the toothpaste on their brush. If children regularly consume higher-than-recommended amounts of fluoride during the tooth-forming years (age 8 and younger), their permanent teeth may develop white lines or flecks called dental fluorosis. Fluorosis is usually mild; in many cases, only a dental professional would notice it. (In children under age 2, dental experts recommend that you do not use fluoride toothpaste unless directed by a doctor or dentist.)

- Until they are 7 or 8 years old, you will need to help your child brush. Young children cannot get their teeth clean by themselves. Try brushing your child's teeth first, then let her finish.

Talk to a Dentist about Sealants

Dental sealants are another good way to help avoid a cavity. Sealants are thin, plastic coatings painted onto the chewing surfaces of the back teeth or molars. Here's why sealants are helpful: The chewing surfaces of back teeth are rough and uneven because they have small pits and grooves. Food and bacteria can get stuck in the pits and grooves and stay there a long time because toothbrush bristles can't easily brush them away. Sealants cover these surfaces and form a barrier that protects teeth and prevents food and bacteria from getting trapped there.

Since most cavities in children and adolescents develop in the molars (the back teeth), it's best to get these teeth sealed as soon as they come in:

- The first permanent molars—called "6 year molars"—come in between the ages of 5 and 7.

- The second permanent molars—"12 year molars"—come in when a child is between 11 and 14 years old.

Take Your Child to the Dentist for Regular Check-Ups (h2)
Visit a dentist regularly for cleanings and an examination. During the visit the dentist or hygienist will:

- Remove dental plaque

- Check for any areas of early tooth decay

- Show you and your child how to thoroughly clean the teeth

- Apply a fluoride gel or varnish, if necessary

- Schedule your next regular check-up

Part Eight

Additional Help and Information

Chapter 50

Glossary of Diet and Nutrition Terms

added sugars: Sugars and syrups that are added to foods during processing or preparation. Added sugars do not include naturally occurring sugars such as lactose in milk or fructose in fruits.

adequate intakes (AI): A recommended average daily nutrient intake level based on observed or experimentally determined approximations or estimates of mean nutrient intake by a group (or groups) of apparently healthy people.

alcoholism: A disease characterized by a dependency on alcohol. Excessive alcohol use can have a negative impact on bone health.

anorexia nervosa: An eating disorder characterized by an irrational fear of weight gain. Individuals with anorexia nervosa can experience nutritional and hormonal problems that negatively impact bone health.

arthritis: A general term for conditions that cause inflammation (swelling) of the joints and surrounding tissues. Some forms of arthritis may occur simultaneously with osteoporosis and Paget's disease.

balance: The ability to maintain your body's stability while moving or standing still. Along with flexibility and strength, improving balance can significantly reduce the risk of falling.

This glossary contains terms excerpted from documents produced by several sources deemed reliable.

blood cholesterol: Cholesterol that travels in the serum of the blood as distinct particles containing both lipids and proteins (lipoproteins). Also referred to as serum cholesterol.

body mass index (BMI): A measure of weight in kilograms (kg) relative to height in meters squared (m2). BMI is considered a reasonably reliable indicator of total body fat, which is related to the risk of disease and death.

bone mineral density (BMD) testing: A test that measures bone strength and fracture risk.

breast cancer: A disease in which abnormal tumor cells develop in the breast. Women who have had breast cancer may be at increased risk for osteoporosis and fracture because of possible reduced levels of estrogen, chemotherapy or surgery, or early menopause.

calcium: A mineral that is an essential nutrient for bone health. It is also needed for the heart, muscles and nerves to function properly and for blood to clot.

calorie balance: The balance between calories consumed through eating and drinking and calories expended through physical activity and metabolic processes.

calorie: A unit commonly used to measure energy content of foods and beverages as well as energy use (expenditure) by the body. A kilocalorie is equal to the amount of energy (heat) required to raise the temperature of 1 kilogram of water 1 degree centigrade.

carbohydrates: One of the macronutrients and a source of energy. They include sugars, starches, and fiber:

cardiovascular disease (CVD): Heart disease as well as diseases of the blood vessel system (arteries, capillaries, veins) that can lead to heart attack, chest pain (angina), or stroke.

celiac disease: An inherited intestinal disorder in which the body cannot tolerate gluten, which is found in foods made with wheat, rye, and barley. Bone loss is a complication of untreated celiac disease.

cholesterol: A natural sterol present in all animal tissues. Free cholesterol is a component of cell membranes and serves as a precursor for steroid hormones (estrogen, testosterone, aldosterone), and for bile acids.

collagen: A family of fibrous proteins that are components of osteogenesis imperfecta is caused by a genetic defect that affects the body's production of collagen.

complex carbohydrates: Large chains of sugar units arranged to form starches and fiber.

constipation: A decrease in frequency of stools or bowel movements with hardening of the stool.

DASH eating plan: The DASH (Dietary Approaches to Stop Hypertension) Eating Plan exemplifies healthy eating. It was designed to increase intake of foods expected to lower blood pressure while being heart healthy and meeting Institute of Medicine (IOM) nutrient recommendations.

diabetes: A disease in which the body does not produce or properly use insulin. Insulin is a hormone that is needed to convert sugar, starches, and other food into energy.

dietary cholesterol: Cholesterol found in foods of animal origin, including meat, seafood, poultry, eggs, and dairy products.

dietary fiber: Nondigestible carbohydrates and lignin that are intrinsic and intact in plants.

dietary reference intakes (DRIs): A set of nutrient-based reference values that are quantitative estimates of nutrient intakes to be used for planning and assessing diets for healthy people.

discretionary calories: The balance of calories remaining in a person's "energy allowance" after consuming sufficient nutrient-dense forms of foods to meet all nutrient needs for a day.

eating behaviors: Individual behaviors that affect food and beverage choices and intake patterns, such as what, where, when, why, and how much people eat.

eating pattern (also called "dietary pattern"): The combination of foods and beverages that constitute an individual's complete dietary intake over time.

energy density: The calories contained in 100 grams of a particular food defines that food's energy density.

energy drink: A beverage that contains caffeine as an ingredient, along with other ingredients, such as taurine, herbal supplements, vitamins, and added sugars.

enrichment: The addition of specific nutrients (i.e., iron, thiamin, riboflavin, and niacin) to refined grain products in order to replace losses of the nutrients that occur during processing.

essential nutrient: A vitamin, mineral, fatty acid, or amino acid required for normal body functioning that either cannot be synthesized by the body at all, or cannot be synthesized in amounts adequate for good health, and thus must be obtained from a dietary source.

estimated average requirements (EAR): The average daily nutrient intake level estimated to meet the requirement of half the healthy individuals in a particular life stage and sex group.

fats: One of the macronutrients and a source of energy.

fiber: Total fiber is the sum of dietary fiber and functional fiber. Dietary fiber consists of nondigestible carbohydrates and lignin that are intrinsic and intact in plants (i.e., the fiber naturally occurring in foods). Functional fiber consists of isolated, nondigestible carbohydrates that have beneficial physiological effects in humans.

flexibility: The range of motion of a muscle or group of muscles. Along with balance and strength, improving flexibility can significantly reduce the risk of falling.

food categories: A method of grouping similar foods in their as-consumed forms, for descriptive purposes. The USDA's Agricultural Research Service (ARS) has created 150 mutually exclusive food categories to account for each food or beverage item reported in What We Eat in America (WWEIA), the food intake survey component of the National Health and Nutrition Examination Survey.

food groups: A method of grouping similar foods for descriptive and guidance purposes. Food groups in the USDA Food Patterns are defined as vegetables, fruits, grains, dairy, and protein foods. Some of these groups are divided into subgroups.

food hub: A community space anchored by a food store with adjacent social and financial services where businesses or organizations can actively manage the aggregation, distribution, and marketing of source-identified food products to strengthen their ability to satisfy wholesale, retail, and institutional demand.

food pattern modeling: The process of developing and adjusting daily intake amounts from each food group and subgroup to meet specific criteria.

foodborne disease: Caused by consuming contaminated foods or beverages. Many different disease-causing microbes, or pathogens, can contaminate foods, so there are many different foodborne infections.

fortification: As defined by the U.S. Food and Drug Administration (FDA), the deliberate addition of one or more essential nutrients to a food, whether or not it is normally contained in the food.

gynecologist: A doctor who diagnoses and treats conditions of the female reproductive system and associated disorders.

high fructose corn syrup (HFCS): A corn sweetener derived from the wet milling of corn.

high-density lipoprotein (HDL-cholesterol): Blood cholesterol often called "good" cholesterol; carries cholesterol from tissues to the liver, which removes it from the body.

high-intensity sweeteners: Ingredients commonly used as sugar substitutes or sugar alternatives to sweeten and enhance the flavor of foods and beverages. People may choose these sweeteners in place of sugar for a number of reasons, including that they contribute few or no calories to the diet.

hydrogenation: A chemical reaction that adds hydrogen atoms to an unsaturated fat, thus saturating it and making it solid at room temperature.

hypertension: A condition, also known as high blood pressure, in which blood pressure remains elevated over time. Hypertension makes the heart work too hard, and the high force of the blood flow can harm arteries and organs, such as the heart, kidneys, brain, and eyes.

inflammatory bowel disease (IBD): Diseases, including ulcerative colitis and Crohn's disease, that cause swelling in the intestine and/or digestive track, which may result in diarrhea, abdominal pain, fever, and weight loss.

lactose intolerance: Inability to digest lactose, the natural sugar found in milk and other dairy products. Individuals with lactose intolerance who avoid dairy products may be at increased risk for osteoporosis.

lean meat: Any meat or poultry that contains less than 10 g of fat, 4.5 g or less of saturated fats, and less than 95 mg of cholesterol per 100 g and per labeled serving size, based on USDA definitions for food label use.

listeriosis: A serious infection caused by eating food contaminated with the bacterium Listeria monocytogenes, which has recently been recognized as an important public health problem in the United States.

low-density lipoprotein (LDL-cholesterol): Blood cholesterol often called "bad" cholesterol; carries cholesterol to arteries and tissues. A high LDL-cholesterol level in the blood leads to a buildup of cholesterol in arteries.

menopause: The cessation of menstruation in women. Bone health in women often deteriorates after menopause due to a decrease in the female hormone estrogen.

micronutrient: An essential nutrient, as a trace mineral or vitamin, that is required by an organism in minute amounts.

mixed dishes: Savory food items eaten as a single entity that include foods from more than one food group. These foods often are mixtures of grains, protein foods, vegetables, and/or dairy.

moderate alcohol consumption: Up to one drink per day for women and up to two drinks per day for men. One drink-equivalent is described using the reference beverages of 12 fl oz of regular beer (5% alcohol), 5 fl oz of wine (12% alcohol), or 1.5 fl oz of 80 proof (40%) distilled spirits.

moderate physical activity: Any activity that burns 3.5 to 7 kcal/min or the equivalent of 3 to 6 metabolic equivalents (METs) (CDC) and results in achieving 60 to73 percent of peak heart rate (ASCM).

nonsteroidal anti-inflammatory drugs (NSAIDs): A class of medications available over the counter or with a prescription that ease pain and inflammation. Includes aspirin, ibuprofen, and naproxen.

nutrient density: Nutrient dense foods are those that provide substantial amounts of vitamins and minerals and relatively fewer calories.

osteoporosis: Literally means "porous bone." This disease is characterized by too little bone formation, excessive bone loss, or a combination of both, leading to bone fragility and an increased risk of fractures of the hip, spine, and wrist.

ounce-equivalent (oz-eq): The amount of a food product that is considered equal to 1 ounce from the grain or protein foods food group.

pathogen: Any microorganism that can cause or is capable of causing disease.

peak bone mass: The amount of bone tissue in the skeleton. Bone tissue can keep growing until around age 30. At that point, bones have reached their maximum strength and density, known as peak bone mass.

physical activity: Any bodily movement produced by the contraction of skeletal muscle that increases energy expenditure above a basal level; generally refers to the subset of physical activity that enhances health.

phytochemicals: Substances found in edible fruits and vegetables that may be ingested by humans daily in gram quantities.

portion size: The amount of a food served or consumed in one eating occasion. A portion is not a standardized amount, and the amount considered to be a portion is subjective and varies.

poultry: All forms of chicken, turkey, duck, geese, guineas, and game birds (e.g., quail, pheasant).

processed meat: All meat or poultry products preserved by smoking, curing, salting, and/or the addition of chemical preservatives.

protein: One of the macronutrients; a major functional and structural component of every animal cell. Proteins are composed of amino acids, nine of which are indispensable (essential), meaning they cannot be synthesized by humans and therefore must be obtained from the diet.

RANK ligand (RANKL) inhibitors: A type of drug approved for the treatment of osteoporosis.

recommended dietary allowances (RDA): The average daily dietary intake level that is sufficient to meet the nutrient requirement of nearly all (97 to 98%) healthy individuals in a particular life stage and sex group.

refined grains: Grains and grain products with the bran and germ removed; any grain product that is not a whole-grain product.

rheumatoid arthritis (RA): An inflammatory disease that causes pain, swelling, stiffness, and loss of function in the joints.

salmonellosis: An infection caused by bacteria called Salmonella. Most persons infected with Salmonella develop diarrhea, fever, and abdominal cramps 12 to 72 hours after infection.

seafood: Marine animals that live in the sea and in freshwater lakes and rivers.

serving size: A standardized amount of a food, such as a cup or an ounce, used in providing information about a food within a food group, such as in dietary guidance.

simple carbohydrates: Sugars composed of a single sugar molecule (monosaccharide) or two joined sugar molecules (a disaccharide), such as glucose, fructose, lactose, and sucrose.

solid fats: Fats that are usually not liquid at room temperature. Solid fats are found in animal foods, except for seafood, and can be made from vegetable oils through hydrogenation.

starches: Many glucose units linked together into long chains. Examples of foods containing starch include vegetables (e.g., potatoes, carrots), grains (e.g., brown rice, oats, wheat, barley, corn), and legumes (beans and peas; e.g., kidney beans, garbanzo beans, lentils, split peas).

sugars: Composed of one unit (a monosaccharide, such as glucose or fructose) or two joined units (a disaccharide, such as lactose or sucrose).

sugar-sweetened beverages: Liquids that are sweetened with various forms of added sugars. These beverages include, but are not limited to, soda (regular, not sugar-free), fruitades, sports drinks, energy drinks, sweetened waters, and coffee and tea beverages with added sugars.

trans fatty acids: Unsaturated fatty acids that are structurally different from the unsaturated fatty acids that occur naturally in plant foods.

variety: A diverse assortment of foods and beverages across and within all food groups and subgroups selected to fulfill the recommended amounts without exceeding the limits for calories and other dietary components.

vitamin A: A family of fat-soluble compounds that play an important role in vision, bone growth, reproduction, cell division, and cell differentiation. Too much vitamin A (in the form of retinol) has been linked to bone loss and an increase in the risk of hip fracture.

vitamin D: A nutrient that the body needs to absorb calcium.

whole fruits: All fresh, frozen, canned, and dried fruit but not fruit juice.

whole grains: Grains and grain products made from the entire grain seed, usually called the kernel, which consists of the bran, germ, and endosperm. If the kernel has been cracked, crushed, or flaked, it must retain the same relative proportions of bran, germ, and endosperm as the original grain in order to be called whole grain. Many, but not all, whole grains are also sources of dietary fiber.

Chapter 51

Government Nutrition Support Programs

Chapter Contents

Section 51.1

Supplemental Nutrition Assistance Program (SNAP)

This section contains text excerpted from documents published by two public domain sources. Text under headings marked 1 is excerpted from "Nutrition Assistance Programs," Social Security Administration (SSA), June 2015; Text under headings marked 2 is excerpted from "Learn How to Apply for Benefits," Food and Nutrition Service (FNS), U.S. Department of Agriculture (USDA), March 21, 2016.

What Is SNAP?[1]

The Supplemental Nutrition Assistance Program (SNAP) helps low-income people buy the food they need for good health. SNAP benefits are not cash. SNAP benefits are provided on an electronic card that is used like an ATM or bank card to buy food at most grocery stores.

Can You Get SNAP Benefits?[1]

You and everyone in your household must meet certain conditions to get SNAP benefits. Your household includes everyone who lives with you, and who buys and prepares food together. If you receive Supplemental Security Income (SSI) payments in California, you aren't eligible for the SNAP because the state includes extra money in the amount it adds to the federal SSI payment.

To get SNAP benefits, households must meet certain tests, including resource and income tests:

Income

There are two income limits: gross and net. Your total income, before taxes or any other subtractions, is called your gross income. However, certain subtractions to your gross income, called deductions, are allowed. These deductions can be for things like housing costs, child support payments, child or dependent care payments, and monthly medical expenses over $35 for people age 60 or older or disabled people. The amount left over after these deductions is called your net income.

Most households must meet both income limits. Households are considered income-eligible if everyone in the household receives Supplemental Security Income (SSI) or Temporary Assistance for Needy Families (TANF).

Resources

In general, households may have $2,250 in resources, such as a bank account or $3,250 in resources if at least one person is age 60 or older or is disabled. However, some states have different resource limits, and not all resources count. If you own your own home, it isn't counted as a resource. In some states, you may have at least one car. The resources of people who receive TANF or SSI do not count.

Work

Generally, able-bodied adults between 18 and 50, who don't have any dependent children, can get SNAP benefits only for 3 months in a 36-month period if they don't work or participate in a workfare or employment and training program, other than their job search. This requirement is waived in some locations.

Immigrants You may get SNAP benefits if you're a legal immigrant. Most legal immigrants must wait five years before getting SNAP benefits.

How to Apply for Benefits?[2]

To apply for benefits or for information about the Supplemental Nutrition Assistance Program, contact your local SNAP office. Local offices are also listed in the State or local government pages of the telephone book. The office should be listed under "Food Stamps," "Social Services," "Human Services," "Public Assistance," or a similar title. You can also call your State's SNAP hotline number. Most are toll-free numbers.

What Amount of SNAP Benefits Can You Get?[1]

If your household is eligible, the amount of SNAP benefits you get depends on your household size, monthly household income, and expenses.

What Can SNAP Benefits Buy?[2]

Households CAN use SNAP benefits to buy:

- Foods for the household to eat, such as:
- breads and cereals;
- fruits and vegetables;
- meats, fish and poultry; and
- dairy products.
- Seeds and plants which produce food for the household to eat.

In some areas, restaurants can be authorized to accept SNAP benefits from qualified homeless, elderly or disabled people in exchange for low-cost meals.

Section 51.2

The Special Supplemental Nutrition Program for Women, Infants, and Children (WIC Program)

This section includes text excerpted from "Women, Infants, and Children (WIC)," Food and Nutrition Service (FNS), U.S. Department of Agriculture (USDA), May 2, 2016.

About WIC

Food, nutrition counseling, and access to health services are provided to low-income women, infants, and children under the Special Supplemental Nutrition Program for Women, Infants, and Children, popularly known as WIC.

WIC provides Federal grants to States for supplemental foods, healthcare referrals, and nutrition education for low-income pregnant, breastfeeding, and non-breastfeeding postpartum women, and to infants and children who are found to be at nutritional risk.

Most State WIC programs provide vouchers that participants use at authorized food stores. A wide variety of State and local organizations cooperate in providing the food and healthcare benefits, and 46,000 merchants nationwide accept WIC vouchers.

WIC is effective in improving the health of pregnant women, new mothers, and their infants. A 1990 study showed that women who participated in the program during their pregnancies had lower Medicaid costs for themselves and their babies than did women who did not participate. WIC participation was also linked with longer gestation periods, higher birthweight and lower infant mortality.

Eligibility for WIC

Pregnant, postpartum and breastfeeding women, infants, and children up to age 5 are eligible. They must meet income guidelines, a State residency requirement, and be individually determined to be at "nutritional risk" by a health professional.

"Nutritional Risk" and WIC Eligibility

Two major types of nutritional risk are recognized for WIC eligibility:

- Medically-based risks (designated as "high priority") such as anemia, underweight, maternal age, history of pregnancy complications or poor pregnancy outcomes.

- Diet-based risks such as inadequate dietary pattern.

Nutritional risk is determined by a health professional such as a physician, nutritionist or nurse, and is based on Federal guidelines. This health screening is free to program applicants.

Beginning April 1, 1999, State agencies use WIC nutrition risk criteria from a list established for use in the WIC Program. WIC nutrition risk criteria were developed by FNS in conjunction with State and local WIC agency experts.

How Many People Does WIC Serve?

During Fiscal Year (FY) 2015, the number of women, infants, and children receiving WIC benefits each month reached approximately 8.0 million. For the first 3 months of FY 2016, States reported average monthly participation over 7.8 million participants per month. In 1974, the first year WIC was permanently authorized, 88,000 people participated. By 1980, participation was at 1.9 million; by 1985, 3.1 million; by 1990, 4.5 million; and by 2000, 7.2 million. Average monthly participation for FY 2014 was approximately 8.3 million.

Food Benefits Received by WIC Participants

In most WIC State agencies, WIC participants receive checks or vouchers to purchase specific foods each month that are designed to supplement their diets with specific nutrients that benefit WIC's target population. In addition, some States issue an electronic benefit card to participants instead of paper checks or vouchers. The use of electronic cards is growing and all WIC State agencies are required to implement WIC electronic benefit transfer (EBT) statewide by October 1, 2020. A few State agencies distribute the WIC foods through warehouses or deliver the foods to participants' homes. Different food packages are provided for different categories of participants.

WIC foods include infant cereal, iron-fortified adult cereal, vitamin C-rich fruit or vegetable juice, eggs, milk, cheese, peanut butter, dried and canned beans/peas, and canned fish. Soy-based beverages, tofu, fruits and vegetables, baby foods, whole-wheat bread, and other whole-grain options were recently added to better meet the nutritional needs of WIC participants.

WIC recognizes and promotes breastfeeding as the optimal source of nutrition for infants. For women who do not fully breastfeed, WIC provides iron-fortified infant formula. Special infant formulas and medical foods may be provided when prescribed by a physician for a specified medical condition.

WIC's Infant Formula Rebate System

Mothers participating in WIC are encouraged to breastfeed their infants if possible, but WIC State agencies provide infant formula for mothers who choose to use this feeding method. WIC State agencies are required by law to have competitively bid infant formula rebate contracts with infant formula manufacturers. This means WIC State agencies agree to provide one brand of infant formula and in return the manufacturer gives the State agency a rebate for each can of infant formula purchased by WIC participants. The brand of infant formula provided by WIC varies by State agency depending on which company has the rebate contract in a particular State.

By negotiating rebates with formula manufacturers, States are able to serve more people. For FY 2014, rebate savings were $1.8 billion, supporting an average of 1.9 million participants each month or 22.5 percent of the estimated average monthly caseload.

Section 51.3

Child Nutrition Programs

This section contains text excerpted from the following sources: Text in this section begins with excerpts from "School Meals," Food and Nutrition Service (FNS), U.S. Department of Agriculture (USDA), February 12, 2016; Text beginning with the heading "National School Lunch Program" is excerpted from "National School Lunch Program," Food and Nutrition Service (FNS), U.S. Department of Agriculture (USDA), September 2013; Text beginning with the heading "The School Breakfast Program (SBP)" is excerpted from "The School Breakfast Program," Food and Nutrition Service (FNS), U.S. Department of Agriculture (USDA), September 2013; Text beginning with the heading "Summer Food Service Program (SFSP)" is excerpted from "Summer Food Service Program (SFSP)," Food and Nutrition Service (FNS), U.S. Department of Agriculture (USDA), June 16, 2016; Text beginning with the heading "Fresh Fruit and Vegetable Program (FFVP)" is excerpted from "Fresh Fruit and Vegetable Program (FFVP)," Food and Nutrition Service (FNS), U.S. Department of Agriculture (USDA), September 2013; Text beginning with the heading "Special Milk Program" is excerpted from "Special Milk Program," Food and Nutrition Service (FNS), U.S. Department of Agriculture (USDA), August 2013.

The Food and Nutrition Service (FNS) administers several programs that provide healthy food to children including the National School Lunch Program, the School Breakfast Program, the Child and Adult Care Food Program, the Summer Food Service Program, the Fresh Fruit and Vegetable Program, and the Special Milk Program. Administered by State agencies, each of these programs helps fight hunger and obesity by reimbursing organizations such as schools, child care centers, and after-school programs for providing healthy meals to children.

National School Lunch Program

The National School Lunch Program (NSLP) is a federally assisted meal program operating in over 100,000 public and nonprofit private schools and residential child care institutions. It provides nutritionally balanced, low-cost or free lunches to more than 31 million children each school day in 2012. In 1998, Congress expanded the National School Lunch Program to include reimbursement for snacks served to children in afterschool educational and enrichment programs to include children through 18 years of age.

The Food and Nutrition Service administers the program at the Federal level. At the State level, the National School Lunch Program is usually administered by State education agencies, which operate the program through agreements with school food authorities.

Nutritional Requirements for School Lunches

School lunches must meet meal pattern and nutrition standards based on the latest *Dietary Guidelines for Americans*. The current meal pattern increases the availability of fruits, vegetables, and whole grains in the school menu. The meal patterns dietary specifications set specific calorie limits to ensure age-appropriate meals for grades K-5, 6-8, and 9-12. Other meal enhancements include gradual reductions in the sodium content of the meals (sodium targets must be reached by SY 2014-15, SY 2017-18, and SY 2022-23). While school lunches must meet Federal meal requirements, decisions about what specific foods to serve and how they are prepared are made by local school food authorities.

How Do Children Qualify for Free and Reduced Price Meals?

Any child at a participating school may purchase a meal through the National School Lunch Program. Children from families with incomes at or below 130 percent of the poverty level are eligible for free meals. Those with incomes between 130 percent and 185 percent of the poverty level are eligible for reduced-price meals, for which students can be charged no more than 40 cents. (For the period July 1, 2013, through June 30, 2014, 130 percent of the poverty level is $30,615 for a family of four; 185 percent is $43,568)

Children from families with incomes over 185 percent of poverty pay a full price, though their meals are still subsidized to some extent. Local school food authorities set their own prices for full-price (paid) meals, but must operate their meal services as non-profit programs.

After school snacks are provided to children on the same income eligibility basis as school meals. However, programs that operate in areas where at least 50 percent of students are eligible for free or reduced-price meals may serve all their snacks for free.

The School Breakfast Program (SBP)

The School Breakfast Program (SBP) is a federally assisted meal program operating in public and nonprofit private schools and residential child care institutions. It began as a pilot project in 1966, and was made permanent in 1975. The School Breakfast Program is administered at the Federal level by the Food and Nutrition Service. At the State level, the program is usually administered by State education agencies, which operate the program through agreements with local school food authorities in more than 89,000 schools and institutions.

Meal Requirements for School Breakfasts

School breakfasts must meet the meal pattern and nutrition standards based on the latest *Dietary Guidelines for Americans*. Most changes to the SBP's meal pattern begin in SY 2013-14 with more whole grains offered, zero grams of trans fat per portion, and appropriate calories for grades K-5, 6-8, and 9-12. More fruit was offered to students beginning SY 2014-15, the first target for reduction of sodium. All school breakfasts must meet Federal meal requirements, though decisions about which specific foods to serve and how they are prepared are made by local school food authorities.

How Do Children Qualify for Free and Reduced Price Breakfasts?

Any child at a participating school may purchase a meal through the School Breakfast Program. Children from families with incomes at or below 130 percent of the Federal poverty level are eligible for free meals. Those with incomes between 130 percent and 185 percent of the poverty level are eligible for reduced-price meals, for which students can be charged no more than 30 cents. (For the period July 1, 2013, through June 30, 2014, 130 percent of the poverty level is $30,615 for a family of four; 185 percent is $43,568) Children from families over 185 percent of poverty pay full price, though their meals are still subsidized to some extent. Schools set their own prices for breakfasts served to students who pay the full meal price (paid), though they must operate their meal services as non-profit programs.

Summer Food Service Program (SFSP)

You know that children who miss school breakfast and lunch are more likely to be sick, absent or tardy, disruptive in class, and inattentive. They also score lower on achievement tests. Good nutrition is essential for learning in school. Summer Food Service Program (SFSP) provides an opportunity to continue a child's physical and social development while providing nutritious meals during long vacation periods from school. It helps children return to school ready to learn.

How Does the Program Operate?

The Food and Nutrition Service, an agency of the U.S. Department of Agriculture (USDA), administers SFSP at the Federal level. State education agencies administer the program in most States. In some areas, the State health or social service department or an FNS regional office may be designated. Locally, SFSP is run by approved sponsors, including school districts, local government agencies, camps or private nonprofit organizations. Sponsors provide free meals to a group of children at a central site, such as a school or a community center. They receive payments from USDA, through their State agencies, for the meals they serve.

Who Is Eligible to Get Meals?

Children 18 and younger may receive free meals and snacks through SFSP. Meals and snacks are also available to persons with disabilities, over age 18, who participate in school programs for people who are mentally or physically disabled.

How Many Meals Do Participants Receive Each Day?

At most sites, children receive either one or two reimbursable meals each day. Camps and sites that primarily serve migrant children may be approved to serve up to three meals to each child, each day.

Fresh Fruit and Vegetable Program (FFVP)

The Fresh Fruit and Vegetable Program (FFVP) is a federally assisted program providing free fresh fruits and vegetables to students in participating elementary schools during the school day. The goal of the FFVP is to improve children's overall diet and create healthier eating habits to impact their present and future health. The FFVP will help schools create healthier school environments by providing healthier food choices; expanding the variety of fruits and vegetables children experience; and increasing children's fruit and vegetable consumption.

How Does the Fresh Fruit and Vegetable Program Work?

Elementary schools participating in the program receive between $50-$75 per student for the school year. The State agency decides the per-student funding amount for the selected schools based on total funds allocated to the State and the enrollment of applicant schools.

With these funds, schools purchase additional fresh fruits and vegetables to serve free to students during the school day. They must be served outside of the normal time frames for the National School Lunch (NSLP) and School Breakfast Program (SBP). The State agency or SFA determines the best method to obtain and serve the additional fresh produce.

Special Milk Program

The Special Milk Program provides milk to children in schools, child care institutions and eligible camps that do not participate in other Federal child nutrition meal service programs. The program reimburses schools and institutions for the milk they serve. In 2012, 3,647 schools and residential child care institutions participated, along with 571 summer camps and 482 nonresidential child care institutions. Schools in the National School Lunch or School Breakfast Programs may also participate in the Special Milk Program to provide milk to children in half-day pre-kindergarten and kindergarten programs where children do not have access to the school meal programs.

The Food and Nutrition Service administers the program at the Federal level. At the State level, the Special Milk Program is usually administered by State education agencies, which operate the program through agreements with school food authorities.

How Does the Special Milk Program Work?

Generally, public or nonprofit private schools of high school grade or under and public or nonprofit private residential child care institutions and eligible camps may participate in the Special Milk Program provided they do not participate in other Federal child nutrition meal service programs, except as noted above. Participating schools and institutions receive reimbursement from the U.S. Department of Agriculture (USDA) for each half pint of milk served. They must operate their milk programs on a non-profit basis. They agree to use the Federal reimbursement to reduce the selling price of milk to all children.

Any child at a participating school or half-day pre-kindergarten program can get milk through the Special Milk Program. Children may buy milk or receive it free, depending on the school's choice of program options.

How Do Children Qualify for Free Milk?

When local school officials offer free milk under the program to low-income children, any child from a family that meets income guidelines for free meals is eligible. Each child's family must apply annually for free milk eligibility.

Section 51.4

Food Distribution Programs

This section contains text excerpted from the following sources: Text in this chapter begins with excerpts from "Food Distribution Programs," Food and Nutrition Service (FNS), U.S. Department of Agriculture (USDA), February 19, 2016; Text beginning with the heading "Commodity Supplemental Food Program" is excerpted from "Commodity Supplemental Food Program," Food and Nutrition Service (FNS), U.S. Department of Agriculture (USDA), January 2016; Text beginning with the heading "Food Assistance in Disaster Situations" is excerpted from "Food Assistance in Disaster Situations," Food and Nutrition Service (FNS), U.S. Department of Agriculture (USDA), July 2, 2014.

Mission of the Food Distribution Program (FDP) is to strengthen the Nation's nutrition safety net by providing food and nutrition assistance to school children and families; and support American agriculture by distributing high quality, 100% American-grown USDA Foods.

Commodity Supplemental Food Program (CSFP)

The Commodity Supplemental Food Program works to improve the health of low income elderly persons at least 60 years of age by supplementing their diets with nutritious USDA Foods. CSFP is administered at the Federal level by the Food and Nutrition Service (FNS), an agency of the U.S. Department of Agriculture. Through CSFP, USDA distributes both food and administrative funds to participating States and Indian Tribal Organizations (ITOs). CSFP food packages do not provide a complete diet, but rather are good sources of the nutrients typically lacking in the diets of the beneficiary population.

Types of Foods Provided to Participants

Food packages include a variety of foods, such as nonfat dry and ultra high-temperature fluid milk, juice, farina, oats, ready-to-eat cereal, rice, pasta, peanut butter, dry beans, canned meat, poultry or fish, and canned fruits and vegetables.

Food Assistance in Disaster Situations

Agencies of USDA help in many ways in a disaster, but perhaps the most immediate is to ensure that people have enough to eat. There are many concerns following a storm, earthquake, civil disturbance, flood or other disaster, but none is more important than providing food in areas where people may find themselves suddenly, and often critically, in need.

Through its Food and Nutrition Service, USDA assists in three ways:

* Provides commodity foods for shelters and other mass feeding sites.

* Distributes commodity food packages directly to households in need.

* Issues emergency SNAP benefits.

Where Does the Commodity Food Come From?

Every State and U.S. territory has on hand stocks of commodity foods that are used for USDA-sponsored food programs. The National School Lunch Program, The Emergency Food Assistance Program and the Food Distribution Program on Indian Reservations are some of the USDA programs for which States maintain stocks of commodity foods.

In an emergency, USDA can authorize States to release these food stocks to disaster relief agencies to feed people at shelters and mass feeding sites. If the President declares a disaster, States can also, with USDA approval, distribute commodity foods directly to households that are in need as a result of an emergency. Such direct distribution takes place when normal commercial food supply channels such as grocery stores have been disrupted, damaged or destroyed or can't function for some reason such as lack of electricity.

How Does USDA Get the Food to Where It's Needed?

Transportation of food donated by USDA for disaster relief efforts is normally handled by commercial carriers. Shipping arrangements are made by the supplier or, if food is being shipped from program inventories, by USDA's Kansas City Commodity Office. In some situations, the military or other public and private emergency assistance agencies are called on to assist in transporting food quickly to where it is needed.

Issue of Emergency SNAP Benefits

USDA can authorize the issuance of emergency SNAP benefits when there is a Presidentially declared emergency or when grocery stores or other regular commercial food supply channels have been restored following a disaster. In order for a disaster Supplemental Nutrition Assistance Program to be established, States must request that USDA allow them to issue emergency SNAP benefits in areas affected by a disaster.

The D-SNAP system operates under a different set of eligibility and benefit delivery requirements than the regular SNAP. People who might not ordinarily qualify for SNAP benefits may be eligible under the disaster Supplemental Nutrition Assistance Program if they have had disaster damage to their homes or expenses related to protecting their homes or if they have lost income as a result of the disaster or have no access to bank accounts or other resources.

People who are already participating in SNAP may also be eligible for certain benefits under the disaster food program. Each household's circumstances must be reviewed by the certification staff to determine whether a particular household is eligible.

Chapter 52

Directory of Nutrition Information Resources

Government Agencies That Provide Information about Diet and Nutrition

Administration on Aging (AOA)
1 Massachusetts Ave., N.W.
Washington, DC 20201
Toll-Free: 800-677-1116
Phone: 202-619-0724
Fax: 202-357-3560
Website: www.aoa.gov
Email: aoainfo@aoa.gov

Center for Nutrition Policy and Promotion (CNPP)
3101 Park Center Dr., 10th Fl.
Alexandria, VA 22302-1594
Toll-Free: 866-632-9992
Phone: 703-305-3300
Fax: 703-305-3300
Website: www.cnpp.usda.gov
Email: john.webster@cnpp.usda.gov

Centers for Disease Control and Prevention (CDC)
1600 Clifton Rd.
Atlanta, GA 30333
Toll-Free: 800-CDC-INFO
(800-232-4636)
Toll-Free TTY: 888-232-6348
Website: www.cdc.gov

Resources in this chapter were compiled from several sources deemed reliable; all contact information was verified and updated in June 2016.

Eunice Kennedy Shriver
National Institute of
Child Health and Human
Development (NICHD)
P.O. Box 3006
Rockville, MD 20847
Toll-Free: 800-370-2943
Toll-Free TTY: 888-320-6942
Fax: 866-760-5947
Website: www.nichd.nih.gov
Email:
NICHDInformationResource
Center@mail.nih.gov

Food and Drug
Administration (FDA)
Consumer Inquiries
10903 New Hampshire Ave.
Silver Spring, MD 20993
Toll-Free: 888-INFO-FDA
(888-463-6332)
Fax: 301-847-8622
Website: www.fda.gov
Email: ConsumerInfo@fda.hhs.gov

Food and Nutrition
Information Center (FNIC)
USDA Agriculture Research
Service
10301 Baltimore Ave.
Beltsville, MD 20705-2351
Toll-Free: 888-624-8373
Phone: 301-504-5414
TTY: 301-504-6856
Fax: 301-504-6409
Website: www.fnic.nal.usda.gov
Email: FNIC@ars.usda.gov

Food Safety and Inspection
Service (FSIS)
United States Department of
Agriculture
1400 Independence Ave.
S.W. Rm.
2932-S
Washington, DC 20250-3700
Toll-Free: 888-MPHotline
(674-6854)
Website: www.fsis.usda.gov
Email: fsis@usda.gov

National Cancer Institute
(NCI)
NCI Public Inquiries Office
6116 Executive Blvd.
Ste. 300
Bethesda, MD 20892-8322
Toll-Free: 800-4-CANCER
(800-422-6237)
Live chat: www.cissecure.nci.
nih.gov/livehelp/welcome.asp
Website: www.cancer.gov

National Center for
Complementary and
Alternative Medicine
(NCCAM)
NCCAM Clearinghouse
9000 Rockville Pike
Bethesda, MD 20892
Toll-Free: 888-644-6226
Phone: 888-644-6226
TTY: 866-464-3615
Fax: 866-464-3616
Website: www.nccih.nih.gov/
health/clearinghouse
Email: info@nccih.nih.gov

National Diabetes Education Program (NDEP)
Rm. 9A06
31 Center Dr.
MSC 2560
Bethesda, MD 20892-2560
Toll-Free: 800–860–8747
Phone: 301-496-3583
Website: www.niddk.nih.gov
Email: healthinfo@niddk.nih.gov

National Diabetes Information Clearinghouse (NDIC)
Rm. 9A06
31 Center Dr.
MSC 2560
Bethesda, MD 20892-2560
Toll-Free: 800–860–8747
Phone: 301-496-3583
Website: www.niddk.nih.gov
Email: healthinfo@niddk.nih.gov

National Heart, Lung, and Blood Institute (NHLBI)
NHLBI Health Information Center
P.O. Box 30105
Bethesda, MD 20824-0105
Toll-Free: 866-359-3226
Phone: 301-592-8573
TTY: 240-629-3255
Fax: 301-592-8563
Website: www.nhlbi.nih.gov
Email: nhlbiinfo@nhlbi.nih.gov

National Institute of Diabetes and Digestive and Kidney Diseases (NIDDK)
Office of Communications and Public Liaison
NIH Bldg. 31 Rm. 9A06
31 Center Dr.
MSC 2560
Bethesda, MD 20892-2560
Toll-Free: 800-860-8747
Phone: 301-496-3583
Website: www.niddk.nih.gov
Email: healthinfo@niddk.nih.gov

National Institute on Aging (NIA)
Bldg. 31 Rm. 5C27
31 Center Dr.
MSC 2292
Bethesda, MD 20892
Toll-Free: 800-222-2225
Phone: 301-496-1752
Toll-Free TTY: 800-222-4225
Fax: 301-496-1072
Website: www.nia.nih.gov
Email: niaic@nia.nih.gov

National Institutes of Health (NIH)
9000 Rockville Pike
Bethesda, MD 20892
Toll-Free: 800-222-2225
Phone: 301-496-4000
TTY: 301-402-9612
Website: www.nih.gov
Email: NIHinfo@od.nih.gov

National Library of Medicine (NLM)
Reference and Web Services
8600 Rockville Pike
Bethesda, MD 20894
Toll-Free: 888-FIND-NLM
(888-346-3656)
Phone: 301-594-5983
Toll-Free TDD: 800-735-2258
(via Maryland Relay Service)
Fax: 301-402-1384;
301-496-2809
Website: www.nlm.nih.gov
Email: custserv@nlm.nih.gov

National Women's Health Information Center
U.S. Department of Health and
Human Services (HHS)
200 Independence Ave.
S.W. Rm., 712E
Washington, DC 20201
Toll-Free: 800-994-9662
Fax: 202-205-2631
Website: www.womenshealth.
gov

Office of Dietary Supplements (ODS)
National Institutes of Health
(NIH)
6100 Executive Blvd.
Rm. 3B01
MSC 7517
Bethesda, MD 20892-7517
Toll-Free: 888-723-3366
Phone: 301-435-2920
Fax: 301-480-1845
Website: ods.od.nih.gov
Email: ods@nih.gov

President's Council on Physical Fitness and Sports (PCPFS)
1101 Wootton Pkwy, Ste. 560
Rockville, MD 20852
Phone: 240-276-9567
Fax: 240-276-9860
Website: www.fitness.gov
Email: fitness@hhs.gov

U.S. Department of Agriculture (USDA)
1400 Independence Ave. S.W.
Washington, DC 20250
Toll-Free: 866-632-9992
Phone: 202-720-2791
Website: www.usda.gov
Email: agsec@usda.gov

USDA Meat and Poultry Hotline
Toll-Free: 888-MPHotline
(888-674-6854)
Website: www.fsis.usda.gov
Email: MPHotline.fsis@usda.gov

U.S. Department of Health and Human Services (HHS)
200 Independence Ave. S.W.
Washington, DC 20201
Toll-Free: 877-696-6775 (Hotline)
Website: www.hhs.gov

Weight-Control Information Network (WIN)
Rm. 9A06
31 Center Dr., MSC 2560
Bethesda, MD 20892-2560
Toll-Free: 800–860–8747
Phone: 301-496-3583
Website: www.niddk.nih.gov
Email: healthinfo@niddk.nih.gov

Private Agencies That Provide Information about Diet and Nutrition

American Academy of Pediatrics
National Headquarters
141 Northwest Point Blvd.
Elk Grove Village,
IL 60007-1098
Toll-Free: 800-433-9016
Phone: 847-434-4000
Fax: 847-434-8000
Website: www.aap.org
Email: kidsdocs@aap.org

American Association of Diabetes Educators (AADE)
200 W. Madison St., Ste. 800
Chicago, IL 60606
Toll-Free: 800-338-3633
Website: www.diabeteseducator.
org
Email: meetings@aadenet.org

American College of Sports Medicine (ACSM)
P.O. Box 1440
Indianapolis, IN 46206-1440
Phone: 317-637-9200
Fax: 317-634-7817
Website: www.acsm.org
Email: jwhitehead@acsm.org

American Council on Exercise (ACE)
4851 Paramount Dr.
San Diego, CA 92123
Toll-Free: 888-825-3636
Phone: 858-576-6500
Fax: 858-576-6564
Website: www.acefitness.org
Email: support@acefitness.org

American Diabetes Association (ADA)
1701 North Beauregard St.
Alexandria, VA 22311
Toll-Free: 800-DIABETES
(800-342-2383)
Phone: 203-639-0385
Website: www.diabetes.org
Email: myada@diabetes.org.

American Dietetic Association (ADA)
120 S. Riverside Plaza
Ste. 2000
Chicago, IL 60606-6995
Toll-Free: 800-877-1600
Phone: 312-899-0040
TTY: 800-514-0383
Fax: 312-899-4899
Website: www.eatright.org
Email: accounting@eatright.org

American Heart Association (AHA)
7272 Greenville Ave.
Dallas, TX 75231-4596
Toll-Free: 800-AHA-USA1
(800-242-8721)
Fax: 414-271-3299
Website: www.americanheart.
org
Email: Tim.Nikolai@heart.org

American Institute for Cancer Research
1759 R St.
N.W.
Washington, DC 20009
Toll-Free: 800-843-8114
Phone: 202-328-7744
Fax: 202-328-7226
Website: www.aicr.org
Email: aicrweb@aicr.org

American Public Health Association (APHA)
800 I St.
N.W.
Washington, DC 20001
Toll-Free: 888-320-APHA
(888-320-2742)
Phone: 202-777-2742
TTY: 202-777-2500
Fax: 202-777-2534
Website: www.apha.org
Email: comments@apha.org

American Society for Metabolic and Bariatric Surgery
100 S.W. 75th St.
Ste. 201
Gainesville, FL 32607
Phone: 352-331-4900
Fax: 352-331-4975
Website: www.asmbs.org
Email: info@asmbs.org

Asthma and Allergy Foundation of America (AAFA)
8201 Corporate Dr.
Ste. 1000
Landover, MD 20785
Toll-Free: 800-7-ASTHMA
(800-727-8462)
Fax: 202-466-8940
Website: www.aafa.org
Email: info@aafa.org

Celiac Disease Foundation
20350 Ventura Blvd.
Ste. 240
Woodland Hills CA 91364
Phone: 818-716-1513
Fax: 818-267-5577
Website: www.celiac.org
Email: gillian.entin@celiac.org

Center for Science in the Public Interest
1220 L St. N.W.
Ste. 300
Washington, DC 20009
Toll-Free: 888-OLESTRA
(888-653-7872)
Phone: 202-332-9110
Fax: 202-265-4954
Website: www.cspinet.org
Email: cspi@cspinet.org

Cleveland Clinic
9500 Euclid Ave.
Cleveland, OH 44195
Toll-Free: 800-223-2273
Phone: 216-444-2200
TTY: 216-444-0261
Website: www.clevelandclinic.
org
Email: sessled@ccf.org

Eating Disorder Referral and Information Center
2923 Sandy Pointe, Ste. 6
Del Mar, CA 92014-2052
Toll-Free: 855-588-3377
Phone: 858-792-7463
Fax: 858-220-7417
Website: www.edreferral.com
Email: edreferral@gmail.com

Food Allergy and Anaphylaxis Network (FAAN)
11781 Lee Jackson Hwy.
Ste. 160
Fairfax, VA 22033
Toll-Free: 800-929-4040
Fax: 703-691-2713
Website: www.foodallergy.org
Email: faan@foodallergy.org

Institute of Food Technologists (IFT)
525 West Van Buren
Ste. 1000
Chicago, IL 60607
Toll-Free: 800-IFT-FOOD
(800-438-3663)
Fax: 312-782-8348
Website: www.ift.org
Email: info@ift.org

International Food Information Council Foundation (IFIC)
1100 Connecticut Ave.
N.W., Ste. 430
Washington, DC 20036
Phone: 202-296-6540
Website: www.foodinsight.org
Email: foodinfo@ific.org

International Foundation for Function Gastrointestinal Disorders (IFFGD)
P.O. Box 170864
Milwaukee, WI 53217-8076
Toll-Free: 888-964-2001
Phone: 414-964-1799
Fax: 414-964-7176
Website: www.iffgd.org
Email: iffgd@iffgd.org

Kidshealth.org
The Nemours Foundation
1600 Rockland Rd.
Wilmington, DE 19803
Toll-Free: 800-222-1222
Phone: 302-651-4046
Website: www.kidshealth.org
Email: PR@KidsHealth.org

National Association of Anorexia Nervosa and Associated Eating Disorders
750 E Diehl Rd.
#127
Naperville, IL 60563
Helpline: 630-577-1330
Website: www.anad.org
Email: anadhelp@anad.org

National Eating Disorders Association (NEDA)
603 Stewart St., Ste. 803
Seattle, WA 98101
Toll-Free: 800-931-2237
Phone: 212-575-6200
Fax: 212-575-1650
Website: www.nationaleatingdisorders.org
Email: info@nationaleatingdisorders.org

The Obesity Society
8757 Georgia Ave.
Ste. 1320
Silver Spring, MD 20910
Toll-Free: 800-974-3084
Phone: 301-563-6526
Fax: 301-563-6595
Website: www.obesity.org
Email: fdea@obesity.org

Shape Up America
506 Brackett Creek Rd.
P.O. Box 149
Clyde Park, MT 59018
Toll-Free: 800-223-2400
Phone: 406-686-4844
Fax: 406-686-4424
Website: www.shapeup.org
Email: askshapeup@shapeup.org

Interactive Tools/Online Interactive Resources

Selected information in this section was compiled from the Food and Nutrition Information Center's Eating Smart resource list at https://fnic.nal.usda.gov/sites/fnic.nal.usda.gov/files/uploads/weight.pdf.

America On the Move

America On the Move Foundation
Description: Allows users to keep track of their physical activity (steps) and dietary progress.

BMI—Body Mass Index Calculator

DHHS, CDC, National Center for Chronic Disease Prevention and Health Promotion
Website: www.cdc.gov/healthyweight/assessing/bmi/index.html
Description: Calculates body mass index (BMI) for adults, children and teens in both English and Metric measurements.

Cyberkitchen

Shape Up America!
Website: www.shapeup.org/kitchen/kitchen_0.html
Description: Shows how to balance food intake with physical activity. Also provides information on how to achieve and maintain a healthy weight through interactive assessment, meal planning, and recipes.

Healthy Body Calculator

Ask the Dietitian - Joanne Larsen, MS, RD, LD

Website: www.dietitian.com/calcbody.php
Description: Calculates body mass index (BMI), and provides information on nutrient composition, body shape, and corresponding disease risk. This Website also gives personalized suggested activities for weight loss.

HealthyDiningFinder.com

Healthy Dining
Website: www.healthydiningfinder.com
Description: Searches for healthier meals at restaurants ranging from fast food to fine dining. Corresponding nutrition information such as calories, fat, and sodium is also provided.

How Active Are You? Calorie Calculator

Center for Science in the Public Interest
Website: www.cspinet.org/nah/09_03/calorie_calc.html
Description: Determines a targeted calorie intake determined by a person's gender, age, height, weight and activity level.

Make Your Calories Count: Use the Nutrition Facts Label for Healthy Weight Management

Food and Drug Administration (FDA), Center for Food Safety and Applied Nutrition
Website: www.accessdata.fda.gov/videos/CFSAN/HWM/hwmintro.cfm
Description: Interactive learning program that provides users with information to help plan a healthful diet while managing calorie intake.

MyPlate – SuperTracker and Other Tools

USDA, Center for Nutrition Policy and Promotion
Website: www.choosemyplate.gov/supertracker-tools.html
Description: Links to various interactive tools and resources to help users plan, analyze, and track food choices and physical activity. Calorie and fats charts, a BMI calculator, and daily food plans are also included.

SuperTracker Website:

Website: www.supertracker.usda.gov
Allows users to compare food choices to recommendations and
nutrient needs, assess personal physical activity, and set a personal
calorie goal.

Nutriinfo Health eTools

Nutriinfo.com, Minu Interactive, Inc.
Website: www.nutrinfo.com
Description: Calculates body mass index, waist-to-hip ratio, daily
caloric needs, calories burned during exercise, and find local health
professionals. Each tool provides information about health status
and weight loss goals. eTools are free to download.

Portion Distortion

DHHS, NIH, National Heart, Lung, and Blood Institute
Website: www.nhlbi.nih.gov/health/educational/wecan/eat-right/
portion-distortion.htm
Description: Interactive Website with two quizzes to compare
portion sizes now and 20 years ago.

USDA National Nutrient Database for Standard Reference

USDA, Agricultural Research Service, Nutrient Data Laboratory
Website: ndb.nal.usda.gov
Description: Provides detailed nutrient analysis for over 8,000 foods.

Brochures, Booklets, and Tools

*Selected information in this section was compiled from the Food
and Nutrition Information Center's Eating Smart resource list
at* https://fnic.nal.usda.gov/sites/fnic.nal.usda.gov/files/uploads/
weight.pdf.

Active at Any Size

Full text: win.niddk.nih.gov/publications/active.htm
Description: Encourages physical activity for individuals of any size.
Suggested physical activities and safety tips are provided, as well as
resources to get started.

Aim for a Healthy Weight

DHHS, NIH, National Heart, Lung, and Blood Institute
NHLBI Publication No. 05-5213
Website: www.nhlbi.nih.gov/health/public/heart/obesity/aim_hwt.
htm

Description: Contains practical, easy-to-use information for losing and maintaining weight, including tips on healthy eating and physical activity, setting weight loss goals, and rewarding success. Also includes portion and serving size information, sample reduced calorie menus, tips on dining out, a sample walking program, and a weekly food and activity diary.
Ordering Information:

NHLBI Health Information Center
P.O. Box 30105
Bethesda, MD 20824-0105
Phone: 301-592-8573 Fax: 240-629-3246
Email: NHLBIinfo@nhlbi.nih.gov
Website: www.nhlbi.nih.gov/index.htm

Better Health and You: Tips for Adults

Full text: win.niddk.nih.gov/publications/better_health.htm
Description: Provides tips for eating right and being active to help individuals reach or maintain a healthy weight.

Cómo Alimentarse y Mantenerse Activo Durante Toda La Vida (Healthy Eating & Physical Activity Across Your Lifespan)

Full text: win.niddk.nih.gov/publications/para_adultos.htm
Description: Discusses how eating well and physical activity contribute to healthy living.

Drawing the Line on Calories, Carbs, and Fats

Roberta Schwartz Wennik, MS, RD
Description: Allows users to track food intake and exercise by connecting a series of dots ("drawing the line"), rather than writing down all foods eaten. Available for purchase in hard copy, downloadable eBook, and DVD from the Website.

Improving Your Health: Tips for African American Men and Women

Full text: win.niddk.nih.gov/publications/improving.htm
Description: Provides tips for making changes to physical activity and eating habits that can improve health.

Just Enough For You: About Food Portions

Full text: win.niddk.nih.gov/publications/just_enough.htm
Description: Discusses the difference between portions and serving sizes, and shows how to identify serving sizes by comparing them to everyday objects.

Let's Eat for the Health of It

U.S. Department of Agriculture; U.S. Department of Health and Human Services
Website: www.cnpp.usda.gov/publications/myplate/dg2010brochure.pdf
Description: Consumer brochure that provides tips for healthful eating and being active based on recommendations from the *2010 Dietary Guidelines for Americans* and MyPlate.

Physical Activity and Weight Control

Full text: win.niddk.nih.gov/publications/physical.htm
Description: Discusses the importance of physical activity and provides tips for a safe physical activity program.

Sisters Together: Move More, Eat Better

Energize Yourself & Your Family
Full text: win.niddk.nih.gov/publications/energize.htm
Fit and Fabulous as You Mature
Full text: win.niddk.nih.gov/publications/mature.htm
Description: Sisters Together: Move More, Eat Better is a national media-based program designed to encourage African American women 18 and over to maintain a healthy weight by becoming more physically active and eating healthier foods.

Weight-control Information Network

DHHS, NIH, National Institute for Diabetes and Digestive and Kidney Diseases

Website: win.niddk.nih.gov/index.htm
Description: Provides the general public, health professionals, the media, and Congress with up-to-date, science-based information on weight control, obesity, physical activity, and related nutritional issues.
Ordering Information:
The Weight-control Information Network
1 WIN Way
Bethesda, MD 20892-3665
Phone: 1-877-946-4627 Fax: 202-828-1028
Publications Order Form: win.niddk.nih.gov/order/orderpub.htm
Email: win@info.niddk.nih.gov

Weight Loss for Life

Full text: win.niddk.nih.gov/publications/for_life.htm
Description: Gives an overview of overweight, the types of programs available for weight loss, portion size, and other weight control strategies.

Index

Index

Page numbers followed by 'n' indicate a footnote. Page numbers in *italics* indicate a table or illustration.

A

acesulfame potassium, sweeteners 340
added sugars
  defined 563
  described 335
  nutrition facts label 38
  weight loss 221
adequate intakes (AI), defined 563
Administration on Aging (AOA),
  contact 585
adolescents
  calcium 34
  calorie needs 21
  dental sealants 559
  diabetes 156
  food allergies 193
  lactose intolerance 207
  obesity 428
adults
  calcium 109
  childhood obesity 428
  common food allergies 177
  energy drinks 361

adults, *continued*
  excessive drinking 324
  food safety 236
  healthy eating 230
  lactose intolerance 516
  mental function 102
  protein 36
  supplements 317
  zinc 120
aflatoxin, described 391
age-related macular degeneration
  (AMD)
  eye disorders 102
  vitamin A 80
  vitamin C 94
  zinc 119
"A Guide to Eating for Sports" (The
  Nemours Foundation/
  KidsHealth®) 310n
alcohol use, overview 322–8
alcoholic drink-equivalent,
  tabulated *323*
alcoholism, defined 563
"All about Oils" (USDA) 54n
"All about the Dairy Group"
  (USDA) 139n
"All about the Fruit Group"
  (USDA) 128n

601

Z